On Call
Neurology

Be ON CALL with confidence!

Successfully managing on-call situations requires a masterful combination of speed, skills, and knowledge. Rise to the occasion with **ELSEVIER's On Call Series!** These pocket-size resources provide you with immediate access to the vital, step-by-step information you need to succeed!

Other Titles in the ON CALL Series

On Call Neurology

RANDOLPH S. MARSHALL, MD, MS
Associate Professor of Clinical Neurology
Co-Director, Levine Cerebral Localization Lab
Columbia University Medical Center
New York, New York

STEPHAN A. MAYER, MD, FCCM
Associate Professor of Clinical Neurology &
    Neurosurgery
Columbia University College of Physicians and
    Surgeons
Director, Neuro-ICU
New York Presbyterian Hospital
Columbia University Medical Center
Neurological Institute
New York, New York

3 rd
edition

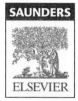

SAUNDERS

ELSEVIER

SAUNDERS
ELSEVIER

1600 John F. Kennedy Blvd.
Ste 1800
Philadelphia, PA 19103-2899   ISBN 13: 978-1-4160-2375-3

On Call Neurology, 3rd ed.

Notice

Knowledge and best practice in this field are constantly changing. As new research and experience broaden our knowledge, changes in practice, treatment and drug therapy may become necessary or appropriate. Readers are advised to check the most current information provided (i) on procedures featured or (ii) by the manufacturer of each product to be administered, to verify the recommended dose or formula, the method and duration of administration, and contraindications. It is the responsibility of the practitioner, relying on their own experience and knowledge of the patient, to make diagnoses, to determine dosages and the best treatment for each individual patient, and to take all appropriate safety precautions. To the fullest extent of the law, neither the Publisher nor the Authors assume any liability for any injury and/or damage to persons or property arising out or related to any use of the material contained in this book.

The Publisher

Previous editions copyrighted 2001, 1997

Library of Congress Cataloging-in-Publication Data

Marshall, Randolph S.
    On call neurology / Randolph S. Marshall, Stephan A. Mayer.—3rd ed.
        p. ; cm.—(On call series)
    Includes index.
    ISBN-13: 978-1-4160-2375-3
  1. Neurology–Handbooks, manuals, etc.   2. Neurological emergencies–Handbooks, manuals, etc.   I. Mayer, Stephan A.   II. Title.   III. Title: Neurology.   IV. Series.
        [DNLM: 1. Emergencies–Handbooks.   2. Nervous System Diseases–therapy–Handbooks.   3. Nervous System Diseases–diagnosis–Handbooks.
  4. Neurology–methods–Handbooks.   WL 39 M369o 2007]

RC355.M37   2007
616.8—dc22

                                                      2006037516

Acquisitions Editor: James Merritt
Editorial Assistant: Nicole DiCicco
Publishing Services Manager: Linda Van Pelt
Project Manager: Priscilla Crater
Cover Designer: Ellen Zanolle
Text Designer: Ellen Zanolle

Working together to grow
libraries in developing countries
www.elsevier.com | www.bookaid.org | www.sabre.org

ELSEVIER   BOOK AID International   Sabre Foundation

Printed in the United States of America

Last digit is the print number: 9   8   7   6   5   4   3

To the New York-Presbyterian neurology residents, past and present, who have helped us teach and learn.

Contributors

Elissa L. Ash, MD, PhD
Clinical Fellow and Assistant Attending Neurologist
Division of Aging and Dementia
Department of Neurology
Columbia University Medical Center
New York, New York

Casilda Balmaceda, MD
Associate Professor of Clinical Neurology and Neurosurgery
Columbia University College of Physicians and Surgeons
Assistant Attending Neurologist
New York-Presbyterian Hospital
The Neurological Institute of New York
Columbia University
New York, New York

Bruce Cree, MD, PhD, MCR
Assistant Professor of Neurology
Department of Neurology
University of California at San Francisco
San Francisco, California

Mark Green, MD
Clinical Professor of Neurology
Director, Columbia University Headache Center
Columbia University College of Physicians and Surgeons
New York, New York

Lawrence J. Hirsch, MD
Associate Clinical Professor of Neurology
Comprehensive Epilepsy Center
Columbia University
Neurological Institute
New York, New York

Elan D. Louis, MD, MS
Associate Professor of Neurology
Associate Chairman for Academic Affairs and Faculty Development
Department of Neurology
College of Physicians and Surgeons
Columbia University
New York, New York

Juan M. Pascual, MD, PhD
Director of Molecular Biophysics
Colleen Giblin Research Laboratories
College of Physicians & Surgeons
Columbia University
Assistant Professor of Neurology and Pediatrics
Neurological Institute of New York
Children's Hospital of New York
Columbia University Medical Center
New York, New York

Jeffrey Joseph Sevigny, MD
Attending Physician
Department of Neurology
Beth Israel Medical Center
New York, New York

Louis H. Weimer, MD
Associate Clinical Professor of Neurology
Department of Neurology
Columbia University College of Physicians & Surgeons
New York Presbyterian Hospital
New York, New York

Preface

This book is meant to serve as a pocket reference for medical students, house officers, and non-neurologist physicians who care for patients in the hospital. Neurologic problems are common and, by their nature, complex. The goal of *On Call Neurology* is to provide the reader with accessible, highly structured protocols for the assessment and management of neurologic disorders in the emergency room, the intensive care unit, the hospital floor, or the clinic. We have tried to emphasize treatment and have attempted to simulate the focused and goal-directed thought processes of an experienced clinical neurologist. This 3rd edition includes updated information to reflect new treatment approaches to various neurological disorders as well as the latest drugs and devices available. New author contributions have enhanced the chapters on Headache, Demyelinating Diseases, Infections of the Central Nervous System, and Dementia.

On Call Neurology is designed to be comprehensive in scope but is admittedly limited in depth. We acknowledge that much of the content reflects our way of doing things. It is our hope that the protocols presented in this book will stimulate the student of neurology (whether a medical student or an attending neurologist) to research the literature, analyze the available data, and reach independent conclusions about optimal patient care. In short, we have intended this book to serve as a starting point for clinical problems in neurology rather than as a definitive reference.

We are grateful to our patients, colleagues, and teachers at The Neurological Institute of New York at New York-Presbyterian Hospital, who taught us most of what we know about neurology. In particular, we would like to thank J.P. Mohr, John Brust, Matthew Fink, and Lewis P. Rowland. Their voices can be heard in many of the pages of this text, and their dedication to teaching and education has served as an inspiration to generations of young physicians.

STEPHAN A. MAYER

RANDOLPH S. MARSHALL

Contents

Introduction

Patient-Related Problems: The Common Calls

Structure of the Book

This book is divided into four main sections:

The first section, Introduction, provides an overview of the clinical approach to the neurologic patient, including the neurologic examination, neuroanatomic localization, and neurodiagnostic testing.

The second section, Patient-Related Problems: The Common Calls, is a symptom-oriented approach to chief complaints that frequently require neurologic consultation in the emergency room, clinic, or hospital floor. Each problem is approached from its inception, beginning with relevant questions that should be asked over the phone, temporary orders that should be given, and the major life-threatening disorders that should be considered as one approaches the bedside:

PHONE CALL

Questions

Pertinent questions to assess the urgency of the situation.

Orders

Urgent orders to stabilize the patient and gain additional information before you arrive at the bedside.

Inform RN

RN to be informed of the time the housestaff anticipates arrival at the bedside.

ELEVATOR THOUGHTS

The differential diagnoses to be considered while the housestaff is on the way to assess the patient (i.e., while in the elevator).

MAJOR THREAT TO LIFE

Neurologic emergencies that can lead to death or neurologic devastation unless immediate action is taken.

BEDSIDE

Quick Look Test

The quick look test is a rapid visual assessment to place the patient into one of three categories: well, sick, or critical. This helps determine the necessity of immediate intervention.

Vital Signs

Selective History and Chart Review

Including pertinent negatives and neurologic review of systems.

Selective Physical and Neurologic Examination

A rapid, focused neurologic examination designed to assess the extent and degree of neurologic dysfunction.

MANAGEMENT

Provides guidelines for neurodiagnostic testing and gives access to indicated medications and dosages. When applicable, checklists and specific management protocols are provided.

The third section, Selected Neurologic Disorders, provides an overview of important neurologic diseases and their management not covered comprehensively in the "common calls" section, such as CNS infections, multiple sclerosis, neuromuscular diseases, movement disorders, and brain tumors.

The fourth section, the Appendices, provides neuroanatomic references and other materials helpful for managing neurologic patients.

The On-Call Formulary is a compendium of medications commonly used to treat neurologic disorders. Drug indications, mechanisms of action, dosages, routes of administration, side effects, and comments for optimal use are provided.

Commonly Used Abbreviations

ABG	arterial blood gas
ACA	anterior cerebral artery
ACE	angiotensin-converting enzyme
ACTH	adrenocorticotropic hormone
AFB	acid-fast bacillus
AIDS	acquired immunodeficiency syndrome
AION	anterior ischemic optic neuropathy
ALS	amyotrophic lateral sclerosis
AMN	adrenomyeloneuropathy
ANA	antinuclear antibody
ANCA	antineutrophil cytoplasmic antibody
APD	afferent pupillary defect
aPTT	activated partial thromboplastin time
AV	arteriovenous
AVM	arteriovenous malformation
BAER	brain stem auditory evoked response
bid	two times a day
BP	blood pressure
BUN	blood urea nitrogen
CAA	cerebral amyloid angiopathy
CBC	complete blood cell count
CBF	cerebral blood flow
CHF	congestive heart failure
CIDP	chronic inflammatory demyelinating polyneuropathy
CK	creatine kinase
CMAP	compound muscle action potential
CMV	cytomegalovirus
CN	cranial nerve
CNS	central nervous system
CPAP	continuous positive airway pressure
CPK	creatine phosphokinase
CPP	cerebral perfusion pressure
CPR	cardiopulmonary resuscitation

CRAO	central retinal artery occlusion
CSF	cerebrospinal fluid
CT	computed tomography
DDAVP	desmopressin acetate
DIC	disseminated intravascular coagulation
D5W	5% dextrose in water
D5WNS	5% dextrose in normal saline
D50W	50% dextrose in water
DVT	deep vein thrombosis
DWI	diffusion-weighted imaging
EBV	Epstein-Barr virus
ECG	electrocardiogram
EEG	electroencephalogram
EMG	electromyography
EP	electrophysiologic
ER	emergency room
ESR	erythrocyte sedimentation rate
EtOH	ethanol
FDA	Food and Drug Administration
FFP	fresh frozen plasma
FNF	finger-nose-finger
GBM	glioblastoma multiforme
GBS	Guillain-Barré syndrome
GCS	Glasgow Coma scale
GI	gastrointestinal
GU	genitourinary
HCG	human chorionic gonadotropin
HEENT	head, eyes, ears, nose, throat
HIV	human immunodeficiency virus
HKS	heel-knee-shin
HR	heart rate
HSE	herpes simplex encephalitis
HSV-1	herpes simplex virus 1
HTLV-1	human T-cell lymphotropic virus type I
Hz	Hertz
ICA	internal carotid artery
ICH	intracerebral hemorrhage
ICP	intracranial pressure
ICU	intensive care unit
IgG	immunoglobulin G
IM	intramuscular
IMV	intermittent mandatory ventilation
INO	internuclear ophthalmoplegia
INR	international normalized ratio
ION	ischemic optic neuropathy
IV	intravenous
IVIG	intravenous immune globulin
IVP	intravenous push

KVO	keep the vein open
LFT	liver function test
LCM	lymphocytic choriomeningitis
LP	lumbar puncture
MABP	mean arterial blood pressure
MAO	monoamine oxidase
MCA	middle cerebral artery
MELAS	mitochondrial encephalomyopathy, lactic acidosis, and stroke
MI	myocardial infarction
MLD	metachromatic leukodystrophy
MLF	median longitudinal fasciculus
MMN	multifocal motor neuropathy
MMSE	Mini Mental State Examination
MRI	magnetic resonance imaging
MS	multiple sclerosis
MSA	multiple-system atrophy
NCS	nerve conduction study
NCV	nerve conduction velocity
NPO	nil per os (nothing by mouth)
NS	normal saline
NSE	neuron specfic enolase
NSAID	nonsteroidal anti-inflammatory drug
OCB	oligoclonal band
OKN	opticokinetic nystagmus
ON	optic neuritis
PCA	posterior cerebral artery
PCNSL	primary central nervous system lymphoma
PCO_2	partial pressure of carbon dioxide
PCR	polymerase chain reaction
PE	pulmonary embolism
PEEP	positive end-expiratory pressure
PET	positron emission tomography
PLED	periodic lateralizing epileptiform discharge
PML	progressive multifocal leukoencephalopathy
PNET	primitive neuroectodermal tumor
PO	per os (by mouth)
PO_2	partial pressure of oxygen
PPD	purified protein derivative
PPRF	paramedian pontine reticular formation
PRN	as needed
PT	prothrombin time
PTT	partial thromboplastin time
PVS	persistent vegetative state
qd	every day
qhs	every day at nighttime
qid	four times a day
RA	rheumatoid arthritis

RAM	rapid alternating movements
RBC	red blood cell
RF	rheumatoid factor
RPR	rapid plasmin reagin
SAH	subarachnoid hemorrhage
SBP	systolic blood pressure
SC	subcutaneous
SFEMG	single-fiber electromyogram
SIADH	syndrome of inappropriate antidiuretic hormone
SIMV	synchronized intermittent mandatory ventilation
SL	sublingual
SLE	systemic lupus erythematosus
SMA	spinal muscular atrophy
SMP	sympathetically maintained pain
SPECT	single photon emission computed tomography
SPEP	serum protein electrophoresis
SSEP	somatosensory evoked potential
SSPE	subacute sclerosing panencephalitis
t-PA	tissue plasminogen activator
TCA	tricyclic antidepressant
TCD	transcranial Doppler
TENS	transcutaneous electric nerve stimulation
TFTs	thyroid function tests
TGA	transient global amnesia
TIA	transient ischemic attack
tid	three times a day
TMB	transient monocular blindness
VDRL	Veneral Disease Research Laboratory
VEP	visual evoked potential
VER	visual evoked response
WBC	white blood cell

Introduction

Approach to the Neurologic Patient On Call: History Taking, Differential Diagnosis, and Anatomic Localization

It's in the early morning hours. You get a call from a resident in the ER. A 48-year-old teacher has headache, neck pain, and urinary incontinence, and, as of this morning, is no longer able to hold a pen in his right hand. How do you proceed? What do you tell the ER resident? What tests should be ordered? How urgent is this situation?

Neurology, perhaps more than any other field in medicine, demands familiarity with a wide spectrum of anatomic details and diagnostic studies. Electrophysiologic, serologic, genetic, pathologic, and a host of imaging techniques have enabled diagnoses to be made with a higher degree of accuracy and certainty than ever before. Yet all diagnostic puzzles, simple or complex, begin with the presentation of a symptom by a patient to a doctor.

It is often said that 90% of the neurologic diagnosis comes from the patient's history. Indeed, it is the exception when a diagnosis is stumbled upon after a "shotgun" approach of ordering diagnostic studies unguided by the patient's initial complaints. In the type of encounter for which this book was written, namely, a rapid response to an acute complaint, the single most important factor in the encounter is the initial interview with the patient. This book aims to guide you through a logical, focused, and effective approach to diagnosis and management of your patient's acute problem. This third edition has updated chapters in all aspects of emergency neurologic care, including the latest pharmacologic and diagnostic options. After a discussion of general principles of managing patients on call, this chapter covers some key points about neurologic history taking along with principles of differential diagnosis and anatomic localization. The neurologic physical examination is outlined in Chapter 2. The basics of the most important initial diagnostic studies are covered in Chapter 3.

PRINCIPLES OF MANAGING PATIENTS WHEN ON CALL

1. **Obtain adequate information from the initial phone contact.**

   Establish the nature of the complaint, understand its acuteness and its severity, and learn what has been done so far (Have vital signs been checked? Has any labwork been sent?).

2. **Establish a working differential diagnosis before you see the patient.**

   Some preparatory thought will produce a more efficient and directed interview and examination of the patient. Prioritize your diagnoses by placing the most potentially dangerous diagnoses at the top of the list, followed by the most likely diagnoses.

3. **Be focused in your bedside assessment.**

   Unlike the comprehensive examination that you perform when admitting a patient to the hospital or when seeing a patient for the first time in the clinic, your history taking and examination of the patient when you are on call needs to be focused and efficient.

4. **Know when to call for additional consultation.**

   Examples would be an ophthalmologic consultation for branch retinal artery occlusion versus anterior ischemic optic neuropathy, or a neurosurgical consultation to place an intracranial pressure monitor.

5. **Be accurate and concise in your documentation of the encounter.**

   Although it will be your responsibility to solve the clinical problem as completely as possible, many times you will be unable to make a diagnosis or complete a treatment during the time you are involved with the patient. You must document the patient's history and physical examination as precisely as possible. Make sure you date and time your note. If there was a delay in arriving at the bedside because of another emergency, document this. Include relevant laboratory data in your note. Your evaluation and formulation of the problem should be well integrated and transparent. The recommendations for treatment should be stated clearly and should be concordant with what was written in the orders. If discussions with family members took place, the content and outcome of the discussions should be documented.

PRINCIPLES OF HISTORY TAKING IN NEUROLOGY

Key features of the neurologic history include the following:
1. **Patient's demographics: age, gender, and race-ethnicity, if relevant**

   Age is often crucial in the initial consideration of the differential diagnosis. Disorders causing ataxia, for instance, would include multiple sclerosis and viral cerebellitis in patients under 45 years of age, whereas cerebral infarction and alcoholic cerebellar degeneration would be higher on the differential diagnosis list for the same syndrome in older patients. Gender-specific neurologic conditions include benign intracranial hypertension and multiple sclerosis, which are more common in women.

   Race-ethnicity differences include the higher incidence of intracranial atherosclerosis in African-American and Hispanic patients, whereas in Caucasians, extracranial atherosclerosis tends to develop with higher frequency.

2. **Temporal course of the disease**

   The temporal pattern of your patient's symptoms is one of the most important pieces of history that you will obtain. Many neurologic disorders can be differentiated by their temporal course. Precipitous onset suggests a vascular or epileptic etiology across a wide spectrum of complaints. Onset over minutes to hours suggests a toxic or infectious cause. Subacute or chronic progression of symptoms prompts investigation of metabolic, neoplastic, or degenerative disorders.

   The subsequent pattern of symptoms is also important. Symptoms that follow a paroxysmal course lead to a limited differential diagnosis: transient ischemic attack, migraine, and seizure are often considered when paroxysmal episodes are relatively short-lived. Myasthenia gravis, multiple sclerosis, and periodic paralysis have a fluctuating or recurrent course as well, but typically with less rapid cycles.

3. **Characterization of the symptoms**

   It may seem excessive or inefficient to obtain a detailed description of your patient's symptoms, yet the initial disqualification of untenable diagnoses can be accomplished with confidence only when you are sure of the symptoms being reported. The mode of onset, prior occurrences, surrounding events, and character of the complaint—including what makes it better or worse—are important in establishing an initial differential diagnosis. You may need to ask more than once or use alternative terminology to elicit the details of a particular symptom. Notoriously ambiguous symptom descriptions in neurology include "heavy," which may mean weak, numb, or clumsy; "numb," which may mean decreased sensation or paresthesias; "dizzy," which may mean vertiginous, lightheaded, or confused; and "confused," which may mean disoriented, agitated, aphasic, or even sleepy. Be wary also of actual diagnoses that are presented in lieu of symptoms. The patient who keeps getting "seizures" in the arm or the one who presents with "trauma" should be redirected to a vocabulary of symptoms alone.

4. **Medical history**

Although a detailed medical history is not necessary in every interview, you will need to obtain information about any disease that could contribute to the patient's present complaint. For example, it is crucial to be aware of cerebrovascular risk factors including cardiac disease, hypertension, diabetes mellitus, and smoking if stroke is in the differential diagnosis. A history of carcinoma would be important if metastasis or paraneoplastic disease is being considered. Some systemic illnesses, such as sarcoidosis, systemic lupus erythematosus, and diabetes mellitus, may be associated with a spectrum of neurologic complaints. Information regarding current medications should be elicited in every case. Travel and occupational history may be relevant, for example, when toxic and infectious etiologies are under consideration. If the patient cannot provide the necessary information, you may need to interview a family member or caretaker or review the patient's medical record.

ESTABLISHING THE INITIAL DIFFERENTIAL DIAGNOSIS

Neurologic complaints lend themselves to categorization of the differential diagnosis based on **anatomic localization.** Acute visual dysfunction, for example, may be divided into unilateral loss of vision (suggesting pathology in the retina or optic nerve), binocular visual field defects (implying disease in the optic tracts or radiations), or diplopia (suggesting either neuromuscular or brain stem dysfunction). Other neurologic complaints are best categorized initially by the **rate of onset.** The likely diagnoses related to acute ataxia, for instance, are different from those associated with chronic or subacute gait failure. The differential diagnosis for many neurologic complaints, however, contains a wide variety of disorders that are not easily sorted until more information is obtained from the history and physical examination. For these complaints, we suggest that you develop a standard method of considering the differential diagnosis. One mnemonic, which appears in many of our patient complaint chapters, may be useful: VITAMINS, representing vascular, infectious, traumatic, autoimmune, metabolic/toxic, iatrogenic/idiopathic or hereditary, neoplastic, and seizure/psychiatric/structural etiologies.

ANATOMIC LOCALIZATION

The neurologic examination is presented in Chapter 2. Certain principles of anatomic localization warrant emphasis here, because establishing the correct diagnosis in neurology is often dependent on localization of the lesion. Listed here in tabular form are general principles of localization of lesions from the brain to the periphery. Most of these localizations are discussed within the pertinent chapters on **patient-related problems**.

Localization in the Upper Motor Neuron (Pyramidal) System
Principle: Tone is increased, causing spasticity and hyperreflexia

Site	Symptoms	Signs
Cortex	• Differential weakness of limbs and face • Sensory symptoms • Language, visual, or attentional alterations	• Fractionated weakness (e.g., arm greater than face and leg) • Aphasia, hemianopia, or hemineglect • Cortical and primary sensory loss • Cognitive dysfunction
Corona radiata Internal capsule	• Differential weakness of limbs and face • Weakness only	• Fractionated weakness • Primary sensory loss • Face, arm, and leg affected equally and densely
Brain stem	• Unilateral or bilateral weakness • Diplopia, vertigo, dysarthria, or weakness	• Dense hemiparesis • Ocular or oropharyngeal dysphagia • Motor posturing • No face involvement
Spinal cord	• Difficulty with gait • Difficulty walking • Urinary incontinence	• Spastic quadriparesis (cervical) or paraparesis (thoracic) • Sensory level

Localization in the Lower Motor Neuron System
Principle: Tone is decreased, causing flaccidity and hyporeflexia

Site	Symptoms	Signs
Anterior horn	• Progressive flaccid weakness	• Wasting, weakness, fasciculations • No sensory loss
Root/plexus	• Single-limb weakness and sensory loss • Pain in the neck, back, or limb	• Weakness in radicular/plexus distribution • Electromyogram (EMG) shows denervation in affected muscles
Nerve	• Focal weakness (mononeuritis) • Distal weakness (polyneuropathy)	• Focal or distal weakness • Atrophy in affected distribution • Fasciculations • Hyporeflexia • Slowing or low amplitude on conduction studies; denervation on EMG
Neuromuscular junction	• Fluctuating weakness • Diplopia	• Positive edrophonium test • Decremental response with repetitive stimulation on EMG
Muscle	• Proximal weakness • Difficulty climbing stairs and brushing hair • Muscle aches	• Proximal weakness • Polyphasic, low-amplitude motor units on EMG

Localization within the Brain Stem
Principle: Specific cranial nerve involvement guides localization (Fig. 1–1)

Site	Signs and Symptoms
Midbrain	• Impaired vertical gaze • **CN 3 palsy** (plus contralateral abduction nystagmus suggests ipsilateral internuclear ophthalmoplegia [INO]) • **CN 4 palsy** • Contralateral motor signs (hemiparesis suggests Weber's syndrome; ataxia suggests Claude's syndrome; tremor or chorea suggests Benedikt's syndrome) • Alterations in consciousness, perception, or behavior (peduncular hallucinosis)

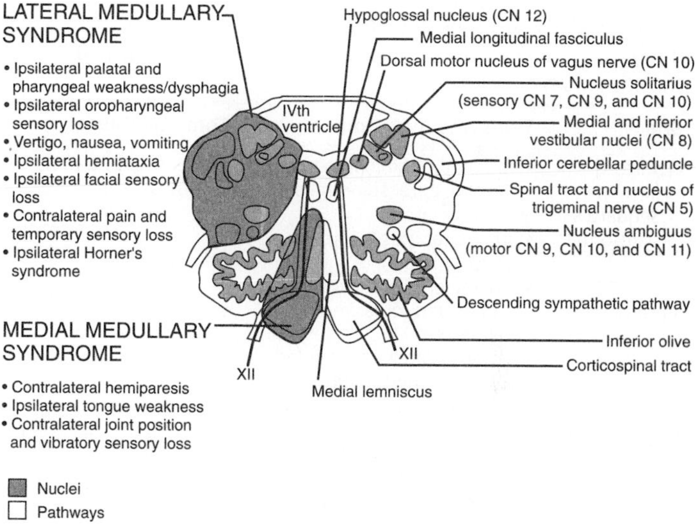
LATERAL MEDULLARY SYNDROME
• Ipsilateral palatal and pharyngeal weakness/dysphagia
• Ipsilateral oropharyngeal sensory loss
• Vertigo, nausea, vomiting
• Ipsilateral hemiataxia
• Ipsilateral facial sensory loss
• Contralateral pain and temporary sensory loss
• Ipsilateral Horner's syndrome
MEDIAL MEDULLARY SYNDROME
• Contralateral hemiparesis
• Ipsilateral tongue weakness
• Contralateral joint position and vibratory sensory loss
Nuclei
Pathways
IVth ventricle
Hypoglossal nucleus (CN 12)
Medial longitudinal fasciculus
Dorsal motor nucleus of vagus nerve (CN 10)
Nucleus solitarius (sensory CN 7, CN 9, and CN 10)
Medial and inferior vestibular nuclei (CN 8)
Inferior cerebellar peduncle
Spinal tract and nucleus of trigeminal nerve (CN 5)
Nucleus ambiguus (motor CN 9, CN 10, and CN 11)
Descending sympathetic pathway
Inferior olive
Corticospinal tract
XII
XII
Medial lemniscus

Figure 1–1 Brain stem sections at the level of the medulla.

Localization within the Brain Stem (continued)

Site	Signs and Symptoms
Pons	• Dysarthria and dysphagia • Contralateral hemiparesis or hemisensory loss • Ipsilateral facial sensory loss **(CN 5)** • Ipsilateral gaze palsy (paramedian pontine reticular formation [PPRF]) or one-and-a-half syndrome (PPRF and median longitudinal fasciculus [MLF]) • Locked-in syndrome (bilateral basis pontis; associated with ocular bobbing) • Horizontal nystagmus (often brachium pontis) • Ataxia
Pontomedullary junction	• Vertigo **(CN 8)** • Dysarthria • Horizontal or vertical nystagmus • Contralateral hemisensory loss and hemiparesis
Lateral medulla (Wallenberg syndrome)	• Ipsilateral Horner's syndrome • Ipsilateral limb ataxia • Ipsilateral face and contralateral body numbness • Gait ataxia • Vertigo, dizziness, nausea **(CN 8)** • Dysphagia **(CN 9, CN 10, and CN 12 palsies)**
Medial medulla (rare)	• Contralateral hemiplegia • Contralateral posterior column sensory loss • Ipsilateral tongue weakness **(CN 12 palsy)**

Localization in the Spinal Cord

Principle: Localization is assisted by the combination of tracts involved

Site	Signs and Symptoms	Common Causes
Hemicord (Brown-Séquard's syndrome)	• Ipsilateral hemiparesis • Contralateral spinothalamic sensory loss • Ipsilateral dorsal column sensory loss • Sphincter dysfunction	• Penetrating trauma • Extrinsic cord compression
Anterior cord	• Upper and lower motor paralysis • Spinothalamic sensory loss • Sphincter dysfunction • Sparing of posterior columns	• Anterior spinal artery infarction (often involves T4 to T8)
Central cord	• Paraparesis • Lower motor paralysis; wasting and fasciculations in arms • Sensory loss in "shawl" distribution (if in cervical region)	• Syringomyelia • Neck flexion-extension injury • Intrinsic tumor
Posterior cord	• Proprioceptive and vibratory sensory loss • Segmental tingling and numbness • Sensation of constricting "bands"	• Vitamin B$_{12}$ deficiency • Demyelination (multiple sclerosis) • Extrinsic compression
Foramen magnum	• Spastic quadriparesis • Neck pain and stiffness • C2 to C4 and upper facial numbness • Ipsilateral Horner's syndrome • Ipsilateral tongue and trapezius muscle weakness	• Tumor (meningioma, chordoma) • Atlantoaxial subluxation
Conus medullaris	• Lower sacral saddle sensory loss (S2 to S5) • Sphincter dysfunction; impotence • Aching back or rectal pain • L5 and S1 motor deficits (ankle and foot weakness)	• Intrinsic tumor • Extrinsic cord compression
Cauda equina	• Sphincter dysfunction • Paraparesis with weakness in the distribution of multiple roots • Sensory loss in multiple bilateral dermatomes	• Extrinsic tumor • Carcinomatous meningitis • Arachnoiditis • Spinal stenosis

The Neurologic Examination

Clinical examination is of primary importance in the practice of neurology, even with the availability of advanced neuroimaging techniques. **This is because the neurologic examination provides critical information that no other test can provide: it tells you whether the patient's nervous system is working normally.** Unfortunately, many clinicians never master the neurologic examination because it is taught in a way that makes it seem time-consuming, excessively complicated, and of questionable relevance. In real on-call situations, however, expert neurologists almost never perform the type of comprehensive, top-to-bottom examination that is taught in medical school; rather, they focus on the problem at hand, eliminate those parts of the examination that are not relevant, and actively test hypotheses suggested by the history.

The intent of this chapter is to acquaint (or reacquaint) the physician with the basic components of the neurologic examination. Suggested problem-oriented examinations for specific clinical presentations (e.g., coma, back pain, or acute weakness) are provided in later chapters.

THE NEUROLOGIC EXAMINATION

The components of the neurologic examination are shown in Box 2-1.

Mental Status

The importance of the mental status examination cannot be overemphasized. In patients with suspected intracranial pathology (e.g., in those experiencing sudden severe headache), a change in mental status signals that the problem is more than just one of pain: it indicates that the brain is not working correctly. The implications for further workup and management are significant.

Human mentation is extraordinarily complex, and students of neurology frequently have difficulty with the mental status

---

BOX 2–1 **Components of the Neurologic Examination**

For the beginner, even remembering all of the components of the neurologic exam can be difficult. Memorizing the first letter of the seven main sections of the exam (M C M C R S G) may be helpful for avoiding omissions when first learning the examination:

- Mental status
- Cranial nerves
- Motor
- Coordination
- Reflexes
- Sensory
- Gait and station

---

examination because they are taught to evaluate a "laundry-list" of mental functions (Table 2–1) without emphasis on how to integrate the findings. To simplify the mental status examination, we advocate a five-step approach that emphasizes five basic elements: (1) alertness and attention, (2) confusion, disorientation, or abnormal behavior, (3) language, (4) memory, and (5) other higher cortical functions.

- **Step One: Examination of level of consciousness, attention, and concentration**

  As illustrated schematically in Figure 2–1, the brain's arousal and attention mechanism (mediated by the diffuse cortical projections of the reticular activating system of the brain stem) serves as the foundation of all higher cognitive function. Level of consciousness, attention, and mental concentration can be conceptualized as three levels of a pyramid, because dysfunction at a more basic level (depressed level of consciousness) almost guarantees that functions at the top of the pyramid (attention and concentration) will be abnormal. Similarly, if a patient cannot remain alert or attend or concentrate, normal functioning of memory, language, or other higher functions cannot be expected. *Delirium* is characterized by severe attentional deficits in a patient with relatively preserved alertness (mildly lethargic to hyperalert).

  1. **Level of consciousness.** *Is the patient alert, lethargic, stuporous, or comatose? Lethargy* resembles sleepiness but with one important difference: the patient cannot be fully and permanently awakened. *Stupor* can be operationally defined by the requirement for painful stimuli to obtain the patient's best verbal or motor response. *Coma* indicates lack of responsiveness even to painful stimuli.

  2. **Attention.** *Is the patient attentive to you?* Global attention is impaired in patients who are lethargic or encephalopathic.

TABLE 2–1 **Mental Status: Emotional and Higher Cognitive Functions**

Behavior	Is the patient's behavior appropriate, hostile, or bizarre?
Abstract reasoning	Can the patient judge similarities and interpret proverbs? Poor abstract reasoning results in "concrete thinking."
Insight	Does the patient have an appropriate understanding of the current medical problem?
Judgment	Is the patient's judgment impaired? Ask what the patient would do if he or she found a wallet or smelled smoke in a theater.
Calculations	Can the patient add, subtract, and multiply?
Visuospatial ability	Can the patient copy figures, draw a clock face, or bisect a line?
Praxis	Does the patient have apraxia—the inability to execute motor tasks (whistle or blow out a match) in response to a verbal command or imitation (ideomotor apraxia) in the absence of a comprehension, sensory, or motor deficit?
Affect	Is the patient's affect (an immediately expressed and observed emotion) depressed, euphoric, restricted, flat, or inappropriate?
Mood	What is the patient's long-term emotional disposition?
Thought form	Does the patient display loosening of associations, flight of ideas, tangentiality, circumstantiality, or incoherence? When seen in the absence of impaired level of consciousness, attention, memory, or language, thought disorders are characteristic of psychiatric illness.
Thought content	Is the patient's thought content characterized by paranoia, delusions, compulsions, obsessions, phobias, or derealization?
Perceptions	Does the patient have hallucinations or illusions?

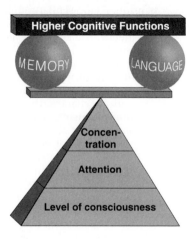

Figure 2–1 Schematic representation of the basic elements of human cognition. Arousal mechanisms (level of consciousness, attention, and concentration) serve as the foundation of all mental activity. Language and memory are anatomically localized, highly developed basic cognitive modalities. All other higher cognitive functions depend on normal function of these three basic elements.

A normally attentive patient looks at you and responds to questions and commands immediately. Inattention is characterized by impaired visual fixation and pursuit, delayed verbal responses requiring multiple prompts, and motor impersistence. *Spatial hemineglect* results from large hemispheric lesions and is almost always associated with impaired global attention as well.

3. **Concentration.** *Can the patient count from 20 to 1 and recite the months in reverse?* These are relatively overlearned tasks and are less susceptible to the effects of prior education than are serial sevens. Abnormal responses include long pauses, omissions, and reversals.

- **Step Two: Assessment for disorientation, confusion, or a behavioral abnormality**

    This step is initially based on observation during history taking. *Behavior* should be assessed in terms of psychomotor activity (agitation versus abulia) and emotional responses (elation, sadness, anger, or flattening).

    1. **Formally test orientation to name, place, time (date, day of week, month, and year), and situation.** Disorientation reflects abnormal *integrative functioning* of the brain. Unlike abnormalities of arousal, memory, or language, disorientation has no implications with regard to anatomic localization—there is no "orientation center" in the brain. *Remember that disorientation typically follows a sequential pattern, first involving situation, then time, place, and name.* Hence, a patient who is oriented to time and place but who does not know his or her own name probably has a psychiatric problem.

- **Step Three: Language testing**

    Focal lesions of the dominant hemisphere may lead to *aphasia,* defined as abnormal language production or comprehension. Four essential components of language should always be tested:

    1. **Fluency.** *Is the rate and flow of the patient's speech production normal?* Dysfluency is defined by reduction in the rate of speech production. Speaking with effort, finding words with difficulty, losing normal grammar and syntax, giving perseverative responses, and making spontaneous paraphasic errors are characteristic.

    2. **Comprehension.** *Can the patient perform one- and two-step commands?* If the patient is attentive, inability to follow commands implies impaired auditory comprehension.

    3. **Naming.** *Can the patient name a watch, a pen, and glasses?* Check for *anomia* and *paraphasic errors.* Listen for *phonemic paraphasias* (substitution of one phoneme for another, e.g., "tadle" for "table") and *semantic paraphasias* (substitution of one semantically related word for another, e.g., "door" for "window").

TABLE 2–2 **Classification of Aphasias**

	Fluency	Comprehension	Naming	Repetition
Broca's aphasia (motor)	0	+	0	0
Wernicke's aphasia (sensory)	+	0	0	0
Transcortical motor aphasia	0	+	0	+
Transcortical sensory aphasia	+	0	0	+
Global aphasia	0	0	0	0
Conduction aphasia	+	+	0	0
Anomic aphasia	+	+	0	+

0, abnormal; +, normal.

4. **Repetition.** *Can the patient repeat "The train was an hour late" and "Today is a sunny day"?* Intact repetition in the presence of serious deficits in fluency or comprehension is diagnostic of *transcortical aphasia,* which implies a good prognosis for recovery.

With the preceding information—fluency, comprehension, naming, and repetition—you can diagnose and classify any aphasia (Table 2–2). Asking the patient to read aloud is also a sensitive screening test for aphasia and alexia. *Broca's aphasia* (localized to the dorsolateral dominant frontal lobe) results in nonfluent, effortful speech and is usually associated with hemiparesis. *Wernicke's aphasia* (localized to the posterior superior temporal lobe) leads to fluent, nonsensical speech with impaired comprehension, and in most cases, the patient is unaware of the problem (anosognosia). If an aphasia is present and more precise characterization of the deficit is desired, check reading and writing in detail. Don't confuse aphasia with *dysarthria,* which is a motor disorder.

- **Step Four: Memory testing**

    Memory is classified as **immediate, short term,** and **long term.** In neurologic patients, impaired immediate recall is usually due to attentional deficits rather than to pure amnesia. Short-term memory can be tested by asking the patient to recall three words (e.g., "Jane, red, elephant") in 3 to 5 minutes. Long-term (remote) memory is best tested by asking about famous politicians (e.g., Richard M. Nixon or John F. Kennedy), twentieth-century historical events (the Watergate crisis or World War II), or sports figures. *Confabulatory (incorrect)* responses occur with severe amnestic disorders.

- **Step Five: Testing for emotional and higher cognitive functions**

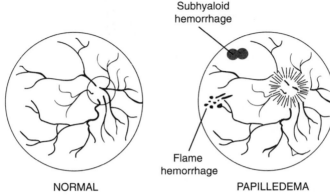

Subhyaloid hemorrhage

Flame hemorrhage

NORMAL   PAPILLEDEMA

Figure 2–2 Common abnormalities found on examination of the optic fundus. Papilledema is characterized by optic disk congestion and the loss of distinct vessels crossing the blurred disk margin.

These components of the mental status exam are listed in Table 2–1 and are usually not anatomically localizable and not essential to test in all cases. They are primarily of value for identifying complex cognitive and neuropsychiatric disorders.

Cranial Nerves

CN 1   **Olfactory nerve**
Testing for olfactory nerve function is rarely needed and is usually omitted.

CN 2   **Optic nerve**
1. **Fundus**
Check for papilledema, optic disk pallor or atrophy, retinal hemorrhages or exudates, spontaneous venous pulsations, and hypertensive microvascular changes (arteriovenous [AV] nicking and copper wiring) (Fig. 2–2).
2. **Visual fields**
Stand facing the patient, instruct him or her to look at your nose, and have the patient count fingers in all four quadrants (Fig. 2–3). Test each eye separately. Check lateralized blink to threat if the patient is inattentive.
3. **Visual acuity**
Test acuity with eyeglasses, one eye at a time, using a "near card."
4. **Color vision**
This is usually tested only by an ophthalmologist. Color desaturation occurs with optic nerve disorders.

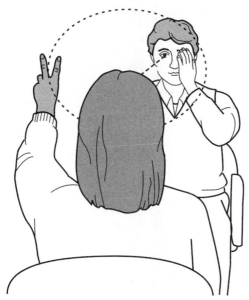

Figure 2–3 Technique for visual field testing.

CN 3,
CN 4,
CN 6

Oculomotor, trochlear, and abducens nerves

1. **Eyelids**

   Check for *ptosis*, defined as a drooping eyelid that does not clear the upper margin of the pupil. Ptosis occurs with oculomotor nerve (CN 3) injury or with *Horner's syndrome* (ptosis, miosis, facial anhidrosis), which results from injury to central or peripheral sympathetic nerve pathways.

2. **Pupils**

   Check for shape, symmetry, reactivity to light, and accommodation. *Anisocoria* (pupillary asymmetry) can result from *miosis* (an abnormally small pupil) or *mydriasis* (an abnormally large pupil), and in some cases, examination in both light and dark conditions is necessary to determine which pupil is abnormal.

   An *afferent pupillary defect* (APD, or Marcus Gunn pupil) results from a lesion of the optic nerve (e.g., optic neuritis in multiple sclerosis). It is elicited using the swinging flashlight test: as the light swings from one eye to the other at 3-second intervals, the abnormal pupil will *dilate* rather than constrict when the light shines on it.

3. Extraocular movements

Ask the patient to fixate on and follow your finger in all directions of gaze. Unilateral impairment of ocular motility usually results from an isolated cranial nerve deficit. Besides checking for limitations of eye movement, look for abnormalities of *fixation* (square wave jerks, nystagmus, opsoclonus), *smooth pursuit* (saccadic pursuit), and *saccadic eye movements* (hypometric saccades, ocular dysmetria). Test saccades by asking the patient to rapidly switch fixation from one hand to the other.

Opticokinetic nystagmus (OKN) is a normal physiologic nystagmus that occurs when the patient is asked to fixate on a series of moving visual stimuli (e.g., striped OKN tape). Asymmetric loss of OKN results from frontal or parietal lobe lesions on the side to which the tape is moving.

CN 5   **Trigeminal nerve**

Sensory function of V1, V2, and V3 is evaluated by testing for deficits to light touch, pinprick, and temperature on the forehead, cheek, and chin, respectively (Fig. 2–4). Motor function can be tested by checking for asymmetry of lateral jaw movements. Lateral pterygoid muscle weakness results in ipsilateral deviation on jaw opening and weakness of lateral movement to the opposite side.

The *corneal reflex* (mediated by V1) is elicited by lightly touching the cornea with a cotton wisp, which results in contraction of the orbicularis oculi (CN 7). It

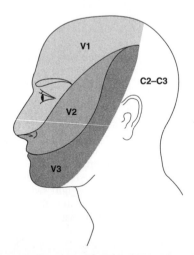

Figure 2–4 **Sensory distribution of the trigeminal nerve.**

usually needs to be tested only in comatose patients, or if focal brain stem or cranial nerve pathology (e.g., an acoustic neuroma) is suspected.

CN 7   **Facial nerve**

A *widened palpebral fissure* and *flattened nasolabial fold* are indicative of facial weakness. Ask the patient to grin and raise the eyebrows, and check the strength of eye and lip closure against active resistance. Upper motor neuron facial weakness tends to spare the contralateral forehead because it has bilateral upper motor neuron innervation, whereas the lower portion of the face does not.

Taste usually requires testing only when there is evidence of facial weakness. Dip a wet cotton swab in sugar or salt and apply it to the tip and side of the tongue with the tongue kept protruded. Absence of taste confirms a peripheral CN 7 lesion proximal to the junction of the chorda tympani.

CN 8   **Vestibulocochlear nerve**

Auditory deficits can be screened for by testing appreciation of *finger rub* in each ear. If unilateral hearing loss is present, sensorineural and conduction deafness can be differentiated using a 512-Hz tuning fork:

- *Weber's test* is performed by striking the tuning fork and placing it against the middle of the forehead. Ask the patient if the tone is equal in both ears. Diminution in the affected ear indicates sensorineural hearing loss. A louder tone in the affected ear results from *conduction deafness* (disease of the ossicles in the middle ear). In conduction deafness, a pure tone transmitted through the skull is appreciated in the affected ear, whereas the tone sounds softer in the normal ear because of competing ambient noise transmitted via the tympanic membrane and ossicles.
- *The Rinne test* is performed to confirm the presence of conduction deafness in the affected ear. Strike the tuning fork, place it on the mastoid process, and ask the patient when the tone can no longer be heard. Then place it over the external auditory meatus— normally, the patient will hear the tone again; if not, conduction deafness is present.

CN 9,   **Glossopharyngeal and vagus nerves**
CN 10   Ask the patient to say "ah," check for symmetry and adequacy of soft palate elevation, and listen for hoarseness or nasal speech (all motor functions of CN 10). The gag reflex, tested by lightly touching the posterior oropharynx with a cotton swab (CN 9 sensory, CN 10 motor), is often absent or depressed in older patients.

Dysphagia and risk for aspiration are best screened for by asking the patient to swallow a small quantity of water (3 oz); coughing indicates aspiration and inability to protect the airway.

CN 11   **Spinal accessory nerve**
Have the patient flex and turn the head to each side against resistance (tests the sternocleidomastoid muscle). Contraction of the left sternocleidomastoid muscle turns the head to the right and vice versa. Have the patient shrug the shoulders against resistance to test the trapezius muscle.

CN 12   **Hypoglossal nerve**
Have the patient stick out the tongue and push it into each cheek. Unilateral CN 12 dysfunction results in deviation of the tongue to the weak side upon protrusion and in inability to push the tongue into the opposite cheek.

Motor

1. **Inspection**
Look for *muscle wasting* (atrophy), *fasciculations,* and *adventitious movements.* Preferential spontaneous movement of the limbs on one side suggests paresis of the unused limbs. If the patient is comatose, check for a preferential localizing response to sternal rub.
Tremor should be evaluated at rest (rest tremor), with sustained posture (postural tremor), and with active movement (action or intention tremor).

2. **Tone**
Have the patient relax; check muscle tone by passively moving the elbows, wrists, and knees.
a. **Hypotonia** occurs with acute paralysis, lower motor neuron disease, ipsilateral cerebellar lesions, and chorea.
b. **Hypertonia** comes in three varieties:
   (1) **Spasticity** develops as a consequence of upper motor neuron lesions. It is generally characterized by a sudden increase in tone (a "catch") as the limb is passively flexed or extended. The clasp-knife phenomenon is a particular form of spasticity sometimes encountered in the legs; muscle tone is greatest at the beginning of movement and slowly decreases until there is a sudden loss of resistance.
   (2) **Rigidity** occurs with disease of the basal ganglia. Increased resistance is present throughout the full range of motion. *Cogwheel rigidity,* characterized by a regular ratchet-like loss of resistance, is especially characteristic of parkinsonism. Cogwheel rigidity at the

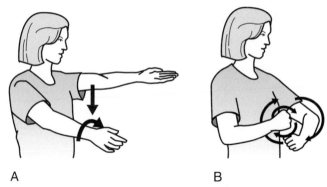

A   B

Figure 2–5 Screening procedures for mild hemiparesis. *A,* Pronator drift: the weaker right arm drifts downward and pronates. *B,* Arm-rolling test: the stronger left arm tends to "orbit" the weaker right arm.

        wrist can often be accentuated if the patient is asked to repeatedly open and close the opposite hand.

   (3) **Gegenhalten** (holding against), or paratonia, occurs with dementia and frontal lobe syndromes. It is characterized by a variably and inconsistently increased tone that alternates with relaxation.

3. **Screening tests for hemiparesis**

    In many instances, cerebral lesions lead to subtle hemiparesis with normal strength against resistance. Check the following to screen for subtle indications of hemiparesis (Fig. 2–5):

a. **Pronator drift**

    Have the patient hold both arms forward, palms up, with eyes closed. Check for pronation and downward drift.

b. **Rapid finger taps**

    Check thumb and forefinger taps in each hand separately. Although often considered a sign of cerebellar dysfunction, slowing of fine rapid finger movements also occurs with corticospinal tract lesions.

c. **Arm-rolling test**

    Have the patient make fists and rotate the forearms around each other. With hemiparesis, the normal arm will tend to orbit the weaker arm.

4. **Power**

    Detailed testing of strength against active resistance in multiple individual muscle groups is usually unnecessary unless a peripheral cause of weakness is suspected. *For screening*

BOX 2–2 **Muscle Strength Grading Scale**

0 No muscle contraction detected
1 A barely detectable flicker or trace of contraction
2 Movement occurs only in the plane of gravity
3 Active movement against gravity but not against resistance
4 Active movement against resistance but less than normal strength
   (may be graded as 4+, 4, or 4−)
5 Normal strength

---

purposes, testing of strength at the shoulders, wrists, hips, and ankles will often suffice. Be aware that estimates of lower extremity strength in bedridden patients are often unreliable and that walking is the best way to screen for leg weakness.

By convention, muscle strength is graded as shown in Box 2–2.

Coordination

Disease of the cerebellar hemispheres leads to limb ataxia, whereas midline cerebellar lesions lead to gait ataxia. The following tests can be used to detect incoordination and ataxia.

1. **Finger-to-nose test**

   Have the patient alternately touch a fingertip to his or her nose and your finger. Check for intention tremor (irregular chaotic movements as the target is approached) and past pointing (often easier to elicit when the eyes are closed). Subtle dysmetria can be detected by holding the cap of a pen and having the patient slowly place the pen into the cap (Fig. 2–6).

2. **Rapid rhythmic alternating movements**

   Have the patient touch each of the fingers to the thumb in rapid succession, turn the hand over and back (pronation-supination) as fast as possible, and touch the toe and the heel to the floor in rapid succession. With cerebellar disease, these movements are slow and awkward *(dysdiadochokinesis)*.

3. **Heel-to-shin test**

   Have the patient slide the heel up and down the front of the shin. Limb ataxia results in a side-to-side "tremor" as the test is performed.

Reflexes

1. **Deep tendon reflexes**

   Striking the muscle tendon with a reflex hammer normally leads to a reflex muscle contraction mediated by the lower motor neuron reflex arc. *Hyper-reflexia* results from upper

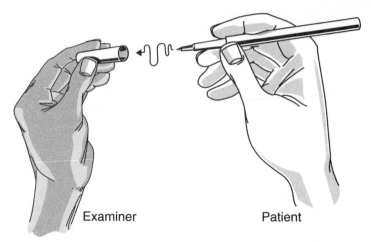

Examiner   Patient

Figure 2–6 Screening procedure for subtle dysmetria. Hold a pen cap, and look for an intention tremor as the patient tries to guide the pen into the cap.

TABLE 2–3 **Deep Tendon Reflexes**

Reflex	Segments
Jaw jerk	Trigeminal nerve (CN 5)
Biceps reflex	C5 and C6
Brachioradialis reflex	C5 and C6
Triceps reflex	C7 and C8
Finger flexion (Hoffman's) reflex	C8 and T1
Knee reflex	L2, L3, and L4
Ankle reflex	S1

motor neuron lesions as a result of release from normal descending inhibition, whereas *hyporeflexia* results from lesions of the lower motor neuron. The principal deep tendon reflexes and their corresponding spinal roots are listed in Table 2–3. Severe hyper-reflexia results in *clonus*—repeated rhythmic contraction elicited by striking a tendon or dorsiflexing the ankle.

By convention, deep tendon reflexes are graded on a scale of 0 to 5 (Box 2–3).

2. **Plantar reflex**

Firmly stroke the sole of the patient's foot with the handle end of your reflex hammer, beginning at the heel and following up the lateral margin and across the ball of the foot to the base of the big toe. Flexion of the big toe at the metatarsophalangeal joint is the normal response; extension *(Babinski's*

> BOX 2–3 **Tendon Reflex Grading Scale**
>
> 0 Absent
> 1 Diminished
> 2 Normal
> 3 Increased (may spread to adjacent muscles)
> 4 Unsustained clonus (a few beats)
> 5 Sustained clonus

sign) occurs with upper motor neuron lesions. If the patient is sensitive, lightly stroking the lateral heel alone is often enough to elicit a normal response.

3. **Cutaneous reflexes**

These reflexes do not require routine testing, but their testing is useful when a spinal cord or a cauda equina lesion is suspected. They are frequently absent in otherwise normal elderly or obese individuals. The presence of these reflexes implies normal function of the spinal cord and corresponding sensory and motor nerves at the level tested.

a. **Abdominal reflexes**

Use a key, wooden stick, or reflex hammer handle to lightly stroke from the lateral to the medial section of the abdomen above (T8-T9) and below (T11-T12) the umbilicus. The normal response is local contraction of the ipsilateral rectus abdominis muscle.

b. **Cremasteric reflex**

Striking the medial thigh (L1-L2) results in ipsilateral retraction of the scrotum (S1).

c. **Bulbocavernosus reflex and anal wink**

Squeezing the head of the penis (S2-S3) or stroking the perianal skin (S3-S4) results in reflex contraction of the external anal sphincter (S3-S4).

4. **Frontal release signs**

These primitive reflexes are typically seen with dementia or frontal lobe disease, but they may also occur in normal individuals.

a. **Snout, suck, and root reflexes**

These reflexes are elicited by lightly tapping the upper lip or the side of the mouth.

b. **Palmomental reflex**

Lightly stroking the palm results in ipsilateral contraction of the mentalis muscle. A unilateral palmomental contraction implies contralateral frontal lobe disease.

c. **Grasp reflex**

Placing two fingers in the palm results in involuntary grasping.

d. **Glabellar reflex**
   Obligatory blinking occurs each time the glabellar area between the eyes is tapped.

Sensory

Sensory testing, because of its subjectivity, is the most difficult and least reliable part of the neurologic examination. In patients with depressed level of consciousness or severe inattention, sensory testing usually provides little useful information and should be omitted. In most cases, testing for signs of sensory loss is unnecessary unless the patient has symptoms of sensory loss. **The key to a successful and efficient sensory examination is to know what you're looking for.** Sensory loss typically occurs in specific patterns, which you should try to rule in or rule out (Box 2–4).

A few simple rules can help make the sensory examination easier and are noted in Box 2–5.

1. **Primary sensory modalities**
   Sensation is mediated by two pathways: the dorsal columns, which mediate vibration and joint position, and the

---

BOX 2–4 Patterns of Sensory Loss

Hemisensory loss (cortical lesions)
Stocking-glove sensory loss (neuropathy)
Spinal level and Brown-Séquard's syndrome (spinal cord lesions)
Dermatomal sensory loss (nerve root lesions)
Peripheral nerve sensory loss (mononeuropathy)
Saddle anesthesia (lesion in cauda equina or conus medullaris)

BOX 2–5 Rules for Sensory Examination

1. *Don't ask leading questions.*
   When testing for hemisensory loss, ask "Does this feel the same on both sides?" If you ask "Which side feels sharper?," you are likely to get inconsistent (and insignificant) lateralizing responses.
2. *When mapping a region of sensory loss, move from the affected into the normal region.*
   Patients are better able to detect when a pinprick turns sharp than when it becomes dull.
3. *Beware of fatigue.*
   Cooperation in the sensory examination takes concentration, and patients may become fatigued. Rather than taking a thorough, top-to-bottom approach, start your sensory examination by getting right to the point.

spinothalamic tracts, which mediate pain and temperature. Touch is mediated by both sensory pathways and is thus usually the last modality to be affected.

a. **Light touch**

Test by lightly touching with fingertips or cotton wool. *Allodynia* refers to pain in response to a normally nonpainful stimulus (e.g., light touch).

b. **Pinprick**

Use a clean safety pin. *Hyperalgesia* refers to an exaggerated painful sensation; *hyperpathia* refers to an abnormal painful sensation (e.g., burning, tingling).

c. **Temperature**

Test with the handle of a reflex hammer or tuning fork submerged under cold tap water.

d. **Vibration**

Apply a 128-Hz tuning fork to the toes, medial malleolus, patella, fingers, wrist, and elbow, and ask when the sensation stops. In the elderly, vibration is commonly absent or reduced in the feet.

e. **Joint position (proprioception)**

Grasp the sides of the digit and ask the patient to identify small (5 to 10 degrees), random, up or down movements. Remember that even with complete proprioceptive loss, 50% of responses will be correct!

2. **Cortical sensory modalities**

If the primary sensory modalities are intact, disturbances of these modalities imply dysfunction of the contralateral parietal lobe. *The main utility of cortical sensory testing is for the detection of subtle hemisensory neglect.*

a. **Double simultaneous stimulation (face-hand test)**

Have the patient close the eyes; quickly touch one cheek and the contralateral hand at the same time. *Extinction* refers to consistent neglect of the hand stimulus on one side and implies a lesion of the contralateral parietal lobe. *Caudal neglect* refers to the tendency to consistently neglect the hand stimulus on either side; it occurs with dementia and frontal lobe disease.

b. **Graphesthesia**

Have the patient close the eyes and identify a number traced on the palm.

c. **Stereognosis**

Ask the patient to close the eyes and identify a key, coin, paperclip, or similar object placed in the palm.

Gait and Station

Disturbances of gait can result from dysfunction in one of many neurologic subsystems, including the motor cortex, corticospinal tracts, basal ganglia, cerebellum, vestibular system, peripheral nerves,

TABLE 2–4 **Some Abnormalities of Gait**

Gait	Features
Hemiparetic	Patient drags or circumducts the affected leg (moves stiffly in a circular motion outward and forward) and has a reduced ipsilateral arm swing
Ataxic	Patient has a wide-based stance with a veering and staggering gait; patient may consistently fall to the same side as the affected cerebellum
Parkinsonian	Patient has a stooped posture, takes small steps (festination), hesitates and freezes, and turns "en bloc"
Steppage	Patient lifts the knee high off the ground because of inability to dorsiflex at the ankle; patient has foot slap (results from peripheral neuropathy)
Waddling	Patient's pelvis drops on non-weight-bearing side with each step (results from myopathy with hip girdle weakness)
Scissor	Patient's gait is stiff, with short steps that cross forward on each other (results from spastic paraparesis)
Apraxic	Patient's gait is slow and unsteady; patient has trouble initiating steps, and the feet barely elevate off the floor (i.e., "magnetic gait") (results from hydrocephalus or frontal lobe disease)
Hysterical	Patient has a bizarre, wild, careening gait but never falls; patient shows excellent balance

muscles, and visual and proprioceptive afferent tracts. **Hence, gait testing is an excellent screening procedure, and many practitioners make it the first part of the neurologic examination.**

Specific components of gait analysis include *posture, width of stance, length of stride, arm swing,* and *balance.* Specific types of gait disturbance are listed in Table 2–4. Test the following:

1. **Natural gait**
2. **Tandem gait**

    Have the patient walk a straight line, touching toe to heel.
3. **Toe walking**
4. **Heel walking**
5. **Sitting to standing**

    To assess proximal leg strength, have the patient stand up from a chair with the arms folded.
6. **Romberg's test**

    Have the patient stand with eyes open and feet together. If the patient cannot do so, suspect a severe cerebellar or vestibular disturbance. *If substantial instability or falling occurs only after the patient closes the eyes, Romberg's test is positive.* A positive test indicates either *proprioceptive* (i.e., neuropathy or dorsal column disease) or *vestibular* dysfunction.

7. **Pull test**

Stand behind the patient and pull back on the shoulders. Normally, the patient should be able to regain balance after one step. Falling or retropulsion (many backward steps) suggests *impaired postural reflexes*, as occurs with parkinsonism.

Diagnostic Studies

A thorough history and examination should enable you to localize the disease process and generate a differential diagnosis. Confirmation of the diagnosis will usually require neurodiagnostic testing. When any of the tests described here is performed, it is essential to know what you are looking for and to understand the sensitivity (likelihood of a true positive result if the disease is present) and specificity (likelihood of a true negative result if the disease is absent) of each test for diagnosing the disease in question. Risks, benefits, and cost must also be considered.

LUMBAR PUNCTURE

Examination of the cerebrospinal fluid (CSF) by lumbar puncture (LP) is essential for diagnosing meningitis and subarachnoid hemorrhage when computed tomography (CT) is negative. It can also be helpful in evaluating peripheral neuropathy, carcinomatous meningitis, pseudotumor cerebri, multiple sclerosis (MS), and a variety of other inflammatory disorders.

- **Technique of LP**

    Proper positioning is the key to success (Fig. 3–1). Position the patient's back at the edge of the bed, with the head flexed and the legs curled up in the fetal position. Place a pillow under the head; it may be helpful to place another pillow between the legs. *Ensure that the shoulders and hips are parallel to each other and perpendicular to the bed* (i.e., not tilted forward). Locate the interspace between L4 and L5, which lies at the intercristal line (across the tops of the iliac crests), and insert the needle one level above, between L3 and L4. After sterilizing the area and locally injecting 2% lidocaine, insert a 20- or 22-gauge needle, parallel to the bed and tilted slightly cephalad. As you enter the subarachnoid space, you will feel a slight "pop." Measure the opening pressure and collect the CSF.

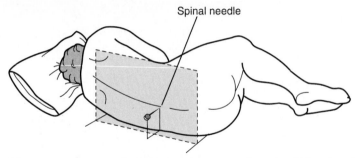

Figure 3–1 Positioning for lumbar puncture. A pillow should be placed beneath the head. Hips and shoulders should be parallel to each other and perpendicular to the bed. The spinal needle should be parallel to the bed.

TABLE 3–1 **CSF Tests**

- Cell count
- Protein and glucose levels
- Gram stain and culture
- VDRL test
- India ink test (for *Cryptococcus neoformans*)
- Wet smear (for fungi and amebae)
- Stain and culture for AFB (for tuberculosis)
- Cryptococcal antigen titers
- pH and lactate levels (abnormal in MELAS)
- Oligoclonal bands (abnormal in multiple sclerosis)
- IgG index (intrathecal IgG production)
- Latex agglutination bacterial antigen tests (for pneumococcus, meningococcus, and *Haemophilus influenzae*)
- Viral isolation studies
- Cytology (requires fixation in formalin)
- Lyme disease antibody titers (compare with serum titers) and Western blot
- Polymerase chain reaction for Lyme disease, tuberculosis, and causes of viral encephalitis
- CSF ACE activity (abnormal with tuberculosis or sarcoidosis)

ACE = angiotensin-converting enzyme; AFB = acid-fast bacteria; CSF = cerebrospinal fluid; HSV-1 = herpes simplex virus 1; IgG = immunoglobulin G; MELAS = mitochondrial encephalomyopathy, lactic acidosis, and stroke; VDRL = Venereal Disease Research Laboratory.

- **Examination of the CSF**
    This examination should always include a cell count (2 ml), protein and glucose analysis (2 ml), a Gram stain and culture (2 ml), and a CSF Venereal Disease Research Laboratory (VDRL) test (1 ml). Additional CSF tests are listed in Table 3–1. If red blood cells (RBCs) are encountered, check for xantho-

chromia, a yellowish tinge that differentiates true subarachnoid hemorrhage (>12 hours old) from a traumatic tap. To evaluate the significance of white blood cells (WBCs) in a traumatic tap, recall that the normal ratio of WBCs to RBCs in peripheral blood is 1 : 700.

● **Complications of LP**

The most frequent complication (in approximately 5% of patients) of LP is *spinal headache*, which results from persistent leakage of CSF from the entry site, leading to low intracranial pressure (ICP) and traction on the pain-sensitive intracranial dura when the patient is upright. The risk is minimized by using a thin (22-gauge) pencil-tipped spinal needle with a side hole (Sprotte, Gertie Marx), as opposed to a conventional bevel-tipped end hole (Quincke) spinal needle. Other complications are rare and occur only in patients with predisposing conditions: (1) *meningitis* can result if the needle is passed through infected tissue (e.g., cellulitis) before penetrating the dura, (2) *epidural hematoma* with compression of the cauda equina can result in patients with coagulopathy, (3) *tentorial herniation* can result in patients who have space-occupying lesions or severe basilar meningitis, and (4) *complete spinal block* and cord compression can result in patients who have a partial spinal block. These predisposing conditions are relative (not absolute) contraindications to LP, and the risk/benefit ratio of performing or not performing the procedure must be considered in each case.

COMPUTED TOMOGRAPHY

CT provides "slice" images of the brain by sending axial x-ray beams through the head. The amount of radiation involved is essentially harmless. Tissues are differentiated by the degree to which they attenuate the x-ray beams:

Low attenuation
(appears **black**)
{
Air (darkest)
Fat
Water

Medium attenuation
(appears **grey**)
{
Edematous or infarcted brain
Normal brain
Subacute hemorrhage
(3 to 14 days old)

High attenuation
(appears **white**)
{
Acute hemorrhage
Intravenous contrast material
Bone or metal (brightest)

● **Intravenous contrast**

When injected, contrast material is normally confined to the cerebral vessels. Hence, *contrast enhancement detects the presence of a disrupted blood-brain barrier*. Contrast is useful in patients with suspected neoplasm, abscess, vascular malformation, or new-onset seizures.

- **CT perfusion imaging**

  Single or multislice CT perfusion scans are obtained after an IV contrast bolus is injected via an 18-gauge IV. The images must be reconstructed using computerized software. Color-coded maps of cerebral blood flow, cerebral blood volume, and mean transit time can be obtained. The main utility of CT perfusion imaging is to demonstrate a region of noninfarcted hypoperfused brain in patients with acute ischemic stroke or subarachnoid hemorrhage.

- **CT angiography**

  After an IV contrast bolus and computerized image reconstruction, these three-dimensional images can provide good to excellent resolution of the cervical and large proximal intracranial arteries. The main utility of CT angiography is for the diagnosis of extracranial carotid stenosis, proximal intracranial stenoses or occlusions, and saccular intracranial aneurysms. But beware: resolution of the distal vasculature for detecting more subtle lesions such as vasculitic beading, a mycotic aneurysm, or a dural arteriovenous fistula is limited.

MAGNETIC RESONANCE IMAGING

MRI provides greater resolution and detail than does CT but takes longer to perform. MRI is superior to CT for evaluating the brain stem and posterior fossa and is superior to myelography for identifying intramedullary spinal cord lesions. Because it uses a powerful magnetic field, there is no exposure to radiation. However, MRI is contraindicated in patients with implanted ferromagnetic objects such as pacemakers, orthopedic pins, and older aneurysm clips.

- **T1 images**

  T1 images (TE <50, TR <100) are best for showing *anatomy*. CSF and bone appear black, normal brain appears gray, and fat and subacute blood (>48 hours old) appears white. Most pathologic processes (e.g., infarction, tumor) are associated with increased water content and hence appear darker than normal brain. *Fat suppression T1 images* are useful for identifying intramural thrombus (appears white) in cases of cervico-cranial arterial dissection.

- **T2 and FLAIR images**

  T2 (TE >80, TR >2000) and FLAIR (fluid attenuation inversion recovery) images are best for showing *pathology*. Most pathologic processes (e.g., infarction, tumor) lead to bright high-signal (white) changes, which reflect increased tissue water content. FLAIR is somewhat more sensitive than T2 in general; the CSF appears dark on FLAIR but bright on T2. Blood

TABLE 3–2 **Evolution of Appearance of Hemorrhage on MRI**

Feature	T1 Image	T2 Image	Metabolic Change
Blood			
4-6 hours	No change	○	Intact RBC with oxyhemoglobin
7-72 hours	No change	●	Intact RBC with deoxyhemoglobin
4-7 days	○	●	Intact RBC with methemoglobin
1-4 weeks	○	○	Free methemoglobin
Months	●	●	Hemosiderin with macrophages
Edema	●	○	Increased water content

● = low signal, appears dark; ○ = high signal, appears bright; MRI = magnetic resonance imaging; RBC = red blood cell.

on T2 varies in signal intensity according to the age of the hemorrhage, as depicted in Table 3–2.

- **Diffusion-weighted imaging**

    Diffusion-weighted imaging (DWI) is useful for detecting *hyperacute ischemia* in patients with acute stroke. Severe cerebral ischemia produces an immediate reduction in the diffusion coefficient of water, resulting in high-intensity (bright) signal changes on these images within minutes. Over several hours, DWI lesions become associated with high-intensity lesions seen on T2 and FLAIR as the ischemic tissue progresses to infarction. "T2 shine-through" refers to the tendency for high-intensity T2 lesions to produce increased signal on DWI, falsely indicating reduced diffusion.

- **Proton density images**

    Proton density images are partway between T1 and T2 images in signal density. Their main utility is for differentiating periventricular pathology (e.g., white matter demyelination) from CSF.

- **STIR sequences**

    STIR (short tau inversion recovery) sequences allow summation of T1 and T2 signals and dropout of fat. They are useful for evaluating mesial temporal sclerosis in patients with epilepsy.

- **Flow voids**

    Flow voids appear black on both T1 and T2 images, and they represent high-velocity blood flow (e.g., normal cerebral vessels or arteriovenous malformation [AVM]).

- **MR angiography**

    MR angiography (MRA) produces images of the extracranial and intracranial cerebral circulation with the brain and skull "subtracted out." The resolution is adequate for the evaluation of large-scale lesions (e.g., internal carotid artery stenosis and large aneurysms) but is inferior to standard angiography for evaluating smaller lesions (e.g., beading, distal spasm).

Time-resolved contrast-enhanced MRA offers improved resolution over conventional MRA, particularly for evaluating high-grade stenosis of the cervical arteries.

- **MR venography**

    MR venography provides subtraction images of the major venous sinuses. It can be useful for diagnosing dural sinus thrombosis but is less sensitive than angiography for detecting cortical vein thrombosis.

MYELOGRAPHY

Myelography consists of injecting radiopaque dye into the spinal canal via either a lumbar or a suboccipital approach. After the patient is tilted, x-rays and axial CT slices allow visualization of the spinal subarachnoid space and can reveal extradural compressive lesions, ruptured intervertebral disks, and vascular malformations on the surface of the cord. In recent years, this test has been largely supplanted by MRI; however, myelography can still be useful if MRI is equivocal, and it remains essential for ruling out cord compression if MRI is not available. Complications are generally the same as those associated with LP.

DOPPLER ULTRASONOGRAPHY

- **Carotid duplex Doppler ultrasonography**

    This imaging technique can provide an accurate and non-invasive estimate of the degree of stenosis of the extracranial internal carotid arteries. B-mode ultrasonography gives a graphic image of the arterial wall and can detect plaques, whereas pulsed Doppler ultrasonography analyzes velocity and turbulence related to stenosis. Results are generally classified as (1) normal, (2) <40% stenosis, (3) 40% to 60% stenosis, (4) 60% to 80% stenosis, (5) 80% to 99% stenosis, and (6) occlusion. If carotid Doppler scans suggest occlusion, confirmation with angiography is required, because high-grade stenosis cannot be ruled out in all cases. Positioning of the transducer over the posterior neck can also differentiate normal, high-resistance, and absent flow in the proximal vertebral arteries.

- **Transcranial Doppler (TCD) ultrasonography**

    This technique measures the velocity of blood flow in the intracranial proximal cerebral arteries (internal carotid artery [ICA] siphon, middle cerebral artery [MCA], anterior cerebral artery [ACA], posterior cerebral artery [PCA], ophthalmic, basilar, and vertebral). The main parameters obtained by TCD ultrasonography are blood flow velocity and pulsatility. TCD ultrasonography can be useful for the following:

1. Diagnosing intracranial stenosis or occlusion
2. Evaluating the hemodynamic significance of carotid stenosis or occlusion (look for blunted poststenotic flow in the MCA and reversed collateral flow in the ACA or ophthalmic artery)
3. Assessing vasospasm in patients with subarachnoid hemorrhage (high-velocity flow)
4. Screening for arteriovenous malformations (high-velocity flow, very low pulsatility)
5. Identifying severely increased ICP (low-velocity flow, high pulsatility)
6. Diagnosing brain death (systolic spikes with absent diastolic flow)

ANGIOGRAPHY

Cerebral angiography provides high-resolution images of the extracranial and intracranial cerebral vasculature (Fig. 3–2). The procedure is performed by threading a small catheter into the cerebral vessels via the femoral artery. Angiography is useful for identifying the following:

1. Occluded or stenotic vessels
2. Arterial dissections
3. Aneurysms
4. Arteriovenous malformations
5. Vasculitic narrowing ("beading")
6. Dural venous sinus thrombosis
- Complications of angiography
    Although infection or bleeding at the puncture site can occur, the most important complication (in 1% to 2% of patients) is stroke, which results from emboli generated by the catheter and which occurs most frequently in older patients with atherosclerotic disease.

ELECTROMYOGRAPHY AND NERVE CONDUCTION STUDIES

Electromyography (EMG) and nerve conduction studies assess the integrity and function of muscle and nerve, respectively, and essentially serve as extensions of the clinical examination.
- **EMG**
    This test can help distinguish neuropathic from myopathic disease, define the precise distribution of muscle involvement, and aid in the diagnosis of specific muscle disorders with unique features (e.g., myotonia). The procedure is performed by inserting a needle electrode into a muscle and analyzing motor unit potentials, both at rest (spontaneous activity) and

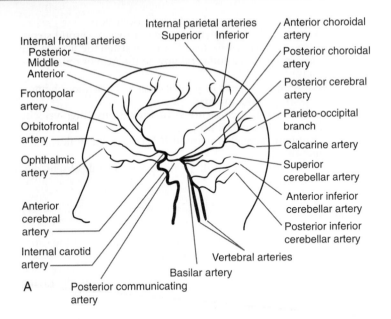

Internal parietal arteries
Superior   Inferior

Anterior choroidal
artery

Internal frontal arteries
Posterior
Middle
Anterior

Posterior choroidal
artery

Posterior cerebral
artery

Frontopolar
artery

Parieto-occipital
branch

Orbitofrontal
artery

Calcarine artery

Ophthalmic
artery

Superior
cerebellar artery

Anterior inferior
cerebellar artery

Anterior
cerebral
artery

Posterior inferior
cerebellar artery

Internal carotid
artery

Vertebral arteries

Basilar artery

A   Posterior communicating
artery

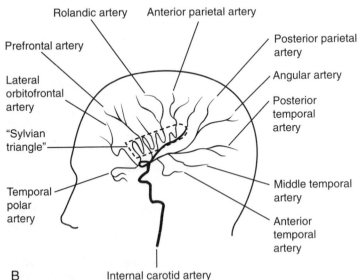

Rolandic artery   Anterior parietal artery

Prefrontal artery

Posterior parietal
artery

Lateral
orbitofrontal
artery

Angular artery

Posterior
temporal
artery

"Sylvian
triangle"

Temporal
polar
artery

Middle temporal
artery

Anterior
temporal
artery

B   Internal carotid artery

Figure 3–2 Diagram of a lateral cerebral angiogram. *A,* Anterior cerebral and posterior cerebral arteries. *B,* Middle cerebral artery.

with varying degrees of muscle contraction. The following parameters are analyzed:

1. **Insertional activity.** Excessive insertional activity is seen in both neuropathic and myopathic disease and hence is nonspecific.

2. **Spontaneous activity.** Normal muscle is electrically silent. Spontaneous muscle fiber contractions (*fibrillation potentials* and *positive sharp waves*) and spontaneous motor unit discharges (*fasciculations*) usually signify muscle denervation. After an acute nerve injury (e.g., disk herniation and nerve root compression), spontaneous activity usually takes 2 weeks to appear. *Paraspinal muscle denervation* implies nerve root injury as opposed to more distal lesions of the plexus or peripheral nerve. *Myotonia* is a special form of continuous motor unit activity characterized by high-frequency waxing and waning discharges, producing a "dive bomber" sound.

3. **Motor unit potential.** This parameter can differentiate myopathy from denervation. Neuropathic features reflect reinnervation of previously denervated motor units, resulting in *high-amplitude, polyphasic potentials*. Myopathic features reflect loss of muscle fiber mass, resulting in *low-amplitude, polyphasic potentials of short duration*.

4. **Recruitment pattern.** Voluntary muscle contraction leads to progressive recruitment of motor units and to a dense interference pattern that completely obliterates the baseline. In neuropathic disease, there are fewer motor units in the affected muscle, resulting in a *reduced* or *discrete recruitment* of motor units. Myopathic disease, with random loss of muscle fibers, leads to *early recruitment* and a *low-amplitude interference pattern*.

5. **Single-fiber EMG (SFEMG).** This technique examines the temporal relationship between firing of single muscle fibers innervated by the same motor neuron. Impaired neuromuscular transmission (e.g., in myasthenia gravis) results in a varying interval, referred to as "jitter."

- **Nerve conduction studies**

  Nerve conduction studies can be performed on motor or sensory nerves. The procedure is performed by applying electrical stimulation to skin sites overlying a peripheral nerve and recording the speed of conduction and amplitude of the "downstream" action potential. The following parameters are analyzed:

  1. **Conduction velocity.** Conduction velocity is generally reduced (<60% of normal) in demyelinating neuropathy. *Conduction block* reflects focal demyelination and is identified when nerve stimulation proximal to the block leads to a compound muscle action potential (CMAP) amplitude

that is less than 50% of that obtained by stimulating distal to the block.

2. **Amplitude.** The amplitude of the CMAP correlates with the number of muscle fibers activated by stimulation of the peripheral nerve. In general, reduced CMAP amplitude with relatively preserved conduction velocity is characteristic of *axonal neuropathy*.

3. **Late responses.** *F waves* result from antidromic conduction followed by orthodromic conduction in the same nerve. Delayed or absent F waves, in combination with normal peripheral nerve conduction, implies disease of the proximal nerve (e.g., root compression, early Guillain-Barré syndrome). The *H reflex* is the electrical counterpart of the ankle jerk and can be performed to assess the integrity of the S1 root; the antidromic potential travels down a sensory nerve, synapses in the spinal cord, and then travels orthodromically down a motor nerve.

4. **Repetitive stimulation.** Muscle responses to repetitive stimulation are useful for assessing neuromuscular junction disease. In myasthenia gravis (see Chapter 15), repetitive stimulation at 2 to 3 Hz produces a characteristic *decremental response* (>10% drop in amplitude between the first and the fifth CMAP).

ELECTROENCEPHALOGRAPHY

EEG provides a multichannel recording of the surface electrical activity of the brain. Background rhythms (Fig. 3–3) are analyzed with regard to amplitude and frequency (delta waves, <4 Hz; theta waves, 4 to 7 Hz; alpha waves, 8 to 13 Hz; and beta waves, >13 Hz). In the

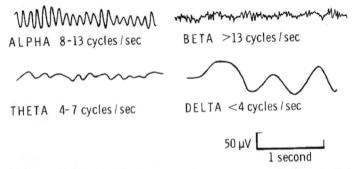

ALPHA   8-13 cycles / sec   BETA   >13 cycles / sec

THETA   4-7 cycles / sec   DELTA   <4 cycles / sec

50 µV
1 second

Figure 3–3 Basic EEG rhythms. (From Solomon GE, Kutt H, Plum F: Clinical Management of Seizures, 2nd ed. Philadelphia, WB Saunders, 1983.)

awake, normal adult, a posterior dominant alpha rhythm is detected when the eyes are closed and the patient is in a relaxed state. Sleep results in characteristic sequential changes (progressive slowing, vertex transients, sleep spindles, and K complexes) that reflect highly organized synchronous activity. The primary utility of a conventional 20- to 40-minute EEG examination is for evaluating epileptiform disorders.

Continuous 24-hour EEG (cEEG) over a period of one or more days is rapidly replacing briefer conventional EEG examinations for hospitalized patients, because it is vastly more sensitive for detecting nonconvulsive electrographic seizure activity. In the intensive care unit, cEEG is mandatory for titrating therapy in stuporous or comatose patients with refractory nonconvulsive status epilepticus. Routine surveillance cEEG is also increasingly being used for the general evaluation of comatose states; with 48 hours of monitoring, otherwise undetectable electrographic seizure activity can be detected in 10% to 30% of patients (see Chapter 5, Stupor and Coma).

- **Seizure disorders**

   The main value of EEG in patients with epilepsy is for detecting *interictal epileptiform activity* (isolated spikes and sharp waves). Focal epileptiform activity reflects a single irritative focus and corresponds with partial-onset seizures, whereas paroxysmal spike-and-wave discharges of diffuse origin correspond with generalized-onset seizures (Fig. 3–4). The absence of epileptiform discharges does not rule out a seizure disorder, however, because 20% to 40% of EEG recordings in patients with epilepsy appear normal. *Sleep, sleep deprivation, hyperventilation,* and *photostimulation* can be used to elicit epileptiform activity or absence seizures, and they are collectively referred to as activation procedures. An *electrographic seizure* is characterized by the distinct onset, evolution, and offset of rhythmic spikes, sharp waves, or ictal-appearing discharges, lasting at least 10 seconds. Electrographic seizures typically evolve with regard to frequency, amplitude, location, or morphology. cEEG is essential for confirming the diagnosis of *nonconvulsive status epilepticus* (complex-partial or absence status) in patients with prolonged postictal or otherwise unexplained impairment of consciousness.

- **Evaluation of stupor and coma**

   Diffuse background slowing (in the range of theta and delta waves) is an almost universal finding in patients with impaired level of consciousness of any cause. In patients with focal lesions (e.g., stroke or brain tumor), the slowing is usually more pronounced in the ipsilateral hemisphere. In patients with coma of unknown etiology, cEEG may be particularly helpful both for detecting nonconvulsive seizure activity or for showing unique background patterns that can point to a specific diagnosis:

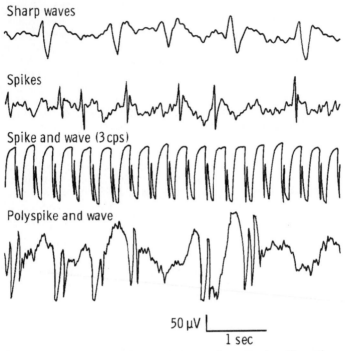

Figure 3–4 Paroxysmal EEG patterns seen in patients with epilepsy. (From Solomon GE, Kutt H, Plum F: Clinical Management of Seizures, 2nd ed. Philadelphia, WB Saunders, 1983.)

1. **Periodic lateralizing epileptiform discharges (PLEDs).** These discharges can occur with large destructive lesions of any type or in the aftermath of focal seizure activity. Although PLEDS are not generally believed to represent ictal activity *per* se, in some cases of prolonged nonconvulsive status epilepticus, PLEDs may reflect ongoing seizures. In patients with encephalitis, bilateral PLEDs are highly suggestive of herpes simplex infection.
2. **Triphasic waves.** Triphasic waves are nonspecific but can occur with high frequency in patients with metabolic encephalopathy (e.g., in hepatic, renal, and pulmonary failure).
3. **Beta activity.** Beta activity combined with diffuse slowing suggests intoxication with barbiturates, benzodiazepines, or other sedative-hypnotic drugs.
4. **Pseudoperiodic discharges.** Pseudoperiodic discharges consisting of repeated but irregular bisynchronous bursts of

high-amplitude, sharp waves are characteristic of subacute sclerosing panencephalitis (SSPE) and Jakob-Creutzfeldt disease.

- **Prognosis in coma**

    In hypoxic-ischemic coma, prognosis for recovery of consciousness is related to the severity of slowing and attenuation of the background rhythm. A *burst-suppression pattern, diffuse low-amplitude attenuation,* and *lack of reactivity* to external stimuli imply a poor prognosis. Keep in mind, however, that prognosis is usually related more to the cause of coma than to the depth of coma. *Alpha coma* and *spindle coma patterns* tend to occur with brain stem coma, are usually associated with lack of reactivity to stimuli, and portend a poor prognosis

- **Brain death**

    Electrocerebral silence can be used as a confirmatory test for brain death (see Chapter 18).

EVOKED POTENTIALS

Evoked potentials provide a recording of electrical activity in central sensory pathways produced by visual, auditory, or sensory stimulation. Signals are recorded by placing electrodes over the scalp or the spine and using a computer to average and amplify the signal, which results in a characteristic pattern of waveform peaks that have approximate anatomic correlates. There are three types of evoked potential studies:

- **Visual evoked responses (VER)**

    The visual stimulus is delivered as an alternating checkerboard pattern or a stroboscopic flash; the waveform corresponds with stimulation of the occipital cortex.

- **Brain stem auditory evoked responses (BAER)**

    Auditory signals are delivered by clicks through earphones. The waveform corresponds with stimulation of CN 8, the cochlear nucleus, pons, and inferior colliculus.

- **Somatosensory evoked potentials (SSEP)**

    Electrical stimuli are delivered to peripheral nerves. The waveform corresponds with stimulation of the lumbosacral or the brachial plexus, the cervicomedullary dorsal column nuclei, and the sensory cortex (the N20 potential).

The uses of evoked potentials in clinical practice are as follows:

1. **Multiple sclerosis.** Evoked potentials can be used to support the diagnosis in a patient with a single symptom by identifying subclinical demyelination at a different anatomic site (e.g., abnormal VERs in a patient with transverse myelitis).

2. **Brain stem lesions.** Brain stem lesions can be verified and localized with BAER.

3. **Acoustic neuroma.** BAER can be used to verify CN 8 injury.
4. **Spinal cord injury.** SSEP can be used for prognosis by differentiating complete from partial injury.
5. **Hypoxic-ischemic coma.** Bilateral absence of the N20 cortical potentials by SSEP on day 5 or later implies with a high degree of certainty that consciousness will not be regained.

MUSCLE AND NERVE BIOPSY

Muscle and nerve biopsy specimens are extremely fragile, and the procedure should be performed only by an experienced surgeon with adequate neuropathology backup for processing and analysis. The sural nerve and gastrocnemius muscle are often examined together, although biopsy of almost any muscle can be performed. Muscle biopsy is essential for diagnosing causes of myopathy such as polymyositis, genetic biochemical deficiencies, mitochondrial disease, sarcoidosis, critical illness myopathy, and infection (e.g., trichinosis). The causes of neuropathy that can be diagnosed by nerve biopsy are listed in Table 19–4.

BRAIN BIOPSY

Brain biopsy can be performed either as an open procedure, usually of the anterior nondominant temporal lobe, or by using stereotactic needle localization. Although stereotactic biopsy is often necessary for deep lesions, the diagnostic yield is better with the open procedure because more tissue can be obtained. Regardless of the condition that is suspected, the diagnostic yield of brain biopsy is always maximized when areas of enhancement or signal abnormality on MR are targeted. The main complication is hemorrhage (in approximately 1% of cases). Brain biopsy is of value for diagnosing brain tumors or abscess, central nervous system (CNS) vasculitis, neurosarcoidosis, encephalitis, heritable metabolic disorders, and Jakob-Creutzfeldt disease.

Patient-Related Problems: The Common Calls

Acute Seizures and Status Epilepticus

Convulsive seizures are dramatic and frightening for all who witness the event—patients, families, and staff—and tend to induce panic, rather than rational thought, even on a neurology service. It is your job to proceed in a logical and thorough manner to identify the cause of the seizures, to stop any ongoing seizures, and to prevent any additional seizures from occurring.

Clinical seizures are caused by an excessive, synchronous, abnormal discharge of cortical neurons that produces a sudden change in neurologic function. Seizures are classified as *simple* if there is no impairment of consciousness or as *complex* if an alteration in consciousness occurs. Seizures may be *focal*, involving a single brain region and causing limited dysfunction, such as clonic movements of a single limb, paresthesias, or abnormal speech or behavior; or they may be *generalized*, involving the whole brain and producing loss of consciousness and convulsions. Although witnessing a generalized tonic-clonic seizure can seem like an eternity, most seizures last seconds to minutes. *Status epilepticus is defined as 10 minutes or more of continuous tonic-clonic seizure activity, or repeated seizures between which the patient fails to fully awaken. Epilepsy* is a chronic condition defined as recurrent, unprovoked seizures and is discussed in Chapter 25.

PHONE CALL

Questions

1. **Is the patient still seizing? If yes, how long has it been going on?**

   Any patient seizing on admission to the ER should be considered to be in status epilepticus until the course of the seizure is known.

2. **What is the patient's level of consciousness?**

   A patient may have a decreased level of consciousness if the seizure is still occurring (nonconvulsive status epilepticus)

45

or if the patient is postictal. The two states are almost impossible to differentiate without an electroencephalogram (EEG).

3. Is this the first known seizure for this patient?

If the patient has a known history of epilepsy, there may be records available regarding anticonvulsants that have worked or failed in the past. Other information regarding past seizures will be gained from taking the patient's history.

4. Is the patient on anticonvulsant medication?

Anticonvulsant levels need to be checked for any seizure patient on medication. Noncompliance with medication in patients with epilepsy is the most common cause of status epilepticus. In some cases anticonvulsants may be epileptogenic at toxic levels.

5. What is the finger stick glucose level?

Focal or generalized seizures may be caused by hyper- or hypoglycemia.

6. Is the patient immunocompromised?

Additional elements in the differential diagnosis need to be considered in immunocompromised patients, particularly opportunistic infections such as toxoplasmosis, fungal meningitides, and tubercular meningitis.

Orders

1. Have two IV setups ready at the bedside.
2. Have oral airway and Ambu bag available at the bedside.
3. Before you arrive, **lorazepam 0.1 mg/kg** should be given by IV push. For most patients, a total of 8 mg given in four repeated 2 mg boluses is required. Although the seizures may stop after the initial 2 mg are given, a full loading dose should be given to minimize the chance of recurrent seizures during the next 6 to 12 hours.
4. Clear any sharp or hard objects from the bed, put the side rails up, and pad the side rails.
5. Perform a finger stick glucose test, and send a calcium and magnesium level in addition to other routine admission lab tests.
6. If the patient has depressed level of consciousness, send an arterial blood gas.

Inform RN

"Will arrive at the bedside in . . . minutes."

If the patient is still seizing, it must be considered a medical emergency. If the patient has stopped seizing, another seizure may occur within a few minutes.

ELEVATOR THOUGHTS

What is the Differential Diagnosis of Seizures?

On your way to the bedside, you should generate a list of probable diagnoses based on the initial information you obtained from your telephone conversation with the nurse.

V (vascular): intracranial hemorrhage, acute or chronic ischemic infarction, subarachnoid hemorrhage, arteriovenous malformation, venous sinus thrombosis, or amyloid angiopathy—chronic ischemic cerebrovascular disease is the most common cause of new onset seizures in adults

I (infectious): meningitis (bacterial, viral, fungal), meningoencephalitis (herpes simplex encephalitis), or abscess (bacterial, fungal, or parasitic)

T (traumatic): new head injury (e.g., from a fall) or old head injury with subdural hematoma

A (autoimmune): systemic lupus erythematosus, central nervous system (CNS) vasculitis, or multiple sclerosis (these are rare)

M (metabolic/toxic): hypo- or hypernatremia, hypo- or hypercalcemia, hypo- or hyperglycemia, hypomagnesemia, hyperthyroidism, uremia, hyperammonemia, ethanol intoxication or withdrawal, and other drugs including cocaine, phencyclidine, and amphetamines

I (idiopathic/iatrogenic): idiopathic epilepsy or medications (Table 4–1 lists common medications that can cause seizures)

N (neoplastic): brain metastasis or primary CNS tumor

S (structural): congenital structural defects (rare in adults)

Beware seizure mimics: Paroxysmal conditions that may mimic seizures include: hypoglycemia, syncope, asterixis, stroke/transient ischemic attack, myoclonus, dystonia, tremor, narcolepsy, complicated migraine, panic attack, transient global amnesia, hyperventilation, malingering.

MAJOR THREAT TO LIFE

- **Aspiration of gastric contents if the airway is not protected**
- **Head injury**
- **Lactic acidosis, hypoxia, hyperthermia, rhabdomyolysis, cerebral edema, or hypotension from a prolonged seizure—** these conditions may produce permanent brain injury

Measures to prevent aspiration and subsequent injury to the patient are described in Management I. The patient should be positioned in the *lateral decubitus* position to prevent aspiration of gastric contents. All hard or sharp objects should be removed from the bed,

TABLE 4–1 Medications That May Cause Seizures

Antidepressants
Imipramine, amitriptyline, nortriptyline, bupropion, maprotiline, clomiprimine
Antipsychotic agents
Clozapine, chlorpromazine, thioridazine, trifluoperazine, perphenazine, haloperidol
Opiod analgesics
Fentanyl, meperidine, pentazocine, propoxyphene
Local anesthetics
Lidocaine, procaine
Sympathomimetics
Terbutaline, ephedrine, phenylpropanolamine
Antimicrobial agents
Penicillin, ampicillin, synthetic penicillins, cephalosporins, imipenem, metronidazole, isoniazid, pytimethamine
Antineoplastic agents
Vincristine, chlorambucil, methotrexate, carmustine (BCNU), cytosine arabinoside
Bronchodilators
Aminophylline, theophylline
Others
Insulin (can cause hypoglycemia), antihistamines, anticholinergics, atenolol, baclofen, flumazenil (benzodiazepine antagonist), lithium (in overdose)

the side rails should be up, and the side rails should be padded. Procedures for aborting an ongoing seizure are described below.

BEDSIDE

Quick Look Test

Is the patient still seizing?

Most seizures will have stopped by the time you arrive at the bedside. If there is still seizure activity when you arrive, you are almost certainly dealing with status epilepticus, and the seizures must be stopped immediately.

If the patient has stopped seizing, assess the patient's level of consciousness.

Is the patient awake and alert? Is he or she interactive and conversing? A period of lethargy or stupor may follow a generalized seizure. Focal deficits such as a hemiparesis may also be apparent from a quick look.

Is there any sign of respiratory distress or agitation?

If there is respiratory distress, labored respirations, or oropharyngeal obstruction, call anesthesia for potential intubation. If

TABLE 4–2 **Seizure Precautions**

- Bed should be at the lowest position
- Side rails should be up
- Side rails should be padded
- Patient should ambulate to bathroom only with supervision
- Only axillary temperatures should be measured
- Patient should be supervised when using sharp objects
- Oral airway, oxygen, and suction should be at bedside

the patient is agitated or delirious, it is very likely that whatever is causing the delirium is also the cause of the seizures.

MANAGEMENT I

Treatment of an Ongoing Seizure

1. **Keep calm.** It is likely that others in the room are reacting with fear or panic. Ask family members to leave the room. Tell them you will speak with them as soon as the situation is evaluated and under control.
2. **Ensure that all measures have been taken to protect the patient from physical injury and aspiration of gastric contents.** Have one or two people maintain the patient in a lateral decubitus position (Table 4–2).
3. **Administer oxygen by nasal cannula or face mask,** particularly if the patient is older or has a history of cardiac disease.
4. **Watch and wait for 2 minutes.** A majority of seizures will stop spontaneously within a short time. There is no immediate risk to the patient, provided the risks of aspiration and physical injury have been addressed. During the waiting period, do the following:
   - Check the **finger stick glucose** level. If there is significant hypo- or hyperglycemia, this may be the first condition to treat.
   - Make sure there are **two IV setups available,** at least one with 0.9% normal saline (NS). If the patient has no IV access, start an IV line. If the seizures stop within 3 minutes, however, IV insertion and blood drawing will be much easier.
   - Draw **lorazepam 8 mg** in a 10-ml syringe, if not already given.
   - **Elicit any further history** not obtained in the initial phone call. Is this a first-ever seizure? Is the patient on anticonvulsants? What is the patient's admitting diagnosis? Is the patient diabetic? Is the patient immunocompromised? Has the patient been febrile in the last 24 hours? Ask for the chart to be brought to the bedside.

- **Observe the seizure type.** Most seizures manifest as one of two types: *convulsive* and *nonconvulsive*. Generalized convulsive seizures are characterized by bilateral tonic-clonic activity and altered level of consciousness. Much more challenging to detect are "nonconvulsive" seizures, which present primarily as a paroxysmal alteration in level of consciousness, with or without subtle motor manifestations such as eyelid blinking, facial twitching, head turning, or motor automatisms (picking at clothes, rubbing movements, etc.).

5. **If the seizure has not remitted in 2 minutes,** ensure that an IV line is available. If the patient has no IV access, have one or two people hold the forearm while the most experienced person available inserts two IV lines and draws blood. Avoid the antecubital area because convulsions may cause flexion of the arm and block off the IV site.

6. Order the following **blood tests:** CBC, electrolytes, glucose, magnesium (Mg), calcium (Ca), ammonia, EtOH level, toxicology screen, and anticonvulsant levels (if applicable).

7. If the patient is hypoglycemic, give **glucose (50 ml of D50W)** by slow, direct injection. If there is any history or suspicion of alcoholism, administer **thiamine 100 mg by slow, direct injection over 3 to 5 minutes** prior to the D50W. The administration of thiamine will prevent susceptible patients from developing Wernicke's encephalopathy. If hypoglycemia is the cause of the seizure, the seizure should stop, and the patient should wake up soon after the glucose administration.

8. If glucose levels are normal or after glucose has been given, administer **lorazepam 0.1 mg/kg in 2-mg increments by IV push over 2 to 3 minutes.** An Ambu bag with face mask should be at the bedside, because benzodiazepines can cause respiratory depression. Alternatives to lorazepam include **diazepam 5 to 10 mg given by IV push in NS or rectally in gel form,** or **midazolam 0.2 mg/kg IV or sublingually.** Lorazepam may be given IM and may be helpful if no peripheral IV access can be achieved.

Evaluation and Initial Management If the Seizure Has Stopped

A single first seizure that has stopped often does not need to be treated acutely. Anticonvulsant therapy should be reserved for patients who have had more than one seizure or who have risk factors that make another seizure more likely (see Chapter 25, Epilepsy and Seizure Disorders, for more details). The potential danger to the patient is not over, however. A patient who has had one seizure may have another seizure within a few minutes. Order "seizure precautions" for the patient (see Table 4–2). Remember also that a seizure is a symptom, not a disease. Your primary job now

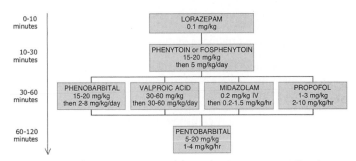

| 0-10 minutes | | LORAZEPAM 0.1 mg/kg | | |

Figure 4–1 Treatment protocol for refractory status epilepticus.

should be to identify the cause of the seizure and to treat the underlying condition.

MANAGEMENT II

Treatment of Status Epilepticus

1. If the seizures have not stopped after a full dose of a benzodiazepine, administer **fosphenytoin** (the prodrug of phenytoin) **15 to 20 mg/kg as a slow IV push or IV infusion** (Fig. 4–1). (This loading dose corresponds to approximately 1500 mg in a 70-kg patient.) The rate of administration should not exceed 200 mg/min because fosphenytoin can cause cardiac arrhythmias, prolongation of the QT interval, and hypotension. The electrocardiogram (ECG) should be monitored continuously, and the blood pressure should be checked periodically during the infusion. The rate of administration should be slowed if ECG changes or hypotension occurs. The usual protocol is to give **500 mg with a slow IV push over 5 minutes, and then repeat twice.** If IV access is unavailable, fosphenytoin can also be given IM. If the patient is known to be on phenytoin already and is suspected of having subtherapeutic levels, **a bolus dose of 10 mg/kg** may be given.

2. Approximately 70% of prolonged convulsive seizures will be brought under control with a combination of lorazepam and fosphenytoin. *The likelihood of success with this combination of therapy is directly correlated to the interval between seizure onset and initiation of treatment:* if the patient has been seizing for greater than 2 hours prior to treatment, the success rate falls to 40%. After the seizure activity stops, the patient should be transferred to an intensive or intermediate-level care unit for observation, because the risk of recurrent seizures during the next 24 hours is very high.

3. The next step is to see if the patient rapidly awakens from a postictal state. **Patients who fail to awaken (i.e., follow commands) after convulsive status epilepticus has been terminated require continuous EEG (cEEG) to detect ongoing nonconvulsive seizure activity.** cEEG will detect additional electrographic seizure activity in 30% to 50% of these patients and ongoing nonconvulsive status epilepticus in approximately 15%. Left unchecked, these seizures can lead to a state of prolonged unconsciousness and progressive cortical injury detectable with diffusion-weighted MRI.

MANAGEMENT III

Refractory Status Epilepticus

Once in the intensive care unit (ICU), if the patient is continuing to seize despite a full lorazepam and fosphenytoin load, the patient is considered to be in refractory nonconvulsive status, which is a true medical emergency, with a mortality rate of 25%. Intubation, if not already done, is required at this point. Continue monitoring the blood pressure, ECG, and oxygen saturation.

The next step is to do whatever is necessary to terminate the seizures. *The number one most common error in the management of status epilepticus is undertreatment.* Patients need to be treated rapidly and aggressively until the seizures have been stopped. At this point, continuous EEG monitoring should be considered mandatory. There are currently four therapeutic options that are reasonable for use as third-line therapy for status epilepticus after loading with lorazepam and phenytoin/fosphenytoin (Fig. 4–1). They are listed below in order of preference at the Columbia University Medical Center Neurological Intensive Care Unit:

1. **Midazolam (Versed) 0.2 mg/kg loading dose,** followed by IV infusion of **0.2 mg/kg/hour.** This short-acting benzodiazepine is the favored agent because it is relatively safe, easy to titrate, and has a rapid offset of sedation once the infusion is discontinued.

2. **Valproic acid (Depacon) IV 30 to 60 mg/kg IV loading dose,** followed by **7.5 to 15 mg/kg IV every 6 hours.** The dose should be adjusted daily to maintain therapeutic levels (70 to 100 mg/dl).

3. **Phenobarbital 15 to 20 mg/kg loading dose** (maximal rate 75 mg/min), followed by **1 to 4 mg/kg/day every 12 hours.** Formerly considered the standard third-line treatment for refractory status epilepticus, this approach is reasonably effective but results in excessive sedation.

4. **Propofol 1 to 3 mg/kg loading dose,** followed by IV infusion of **2 to 10 mg/kg/hour.** Advantages include ease of dose titration and rapid offset of sedation, but the prolonged high doses

needed to control seizures can provoke a rare, idiosyncratic, and often fatal complication called "propofol infusion syndrome" (metabolic acidosis, rhabdomyolysis, and renal failure).

If there is no response to full doses of a benzodiazepine and two additional anticonvulsants, definitive therapy in the form of total barbiturate anesthesia is required. Administer **pentobarbital 5 to 20 mg/kg loading dose and then 1 to 4 mg/kg per hour as a maintenance infusion.** Monitor the EEG continuously to keep the patient in a burst suppression pattern. Hypotension is nearly always encountered with pentobarbital, and pressors (such as phenylephrine 40 to160 µg/min) are usually required. General anesthesia with halothane and neuromuscular blockade has been used in some cases to avoid rhabdomyolysis, but the need for this is extremely rare.

MANAGEMENT IV

Remember that a seizure is a symptom, not a disease. Although nearly all seizures may be brought under control with anticonvulsant therapy (Table 4–3), continued control may be impossible until the underlying cause is identified and treated. Your primary job now should be to identify any acute neurologic illness causing the seizures and to treat the underlying condition.

1. **Review routine blood tests:** CBC, electrolytes, glucose, Mg, Ca, ammonia, EtOH level, toxicology screen, and anticonvulsant levels.
2. **Ensure that there is adequate intravenous access.** A central line may be desirable. Give a baseline infusion of 0.9% normal saline.
3. **Review the chart** and perform a selective physical examination.

TABLE 4–3 **Drugs Used for the Treatment of Status Epilepticus**

Drug	Loading Dose	Maximum Loading Rate	Continuous Infusion Dose
Lorazepam	0.1 mg/kg IV	2 mg/min to max 8 mg	N/A
Fosphenytoin or phenytoin	20 mg/kg IV	200 mg/min or 50 mg/min for phenytoin	N/A
Phenobarbital	20 mg/kg IV	75 mg/min	N/A
Valproic acid	15-60 mg/kg	20 mg/min	N/A
Midazolam	0.2 mg/kg IV	N/A	0.1-0.4 mg/kg/hour
Propofol	1-2 mg/kg IV	N/A	2-10 mg/kg/hour
Pentobarbital	5-20 mg/kg IV	N/A	1-4 mg/kg/hour

Selective Physical Examination

Initial physical examination of a patient who has had a seizure should take no more than 5 minutes. Important clues to the etiology of the seizure may emerge. Pay particular attention to unilateral focal deficits that could indicate a structural lesion.

General Physical Examination

Vital signs	Fever could be a clue to an infectious cause, although a prolonged seizure may cause hyperpyrexia. Dyspnea may suggest hypoxia. Cardiac arrhythmia or tachycardia could suggest a cardioembolic or syncopal event. Hypertensive encephalopathy may present with seizures.
HEENT	Look for evidence of bites on the tongue, lips, or buccal mucosa. Look for any evidence of new or old head injury. Check the fundi for papilledema.
Neck	Look for neck stiffness (meningismus).
Skin	Look for cafe au lait spots or port-wine stains as a sign of neurocutaneous disorders (e.g., neurofibromatosis or Sturge-Weber syndrome). Hematomas, lacerations, or even fractures may have been produced as a consequence of the seizure.
Chest	Focal decreased breath sounds or rales may be a clue to aspiration. Cardiac murmur or arrhythmia may suggest a cardioembolic event.
GU	Incontinence, particularly urinary, may accompany a generalized seizure.

Focused Neurologic Examination

Assess for new or residual focal deficits:
- The *level of consciousness* may be decreased after a seizure. A period of lethargy, stupor, or inattentiveness may follow a generalized seizure. If the patient is awake, have him or her count backward from 20 to 1 as a screening test for attentiveness.
- *Aphasia* has been partially screened for by asking the patient to count backward from 20 to 1. If the patient is unable to do this task, he or she may be either too inattentive, in which case aphasia testing will be futile, or aphasic. Ask the patient to show two fingers, then to repeat an unfamiliar phrase (e.g., "The spy fled to Greece").
- *Hemiparesis* may be obvious, as evidenced by an inability to lift an arm or leg, or it may be subtle, as detected by a widened palpebral fissure, a flattened nasolabial fold, or a pronator drift when arms are extended with palms up.

- *Reflex asymmetry* or a unilateral Babinski's sign may be indicative of a focal lesion.

Selective History and Chart Review

Reassess the timing, circumstances, and duration of the seizures. Try to establish with the patient or with witnesses whether this was indeed a seizure. An aura is often present at the onset of a seizure, which is thought to represent the beginning of the abnormal epileptic discharges. Auras are most commonly olfactory, gustatory, or other visceral sensations that precede motor or sensory activity. Were there rhythmic, synchronous movements of more than one body part? Identify a "focal signature" if present; that is, did the seizure begin in one part of the body and then progress or become generalized? Were there head and eye deviations at the beginning? A seizure that begins focally can aid in the localization of the underlying pathology. If both sides of the body were involved, did the patient lose consciousness, become incontinent, or bite the tongue or mouth?

From the chart, look for clues to the underlying cause. Check for the following:

1. Medications the patient is on that are potentially epileptogenic (see Table 4–1)
2. History of alcohol or drug use
3. Underlying medical problems that could cause seizures, including hepatic or renal disease, prior head injury, cerebrovascular disease, connective tissue diseases, porphyria, or carcinoma (lung, breast, and colon cancer are the most common tumors that metastasize to the brain)
4. HIV infection. Patients who are immunocompromised, particularly patients with AIDS, are predisposed to opportunistic infections such as toxoplasmosis, tubercular meningitis, and cryptococcal meningitis and to CNS lymphoma
5. Recent laboratory results: electrolyte, glucose, Ca and Mg levels, thyroid and liver function tests, toxicology screen, EtOH levels, and anticonvulsant levels

MANAGEMENT ▼

Having accumulated information from the history, the physical examination, and the laboratory, a working differential diagnosis should be generated. As always, in an acute situation, the differential diagnosis should include the most dangerous diagnosis as well as the most likely. Management should proceed from the differential diagnosis.

1. If a **metabolic cause** is identified or suspected, the underlying cause should be treated appropriately.
2. If the examination reveals a focal deficit, if the onset of the seizure appeared to be focal, or if the patient has new-onset

seizures, a **CT or MRI scan** should be obtained. If there is no renal insufficiency, CT contrast should be administered. Keep in mind that a cerebral infarction may not be detectable by CT within the first 6 hours.

3. If there is no evidence of obvious focal pathology on imaging and an infectious etiology such as meningitis or encephalitis is suspected, a **lumbar puncture** may be performed so that antibiotic or antiviral therapy may be targeted as specifically as possible. If infection is suspected, other supportive evidence should be sought as well, such as blood and urine cultures, viral serologies, and chest x-ray.

4. If treatment was given to correct abnormal laboratory results, those tests should be repeated, including electrolytes, Mg, Ca, and glucose. For all anticonvulsant drugs administered, a blood level should be ordered for the next morning.

5. If not already performed, an **EEG** should be obtained if the diagnosis of seizure is at all uncertain; it also serves the purpose of guiding long-term management. The finding of interictal epileptiform activity implies an increased risk of seizures.

6. If **no underlying cause** for seizures is determined, idiopathic epilepsy may be the diagnosis. An EEG is often helpful in differentiating specific epileptic syndromes. Treatment with an appropriate anticonvulsant would then be indicated. See Chapter 25 for treatment of epilepsy.

Stupor and Coma

Stupor and coma refer, respectively, to moderate and severe depression of the level of consciousness. The acute onset of stupor or coma is a medical emergency. A wide variety of metabolic and structural disorders can produce this state. Management should focus on stabilizing the patient, establishing a diagnosis, and treating the underlying cause.

PHONE CALL

Questions

1. **What are the vital signs?**
2. **Is the airway protected?**

    Stuporous and comatose patients are at high risk for *aspiration*, because of impaired cough and gag reflexes, and *hypoxia*, which results from diminished respiratory drive. Endotracheal intubation is the most effective method for securing the airway and ensuring adequate oxygenation.

3. **Is there any history of trauma, drug use, or toxin exposure?**

    Obtain a quick description of recent events and pre-existing medical or neurologic conditions. Check the Emergency Medical Service sheet.

4. **Is someone available to provide further history?**

    Relatives, friends, ambulance personnel, or anyone else who has had recent contact with the patient should be identified and instructed to wait for further questioning.

Orders

1. **Call the anesthesiology service for intubation if the patient is deeply comatose or exhibiting signs of respiratory compromise.**

    In stuporous patients with normal respirations, give 100% oxygen via face mask until hypoxemia is ruled out.

2. **Order an intravenous line.**
3. **Order a finger stick glucose measurement.**

This should always be checked immediately, because hypoglycemia is a rapidly treatable cause of stupor or coma that can coexist with other diagnoses (e.g., sepsis, cardiac arrest, or trauma).

4. **Order diagnostic blood tests.**
   - Serum chemistries (glucose, electrolytes, blood urea nitrogen [BUN], creatinine)
   - CBC
   - Arterial blood gas
   - Calcium, magnesium
   - PT/PTT

5. **If the etiology of stupor or coma is unclear,** order toxicology screen, thyroid function tests, liver function tests, serum cortisol, and ammonia level.

6. **Insert a Foley catheter.**

7. **Order urinalysis, ECG, and chest x-ray.**

8. **Give emergency treatment.** These measures are often given in the field, or whenever the cause of stupor or coma is unclear.
   - **Thiamine 100 mg IV**

     Thiamine reverses stupor or coma resulting from acute thiamine deficiency (Wernicke's encephalopathy). It must be given *before* dextrose because hyperglycemia can lead to consumption of thiamine and acute worsening of Wernicke's encephalopathy.
   - **50% dextrose 50 ml (1 ampule) IV**
   - **Naloxone (Narcan) 0.4 to 0.8 mg IV**

     Naloxone reverses coma caused by opiate intoxication. Up to 10 mg may be required to reverse severe intoxication.
   - **Flumazenil (Romazicon) 0.2 to 1.0 mg IV**

     Flumazenil reverses stupor or coma caused by benzodiazepine intoxication. Up to 3 mg may be required. Do not give flumazenil if seizures have occurred, because flumazenil may precipitate further seizures.

ELEVATOR THOUGHTS

What causes stupor or coma?

The causes of stupor and coma (Table 5–1) can be broadly grouped into three categories:

1. **Structural intracranial disorders (33%)**

   In most cases, these disorders are diagnosed by positive brain imaging (CT or MRI) or by lumbar puncture (LP).

2. **Toxic or metabolic disorders (66%)**

   Abnormal blood tests usually, but not always, confirm these disorders.

3. **Psychiatric disorders (1%)**

   Stupor and coma result from diseases affecting either both of the cerebral hemispheres or the brain stem. As a rule,

TABLE 5–1 Causes of Stupor and Coma

1. Structural intracranial disorders
   a. Trauma
      (1) Epidural, subdural, intracerebral, or subarachnoid hemorrhage
      (2) Diffuse axonal injury
      (3) Concussion
   b. Cerebrovascular events
      (1) Intracerebral or subarachnoid hemorrhage
      (2) Hemispheric or brain stem infarction
      (3) Dural sinus thrombosis
      (4) Hypertensive encephalopathy
   c. Infection
      (1) Meningitis
      (2) Encephalitis
      (3) Abscess
   d. Inflammatory disorders
      (1) Autoimmune vasculitis or cerebritis
      (2) Demyelinating disease (e.g., multiple sclerosis)
   e. Neoplasm
   f. Hydrocephalus
2. Toxic or metabolic disorders
   a. Global hypoxia-ischemia
   b. Electrolyte or acid-base disorders
      (1) pH disturbances
      (2) Hyper- or hyponatremia
      (3) Hyper- or hypoglycemia
      (4) Hyper- or hypocalcemia
   c. Drug intoxication or withdrawal
   d. Temperature disorder (hyper- or hypothermia)
   e. Organ system dysfunction
      (1) Liver (hepatic encephalopathy)
      (2) Kidney (uremia)
      (3) Thyroid (myxedema, thyrotoxicosis)
      (4) Adrenal (hyper- or hypoadrenalism)
      (5) Multisystem organ failure
   f. Seizure and postictal states
   g. Thiamine or vitamin B_{12} deficiency
3. Psychogenic coma

unilateral hemispheric lesions do not produce stupor or coma unless there is mass effect sufficient to raise the intracranial pressure, or compress either the contralateral hemisphere or the brain stem. *Focal brain stem lesions* produce coma by disrupting the reticular activating system. *Metabolic disorders* impair consciousness by diffuse effects on both the reticular formation and the cerebral cortex.

MAJOR THREAT TO LIFE

Three common and treatable causes of coma can rapidly lead to death:

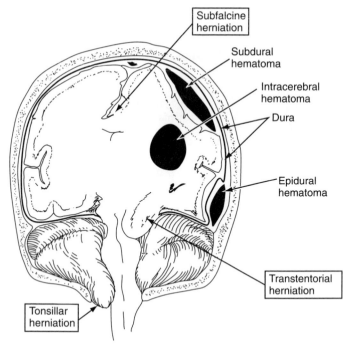

Figure 5–1 Types of brain herniation that can occur in patients with compartmentalized intracranial pressure.

- **Herniation and brain stem compression**
  Space-occupying mass lesions that produce stupor or coma are a neurosurgical emergency (Fig. 5–1).
- **Increased intracranial pressure (ICP)**
  Increased ICP can lead to impaired cerebral perfusion and global hypoxic-ischemic injury (see Chapter 12).
- **Meningitis or encephalitis**
  Death from bacterial meningitis or herpes encephalitis can be prevented with early treatment (see Chapter 21).

BEDSIDE

Selective History

The cause of coma can frequently be determined by the history. Ask family, friends, ambulance personnel, or others who have had recent contact with the patient about the following:

1. *Recent events*

    When was the patient last seen? How was the patient discovered? Were there any preceding neurologic complaints? Was there any recent trauma or toxin exposure?

2. *Medical history*
3. *Psychiatric history*
4. *Medications*
5. *Use of drugs or alcohol*

SELECTIVE PHYSICAL EXAMINATION

With or without history, clues to the etiology of coma can be elicited from the physical examination.

General Physical Examination

Vital signs	*Severe hypertension* suggests a structural CNS lesion with increased ICP or hypertensive encephalopathy.
Skin	Look for external signs of trauma, needle marks, rashes, cherry redness (suggests carbon monoxide poisoning), or jaundice.
Breath	Alcohol, acetone, or fetor hepaticus (from liver failure) can lead to a pungent or "fruity" smell.
Head	The skull should be inspected for fractures, hematomas, and lacerations.
Ear, nose, and throat	*CSF otorrhea or rhinorrhea* results from skull fracture with disruption of the dura (a positive dextrose stick test, indicating a high level of glucose, differentiates CSF from mucus). *Hemotympanum* is also highly suggestive of skull fracture. *Tongue biting* suggests an unwitnessed seizure.
Neck (do not manipulate the neck if there is suspicion of cervical spine fracture)	Stiffness suggests meningitis or subarachnoid hemorrhage.

Neurologic Examination

The goals of the neurologic examination are (1) to determine the depth of coma and (2) to localize the process leading to coma.

1. **General appearance**

    Open eyelids and a slack jaw indicate deep coma. Head and gaze deviation suggest a large ipsilateral hemispheric

TABLE 5–2 **Glasgow Coma Scale**

Parameter	Patient Response	Score
Eye opening	Spontaneous	4
	To voice	3
	To pain	2
	None	1
Best motor response	Obeys commands	6
	Localizes to pain	5
	Withdraws to pain	4
	Flexor posturing	3
	Extensor posturing	2
	None	1
Best verbal response	Conversant and oriented	5
	Conversant and disoriented	4
	Uses inappropriate words	3
	Makes incomprehensible sounds	2
	None	1
Total score		3-15

lesion. Observe for *myoclonus* (which suggests a metabolic process), *rhythmic muscle twitching* (which is indicative of seizure activity), or *tetany* (spontaneous, prolonged muscle spasms).

2. **Level of consciousness**

Many inexact terms are used to describe depressed level of consciousness (e.g., somnolent, clouded, drowsy, obtunded). Because of the lack of precision associated with these terms, it is much more useful to document **the response of the patient to a specific stimulus;** for example, "opens eyes temporarily and responds with brief phrases to repeated questioning," or "moans and localizes to sternal rub." Responses to verbal and noxious stimuli can be used to generate a **Glasgow Coma Scale score** (Table 5–2), a reproducible and widely used method for quantifying level of consciousness. For the sake of simplicity, we advocate describing nonalert patients as *lethargic, stuporous,* or *comatose.*

a. **Lethargy**

Lethargy resembles sleepiness, except that the patient is incapable of becoming fully alert. These patients are conversant but inattentive and slow to respond. They are unable to adequately perform simple concentration tasks, such as counting from 20 to 1 or reciting the months in reverse.

b. **Stupor**

Stupor is defined by a state in which the best motor or verbal response requires a painful stimulus. There is little or no response to verbal commands. Painful stimulation

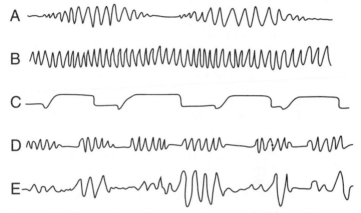

Figure 5–2 Abnormal respiratory patterns associated with coma. Tracings represent chest wall excursion; upward deflections represent inspiration. *A,* Cheyne-Stokes respiration. *B,* Central neurogenic hyperventilation. *C,* Apneustic breathing. *D,* Cluster breathing. *E,* Ataxic breathing.

results in brief responses to questions, exclamations ("ouch"), or moaning. The patient may obey commands temporarily when aroused by noxious stimuli but more often only localizes to pain.

c. **Coma**

Coma is defined by the absence of verbal or complex motor responses to any stimulus. *A Glasgow Coma Scale score of 8 or lower is frequently used to define coma.*

3. **Respirations**

Abnormal respiratory patterns (Fig. 5–2) occur frequently with coma and can aid in localization. Respirations in intubated patients can be observed by briefly disconnecting the endotracheal tube from the ventilator.

a. **Patterns without localizing value**

(1) **Depressed respirations** can occur with severe coma of any cause.

(2) **Cheyne-Stokes respiration** is characterized by alternating periods of hyperventilation and apnea. It usually occurs with bihemispheric lesions or metabolic encephalopathy. *Slow-cycling Cheyne-Stokes respirations are considered to represent a "stable" breathing pattern that does not imply impending respiratory arrest.* Rapid-cycling Cheyne-Stokes respirations may be more ominous.

(3) **Hyperventilation** in comatose patients is most often due to systemic disease. Hyperventilation associated

with *metabolic acidosis* can result from lactic acidosis, ketoacidosis, uremia, or organic acid poisoning. An association with *respiratory alkalosis* can result from hypoxia or hepatic encephalopathy. **Central neurogenic hyperventilation** is sometimes associated with CNS lymphoma or brain stem damage from tentorial herniation.

b. **Patterns with localizing value**

(1) **Apneustic breathing** is characterized by a prolonged inspiratory phase (the inspiratory cramp) followed by apnea. It implies pontine damage.

(2) **Cluster breathing** consists of brief cycles of shallow hyperventilation with periods of apnea. It has less of a crescendo-decrescendo quality than Cheyne-Stokes respiration and is often a sign of pontine or cerebellar damage.

(3) **Ataxic (Biot's) breathing**, an irregular, chaotic breathing pattern, implies damage to the medullary respiratory centers and is usually seen in association with posterior fossa lesions. *Progression to apnea occurs frequently.*

4. **Visual fields**

Visual fields should be tested with threatening movements, which normally evoke a blink. Asymmetry of this response implies hemianopia.

5. **Fundoscopy**

Papilledema occurs after prolonged (>12 hours) elevation of ICP, and only rarely does it develop acutely. Thus, the absence of papilledema does not rule out increased ICP. *Spontaneous venous pulsations* are difficult to identify, but their presence implies normal ICP. *Subhyaloid hemorrhages* appear as globules of blood on the retinal surface and are commonly associated with subarachnoid hemorrhage.

6. **Pupils**

The shape, size, and reactivity to light of the pupils should be noted.

a. **Symmetry and normal reactivity to light** implies structural integrity of the midbrain. *Reactive pupils in conjunction with absent corneal and oculocephalic responses are highly suggestive of metabolic coma.*

b. **Midposition (2 to 5 mm) fixed or irregular pupils** imply a focal midbrain lesion.

c. **Pinpoint reactive pupils** occur with pontine damage. Opiates and cholinergic intoxication (e.g., with pilocarpine) also produce small reactive pupils.

d. **A unilateral dilated and fixed pupil** usually occurs with CN 3 compression in the setting of uncal herniation. Ptosis and exodeviation of the eye are also seen. *An acutely* "blown" pupil represents an immediate threat to life and requires urgent intervention.

  e. **Bilateral fixed and dilated pupils** can reflect central herniation, global hypoxia-ischemia, or poisoning with barbiturates, scopolamine, atropine, or glutethimide.

7. **Ocular movements**

Horizontal conjugate gaze is mediated by the *frontal eye fields* and the *pontine gaze centers*. The frontal eye fields, when activated, drive gaze to the opposite side. The pontine gaze centers, when activated, drive gaze to the same side. Vertical conjugate gaze is mediated by centers in the *midbrain tegmentum and lower diencephalon.* In unresponsive patients, conjugate eye movements can be actively elicited by testing the **oculocephalic and oculovestibular reflexes** (Fig. 5–3). Both reflexes are mediated by stimulating the semicircular canals, with CN 8 input to the vestibular nuclei and bilateral connections to the third, fourth, and sixth nuclei. *Thus, intact eye movements indicate brain stem integrity from the level of CN 3 to CN 8 (midbrain and pons).*

  a. **The position of the eyes at rest** should be noted.

      (1) **Gaze deviation away from the hemiparesis** results from hemispheric lesions contralateral to the hemiparesis.

      (2) **Gaze deviation toward the hemiparesis** can result from the following:

          (a) Pontine lesions contralateral to the hemiparesis

          (b) "Wrong-way gaze" from thalamic lesions contralateral to the hemiparesis

          (c) Seizure activity in the hemisphere contralateral to the hemiparesis

      (3) **Forced downward eye deviation** results from lesions of the midbrain tectum. Association with impaired pupillary reactivity and refractory nystagmus is known as *Parinaud's syndrome.*

      (4) **Slow roving eye movements** may be conjugate or dysconjugate and are not of localizing value. They are most frequently associated with bilateral hemispheric dysfunction and active oculocephalic reflexes.

      (5) **Ocular bobbing** consists of fast downward "bobbing" with slow return to the primary position. It results from bilateral damage to the pontine horizontal gaze centers.

      (6) **Saccadic (fast) eye movements** are not seen in coma and imply psychogenic unresponsiveness.

  b. **The oculocephalic (doll's eye) reflex** should be noted.

      This reflex is elicited by briskly turning the head side to side. In alert patients, supranuclear cortical inputs to the oculomotor nuclei control eye movement, and the

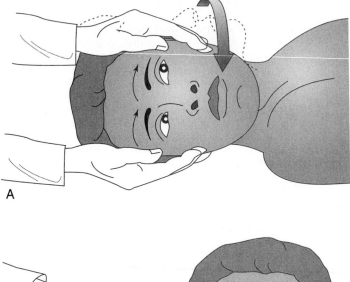

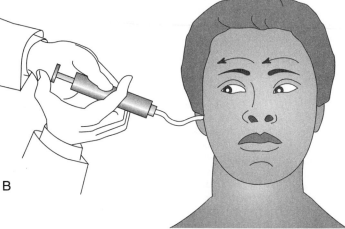

Figure 5–3 *A,* "Doll's eye" maneuver (oculocephalic reflex): with an intact brain stem (cranial nerves 3 through 8), the eyes move opposite to the direction of head turning. *B,* Cold caloric test (oculovestibular reflex): with an intact brain stem, injecting cold water in the auditory canal results in tonic conjugate eye deviation toward the cold ear.

response cannot be elicited. *An intact response consists of full conjugate eye movement opposite to the direction of head movement.*

A full and easy-to-elicit reflex ("ball-bearing eyes") implies bilateral cerebral hemisphere dysfunction and structural integrity of the brain stem, as seen with metabolic coma.

c. **The oculovestibular (cold caloric) reflex** should be tested.

This reflex is a more potent method for eliciting conjugate eye movements. The head is tilted 30 degrees above horizontal, and the ear is lavaged with 30 to 60 ml of ice water using butterfly tubing attached to a syringe. *A normal response consists of tonic eye deviation toward the cold ear and fast nystagmus away from the cold ear (mediated by the frontal lobe contralateral to the direction of the fast component).*

(1) **Tonic phase bilaterally intact, with absent fast responses** suggests coma from bihemispheric dysfunction.

(2) **Conjugate gaze paresis** can result from unilateral hemispheric or pontine lesions.

(3) **Asymmetric eye weakness** implies a brain stem lesion. CN 3 paresis, CN 6 paresis, and internuclear ophthalmoplegia are the most commonly identified abnormalities.

(4) **Absent oculovestibular responses** are seen with deep coma of any cause and imply severe depression of brain stem function.

8. **Corneal reflex**

Stroking the cornea with sterile gauze or cotton normally results in bilateral eye closure. The afferent limb of the reflex is mediated by CN 5, and the efferent limb by CN 7.

9. **Gag reflex**

In intubated patients, this reflex can be tested by gently manipulating the endotracheal tube.

10. **Motor responses**

Motor responses are the single best indicator of the depth and severity of coma.

a. **Spontaneous movements** should be observed for symmetry and purpose. Preferential movement on one side indicates weakness of the unused limbs.

b. **Limb tone** should be tested for symmetry.

Tone in the upper extremities is tested by passive motion at the elbow and wrist. Lower extremity tone is tested by a quick lifting motion under the thigh; if the heel elevates off the bed, tone is abnormally increased. *Bilaterally increased lower extremity tone is an important sign of herniation.*

c. **Induced movements** should be tested systematically by observing responses to stimuli of increasing intensity, in the following order:

(1) **Verbal command.** Ask the patient to open the eyes, protrude the tongue, raise one arm, and show two

fingers. *Hand squeezing often occurs as an automatic response and, in isolation, should not be taken as evidence of the patient's following commands.*

(2) **Sternal rub.** Apply gentle pressure with fingertips. Proceed to deep knuckle pressure if there is no response.

   (a) **Fending off responses** consist of precise hand movements and active attempts to ward off the examiner.

   (b) **Gross localizing responses** are slower and less accurate. They occur with deepening coma or with nondominant hemispheric lesions, causing impaired spatial discrimination.

(3) **Nailbed pressure.** Use the handle of the reflex hammer and gradually increase the pressure on each extremity.

   (a) **Withdrawal** is mediated by the motor cortex. The movements are sudden, nonstereotyped, and variable in intensity.

   (b) **Flexor (decorticate) posturing** (Fig. 5–4) results from damage to the corticospinal tracts at the level of the *deep hemisphere or upper midbrain.* The full response consists of flexion with adduction of the arms and extension of the legs.

   (c) **Extensor (decerebrate) posturing** (see Fig. 5–4) consists of extension, adduction, and internal rotation of the arms and extension of the legs. It results from corticospinal tract damage at the level of the *pons or upper medulla.*

11. **Sensory responses**
    Asymmetry of response to noxious stimulation suggests a lateralizing sensory deficit.

12. **Reflexes**
    a. **Deep tendon reflexes**
       Asymmetry indicates a lateralizing motor deficit caused by a structural lesion.
    b. **Plantar reflexes**
       Bilateral Babinski's responses can occur with structural or metabolic coma.

DIAGNOSTIC TESTING

Once the history and neurologic examination are completed, a differential diagnosis should be generated. Most patients in stupor or coma can be placed into one of three categories on the basis of neurologic findings:

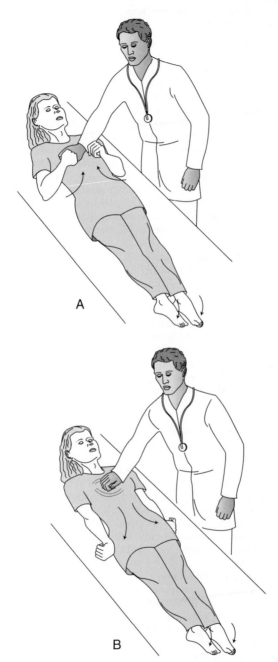

Figure 5–4 *A,* Decorticate (flexor) posturing. *B,* Decerebrate (extensor) posturing.

1. **Nonfocal examination with brain stem intact**

   This category is characterized by reactive pupils, full eye movements, and symmetric motor responses and suggests a toxic-metabolic etiology, CNS infection, or hydrocephalus.

2. **Focal hemispheric signs**

   These signs are characterized by contralateral hemiparesis and gaze paresis and suggest a structural CNS lesion such as stroke, subdural hematoma, or neoplasm.

3. **Focal brain stem signs**

   These signs are characterized by abnormal pupil reactivity, cranial nerve signs, and motor posturing and suggest a brain stem lesion or a space-occupying lesion associated with herniation.

Because it is important to quickly rule out life-threatening conditions in patients with coma, diagnostic testing should generally proceed in the following order in all patients until a diagnosis is established:

1. **Head CT (or MRI) scan**

   Intravenous contrast material should be given if a tumor or an abscess is suspected. Order bone windows if there is a history of trauma.

2. **Lumbar puncture**

   LP should be performed to rule out meningitis, encephalitis, or subarachnoid hemorrhage if the diagnosis is not established by CT or MRI. *Never postpone treatment for meningitis or encephalitis if there is a delay in obtaining the CSF.*

3. **EEG**

   An EEG may be necessary to rule out *nonconvulsive status epilepticus*, a postictal state, or metabolic coma if the diagnosis is not established by CT and LP.

   Pseudocoma states should be considered if the cause of coma remains unclear after diagnostic testing.

   - **Psychogenic coma**

     Psychogenic coma occurs in patients who are physiologically awake but unresponsive. Clues to the diagnosis include negativistic behavior (active resistance to eye-opening or passive limb movement), avoidance behavior (the hand avoids the face when dropped from above the head), intact saccadic eye movements and nystagmus on cold caloric testing, and recovery of alertness in response to very painful stimuli.

   - **Locked-in syndrome**

     Locked-in syndrome refers to bilateral pontine damage (usually from infarction) that renders the patient awake but completely paralyzed except for vertical eye movements. *Ocular bobbing* is a common finding.

   - **Akinetic mutism**

     Akinetic mutism refers to states of extreme psychomotor retardation (abulia) resulting from extensive thalamic or frontal lobe damage. These patients appear awake but demonstrate reduced spontaneity and exhibit only limited responses after extremely long delays.

MANAGEMENT

Emergency Treatments for Patients in Coma

1. **Space-occupying lesions** require prompt neurosurgical evaluation because emergent decompression may be lifesaving.
2. **Increased intracranial pressure,** if suspected, should be treated immediately. Stepwise treatment includes
   a. *Head elevation*
   b. Intubation and *hyperventilation*
   c. *Sedation* if severe agitation is present (**midazolam 1 to 2 mg IV** is an effective, short-acting agent)
   d. *Osmotic diuresis* with **20% mannitol 1.0 to 1.5 g/kg via rapid IV infusion.** If the patient is hypotensive, a suitable alternative is **0.5 to 2.0 ml/kg of 23.4% hypertonic saline** infused via a central venous line.

      These therapies can be used to "buy time" before definitive neurosurgical intervention. **Dexamethasone 10 mg IV every 6 hours** may also be of benefit for reducing edema associated with tumor or abscess. After these emergency treatments, an ICP monitor should be inserted to further guide management (see Chapter 12).
3. **Encephalitis** from herpes virus infection, if suspected, should be treated empirically with **acyclovir 10 mg/kg IV every 8 hours.** Further diagnostic testing should proceed as outlined in Chapter 21.
4. **Bacterial meningitis,** if suspected, should be treated empirically. Pretreat with **dexamethasone 6 mg IV** before starting **ceftriaxone 1 g IV every 12 hours** and **vancomycin 1 g IV every 12 hours** pending CSF culture results.

General Care of the Comatose Patient

1. **Airway protection**
   Adequate oxygenation and ventilation and prevention of aspiration are the goals. Most patients will require endotracheal intubation and frequent orotracheal suctioning. *Nonintubated stuporous patients should always be designated to receive NPO.*
2. **Intravenous hydration**
   Use only isotonic fluids (e.g., normal saline) in patients with cerebral edema or increased ICP.
3. **Nutrition**
   Administer enteral feeds via a small-bore nasoduodenal tube. Nasogastric tubes impair the integrity of the upper and

lower esophageal sphincters and increase the risk of gastro-esophageal reflux and aspiration.

4. **Skin**

   Order that the patient be turned every 1 to 2 hours to prevent pressure sores. An inflatable or foam mattress and protective heel pads may also be beneficial.

5. **Eyes**

   Prevent corneal abrasion by taping the eyelids shut or by applying a lubricant.

6. **Bowel care**

   Constipation can be avoided by giving a stool softener (docusate sodium 100 mg three times a day). Intubation and steroids may predispose to gastric stress ulceration, and this should be prevented by giving an H_2 blocker (ranitidine 50 mg IV every 8 hours).

7. **Bladder care**

   Indwelling urinary catheters are a common source of infection and should be used judiciously. Use intermittent catheterization every 6 hours when possible.

8. **Joint mobility**

   Order daily passive range-of-motion exercises to prevent contractures.

9. **Deep vein thrombosis (DVT) prophylaxis**

   Immobility is a major risk factor for DVT and subsequent pulmonary embolism. Order heparin 5000 U SC every 12 hours or enoxaparin 40 mg SC once a day. External pneumatic compression stockings should also be used.

PROGNOSIS

The prognosis for recovery from coma depends primarily on the cause, rather than on the depth, of coma. Coma from drug intoxication and metabolic causes carries the best prognosis; patients with coma from traumatic head injury fare better than those with coma from other structural causes; and coma from global hypoxia-ischemia carries the least favorable prognosis. Simple bedside testing can be used to prognosticate outcome as early as 3 days after hypoxic-ischemic coma (Fig. 5–5). Confirmation of a hopeless situation in patients with hypoxic-ischemic coma can be attained with somatosensory evoked potential testing. Bilaterally absent cortical responses with medial nerve stimulation 5 days or more after the onset of coma implies a 100% likelihood of a vegetative outcome. This information may be useful for helping families to decide whether to withdraw life support.

Persistent vegetative state (PVS) refers to a state of "eyes-open unresponsiveness" that is applied to patients in coma for 30 days or more. These patients regain normal sleep-wake cycles and display

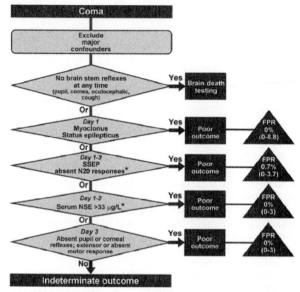

Figure 5–5 Decision algorithm for use in prognostication of comatose survivors after cardiopulmonary resuscitation. The numbers in the triangles are percentages; FPR indicates false positive rate (with 95% confidence percentages in parentheses), or the chance that the presence of a given finding can be associated with recovery from coma. Major confounders can include the use or prior use of sedatives or neuromuscular blocking agents, induced hypothermia therapy, presence of organ failure, or shock.

*These test results may not be available on a timely basis. Serum NSE testing may not be sufficiently standardized. (Reproduced with permission from Wijdicks EFM, et al: Prediction of outcome in comatose survivors after cardiopulmonary resuscitation an evidence-based review: Report of the Quality Standards Subcommittee of the American Academy of Neurology. Neurology 2006 67: 203-210.)

primitive responses to stimuli, such as chewing, sucking, and grasping, but demonstrate no evidence of conscious awareness. Prognostication is important, because this information may influence decisions to withhold life-sustaining measures such as cardiopulmonary resuscitation (CPR) or intensive care unit (ICU) care. Recovery of consciousness from PVS is generally defined as return of the ability to communicate or follow commands. By this criterion, 15% of adult patients with nontraumatic injury and 50% of patients with traumatic injury who are still in a vegetative state after 1 month will recover consciousness by 12 months. Recovery of consciousness after 12 months in a PVS is exceedingly rare.

Acute Stroke

Stroke should be suspected whenever a patient presents with the characteristic sudden onset of focal neurologic signs, such as hemiparesis, hemisensory loss, hemianopia, aphasia, or ataxia (Table 6–1). Time is of the essence for treating stroke, because the "therapeutic window" is only 3 to 6 hours. Because of the importance of early intervention in acute stroke, the emphasis of ER management should not be on identifying subtle, unusual, or interesting neurologic signs but on the following:

1. **Stabilizing the patient**
2. **Obtaining blood tests, an ECG, and a chest radiograph**
3. **Establishing the diagnosis by history and physical examination**
4. **Obtaining a head CT or MRI scan as soon as possible**

It should be kept in mind that mortality is reduced and the likelihood of a good recovery is increased when stroke patients are cared for in a dedicated stroke unit. If your patient is unusually complex or critically ill, consideration should be given to transferring the patient to the nearest comprehensive stroke center once he or she has been stabilized.

This chapter focuses on the emergency management of stroke. Additional information regarding hospital care and long-term management can be found in Chapter 23.

PHONE CALL

Questions

1. What were the presenting symptoms?
2. Exactly when did the symptoms begin?
3. Have the symptoms worsened, fluctuated, or improved since onset?
4. What are the vital signs?
5. Does the patient have a history of hypertension, diabetes, or cardiac disease?
6. Is the patient taking aspirin or warfarin?

    It is particularly important to perform an urgent CT scan in patients taking warfarin, in order to rule out intracerebral

TABLE 6–1 **Presentations of Acute Stroke**

- Abrupt onset of facial or limb weakness (usually hemiparesis)
- Sensory loss in one or more extremities
- Sudden change in mental status (confusion, delirium, lethargy, stupor, or coma)
- Aphasia (incoherent speech, lack of speech output, or difficulty understanding speech)
- Dysarthria (slurred speech)
- Loss of vision (hemianopic or monocular) or diplopia
- Ataxia (truncal or limb)
- Vertigo, nausea and vomiting, or headache

hemorrhage, because early treatment with fresh frozen plasma (FFP) and vitamin K can be lifesaving.

Orders

1. Establish an intravenous line with **0.9% normal saline (NS) at 1 ml/kg/hour.** Hypotonic fluids such as D5W and half-normal saline aggravate cerebral edema.
2. Provide oxygen via a nasal cannula and obtain a chest radiograph if the patient is tachypneic.
3. Keep the patient NPO.
4. Obtain an ECG.
5. Obtain a stat noncontrast head CT scan.
7. Perform the following diagnostic blood tests:
   - CBC and platelet count
   - Serum chemistries (glucose, electrolytes, BUN, creatinine)
   - PT/PTT
   - Cardiac troponin level
8. If indicated, perform the following tests:
   - Alcohol level
   - Liver function tests
   - Arterial blood gases
   - Toxicology screen

ELEVATOR THOUGHTS

What are the causes of stroke?
1. **Infarction: causes 80% of all strokes**
   a. Embolic
      (1) Cardiogenic embolism
         (a) Atrial fibrillation or other arrhythmia
         (b) Left ventricular mural thrombus
         (c) Mitral or aortic valve disease
         (d) Endocarditis (infectious or noninfectious)
      (2) Paradoxical embolism (patent foramen ovale)

(3) Aortic arch embolism
   b. Atherothrombotic (large- or medium-vessel disease)
      (1) Extracranial disease
         (a) Internal carotid artery
         (b) Vertebral artery
      (2) Intracranial disease
         (a) Internal carotid artery
         (b) Middle cerebral artery
         (c) Basilar artery
   c. Lacunar (small penetrating artery occlusion)
2. **Intracerebral hemorrhage (ICH): causes 15% of all strokes**
   a. Hypertensive
   b. Arteriovenous malformation
   c. Amyloid angiopathy
3. **Subarachnoid hemorrhage (SAH): causes 5% of all strokes**
   a. Aneurysmal (80%)
   b. Nonaneurysmal (20%)
4. **Miscellaneous causes (can lead to infarction or hemorrhage)**
   a. Dural sinus thrombosis
   b. Carotid or vertebral artery dissection
   c. CNS vasculitis
   d. Moyamoya disease (progressive intracranial large artery occlusion)
   e. Migraine
   f. Hypercoagulable state
   g. Drug abuse (cocaine or other sympathomimetics)
   h. Hematologic disorders (sickle cell anemia, polycythemia, or leukemia)
   i. MELAS (mitochondrial encephalopathy, lactic acidosis, and stroke)
   j. Atrial myxoma

MAJOR THREAT TO LIFE

- **Transtentorial herniation**
   Occurs primarily in the following presentations:
   1. Massive hemispheric infarction or hemorrhage
   2. Intraventricular extension of ICH or SAH
- **Cerebellar infarction or hemorrhage**
   All patients with large cerebellar lesions require neurosurgical evaluation because emergent decompression can be lifesaving.
- **Aspiration**
   Aspiration pneumonia is a common cause of death in stroke patients. All patients should be considered to have impaired swallowing until proven otherwise.

- **Myocardial infarction (MI)**
    Acute MI complicates approximately 3% of acute ischemic strokes.

BEDSIDE

Quick Look Test

What is the patient's level of consciousness?
    The urgency of the situation can be assessed immediately by evaluating the level of consciousness. Patients in stupor or coma are at the highest risk for further deterioration and are most likely to benefit from urgent intervention.

Airway and Vital Signs

Is the patient in respiratory distress?
    If the patient's breathing appears labored, check arterial blood gas levels and start oxygen. **Patients with severe dyspnea or depressed level of consciousness (stupor or coma) should be intubated prior to CT scanning.** Failure to control the airway in either setting can lead to massive aspiration or to respiratory arrest.

What is the blood pressure?
    Hypertension occurs frequently after stroke as a nonspecific response to cerebral injury. In ischemic stroke, this response may be advantageous, because increased cerebral perfusion pressure improves blood flow in regions of marginally perfused brain (the ischemic penumbra) that have lost the capacity to autoregulate. As a result, *overly aggressive BP reduction in acute ischemic stroke patients can lead to increased infarction and neurologic deterioration.* For this reason, only severe hypertension should be treated prior to CT scanning unless there is a non-neurologic indication (Box 6–1).
    If the patient meets one of the criteria listed in Box 6–1 and needs urgent BP control, start with IV labetalol.
1. Order 100 mg of IV labetalol in a 20-ml syringe (5 mg/ml) to the bedside.
2. Order a labetalol drip to the bedside (200 mg in 200 ml NS).
3. IV push 20 mg of labetalol over 2 minutes; then repeat 40, 60, and finally 80 mg at 5- to 10-minute intervals until the desired BP is attained, up to a total dose of 200 mg.
4. Once the desired BP is attained, start infusion of 2 mg/min (120 ml/hr) and titrate to keep BP less than 180/110 mm Hg.
    If labetalol fails to control hypertension, start **nicardipine 5 mg/hr (1 mg/10 ml)** and infuse in addition to labetolol. The dose can be titrated up to a maximum of 15 mg/hr.

> ### BOX 6–1 Guidelines for ER Treatment of Hypertension in Acute Stroke
>
> *Treat hypertension if a nonneurologic hypertensive emergency exists:*
> 1. Acute myocardial ischemia
> 2. Cardiogenic pulmonary edema
> 3. Malignant hypertension (retinopathy)
> 4. Hypertensive nephropathy or encephalopathy
> 5. Aortic dissection
>
> *Also treat hypertension if the BP is highly elevated on three repeated measurements 15 minutes apart:*
> 1. Systolic BP >220 mm Hg
> 2. Diastolic BP >120 mm Hg
>
> **Otherwise, systolic BPs of 160 to 220 mm Hg should *not* be treated prior to CT scanning.** If hemorrhage is identified by CT, reduction of the systolic BP to 150 to 180 mm Hg should be considered.

Low BP in acute stroke is unusual. Hypotension that is severe enough to precipitate cerebral infarction is rare but can occur in patients with severe carotid artery or intracranial artery stenosis.

What is the heart rate?

Rapid atrial fibrillation may require treatment with **diltiazem 20 to 25 mg** or **verapamil 5 to 15 mg IV push** for rate control prior to CT scanning.

What is the temperature?

The most common cause of fever at onset after stroke is aspiration pneumonia. If fever is present, give acetaminophen 650 mg PO, and order a cooling blanket and blood and urine cultures. If respiratory distress is present or the patient looks especially sick, consider administering antibiotics empirically **(amopxicillin/ clavulanate [Unasyn] 1.5 g IV every 6 hours** or **clindamycin 600 mg IV every 8 hours).**

Selective History

If possible, obtain an eyewitness to corroborate the patient's account. Be sure to check the following:

1. **Exactly what time did the stroke begin?**

   If the symptoms began within 6 hours and an ischemic stroke is confirmed by CT, intravenous or intra-arterial reperfusion therapy may be possible, and the evaluation should proceed as quickly as possible.

2. **What were the initial symptoms?**

   A maximal deficit at onset in a fully alert patient supports cerebral infarction and suggests embolism in particular. Loss of consciousness, headache, or vomiting supports intracerebral hemorrhage. Inquire specifically about the following:

- Headache or neck pain (hemorrhage or dissection)
- Loss of consciousness
- Confused or slurred speech
- Visual disturbances
- Dizziness or vertigo (brain stem ischemia)
- Weakness or clumsiness
- Numbness or paresthesias
- Gait instability
3. **Were there any antecedent attacks consistent with transient ischemic attack (TIA)?**
4. **Was any seizure activity observed?**
5. **What is the patient's medical history?**
6. **Has the patient used drugs or alcohol recently?**
   Cocaine can precipitate infarction or hemorrhage.
7. **What medications is the patient taking?**

Selective Physical Examination
General Physical Examination

Neck	Auscultate for carotid bruits. Neck stiffness suggests subarachnoid hemorrhage.
Lungs	Check for aspiration pneumonia or congestive heart failure.
Heart	Murmurs suggest valvular heart disease and a possible source of embolism.

Neurologic Examination

Because time is of the essence, the initial neurologic examination needs to be systematic and efficient. The goal is to simply localize and characterize the severity of the deficit. An experienced examiner can accomplish this in 10 to 15 minutes; a more detailed examination should be carried out later.

- **Mental status**
  1. **Level of consciousness and attentiveness**
  2. **Concentration.** Ask the patient to count from 20 to 1 or to recite the months in reverse.
  3. **Orientation**
  4. **Aphasia.** Check the fluency of spontaneous speech, naming, repetition, and paraphasic errors (word or syllable substitutions).
  5. **Hemispatial neglect.** Forced head and gaze deviation implies a large hemispheric lesion.
- **Cranial nerves**
  1. **Fundus.** Check for papilledema.
  2. **Visual fields.** Ask the patient to count fingers in all four quadrants. Check the patient's blink-to-threat if the patient is inattentive.

3. **Pupils**
4. **Extraocular movements**
5. **Face.** A widened palpebral fissure and flattened nasolabial fold are indicative of facial weakness.
6. **Palate and tongue.** Check for symmetry and adequacy of the gag reflex.

- **Motor**
  1. **Spontaneous movements.** Preferential movement of the limbs on one side indicates paresis of the unused limbs. If the patient is unresponsive, check for a preferential localizing response to sternal rub.
  2. **Limb tone.** Increased tone occurs with deep lesions in the internal capsule or brain stem.
  3. **Arm (pronator) drift.** If the patient is unable to follow commands, passively elevate both arms and check whether one falls preferentially.
  4. **Power.** Check strength against active resistance at the shoulders, wrists, hips, and ankles.

- **Reflexes**
  1. **Deep tendon reflexes**
  2. **Plantar reflexes**

     Proceed with the following elements of the neurologic examination only if the patient's level of consciousness allows:

  - **Sensory**
    1. **Pinprick or pinch test** identifies a lateralizing deficit.
  - **Coordination**
    1. **Finger-to-nose test** identifies intention tremor and past pointing.
    2. **Gait and station.** Check for reduced arm swing on the paretic side. A wide base is indicative of truncal ataxia.

MANAGEMENT I: ACUTE MANAGEMENT

Once the history and examination are completed, you should be able to localize the lesion clinically. **The main differential diagnoses are infarction and hemorrhage, which can be accurately diagnosed only by CT or MR.** Hence, all further management decisions (thrombolysis, BP management, or further workup) will depend on the results of brain imaging.

Hemorrhage

Radiographic Assessment

Blood is readily identified by the presence of a high-density (bright) signal (Fig. 6–1). If ICH is present, be sure to check for the following radiographic findings:

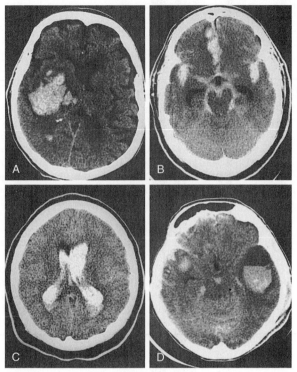

Figure 6–1 CT scans of brain hemorrhage. *A*, Intracerebral hemorrhage. *B*, Subarachnoid hemorrhage. *C*, Intraventricular hemorrhage. *D*, Acute hemorrhage with fluid/fluid level, indicative of a clotting disturbance.

- *Subarachnoid hemorrhage* (Fig. 6–1*B*) in association with intraparenchymal hemorrhage suggests a ruptured aneurysm and requires angiography.
- *Intraventricular hemorrhage* (Fig. 6–1*C*) in association with ventricular enlargement requires neurosurgical evaluation for possible emergent ventriculostomy.
- *Fluid/fluid levels* within a hematoma (Fig. 6–1*D*) result from separation of red blood cells and plasma and are indicative of a coagulopathy.
- *Edema and mass effect* usually lead to delayed neurologic deterioration when associated with a large hemorrhage (>30 ml). An abnormally large or an irregular amount of edema associated with hemorrhage suggests (1) hemorrhagic infarction, (2) bleeding associated with neoplasm, or (3) venous infarction from dural sinus thrombosis.

Checklist for Acute Management of Intracerebral Hemorrhage

1. **Rule out coagulopathy**

   Confirm that the PT/international normalized ratio (INR) and PTT are normal. If the PT is elevated or the patient is actively taking warfarin or another form of oral anticoagulant therapy, give **FFP 15 ml/kg (200 ml units, usually 4 to 6) every 4 hours** and **vitamin K 15 mg by IV push, then SC three times a day** until the INR is normalized to <1.4. Reverse heparin anticoagulation with **protamine sulfate 10 to 50 mg by slow IV push** (1 mg reverses approximately 100 units of heparin). **Recombinant activated factor VII 40 to 80 µg/kg,** which can normalize the INR within minutes of a single IV dose, is a newer treatment for the emergency reversal of coagulopathic ICH, but experience for this indication is limited (Box 6–2).

2. **Control severe hypertension**

   In contrast to the approach taken with acute cerebral infarction, a somewhat more aggressive approach to BP control is suggested for patients with acute ICH, because high levels may lead to worsening of perilesional edema. Although the optimal management has yet to be established, we advocate reduction of systolic BPs that are higher than 180 mm Hg to levels between 150 and 180 mm Hg using a **labetalol** or **nicardipine** infusion (see Airway and Vital Signs).

BOX 6–2 Ultraearly Hemostatic Therapy for ICH: A Promising Treatment Paradigm

Even in noncoagulopathic patients, the period of active bleeding in acute ICH may extend for up to 4 to 6 hours. In February of 2005, a phase II clinical trial of 399 ICH patients scanned with CT within 3 hours of onset found that a single IV dose of recombinant activated factor VII (Novo Seven, Novo Nordisk A/S) ranging from 40 to 160 µg/kg resulted in a 5 ml absolute reduction in subsequent hemorrhage growth relative to placebo. This reduction in bleeding was associated with a 38% relative reduction in mortality and a significant increase in the proportion of patients alive with minimal or no disability at 3 months. Risks included a 7% frequency of serious thromboembolic adverse events (primarily non-ST-elevation myocardial infarction and ischemic stroke), compared with a 2% rate in placebo. Routine use of this agent cannot currently be recommended on the basis of a single trial. However, a confirmatory phase III trial (The FAST Trial) will be completed in early 2007.

3. **Consider emergent hematoma evacuation**

The criteria for emergent evacuation of intracerebral hemorrhage are controversial. It is generally accepted that cerebellar hemorrhages greater than 3 cm in diameter should be evacuated when there is depressed level of consciousness with clinical signs and radiographic evidence of posterior fossa mass effect. A recent randomized controlled trial (STICH: Surgical Trial in Intracerebral Hemorrhage) found no benefit when craniotomy was performed for supratentorial ICH within 72 hours of onset compared to best medical therapy. Despite this, patients classically considered good candidates for emergency surgery, such as younger patients with early deterioration caused by symptomatic mass effect from a large lobar hemorrhage, were excluded from the trial, and in selected cases might still benefit from surgery.

Consideration should also be given to inserting a *ventricular drain* in stuporous or comatose patients with intraventricular hemorrhage and obstructive hydrocephalus, or a *parenchymal* ICP monitor in patients with large, deep hemorrhages who are not candidates for surgery.

4. **Consider angiography**

Angiography can rule out an aneurysm or AVM. This is particularly important when subarachnoid hemorrhage is present, in young nonhypertensive patients when a lobar hemorrhage is present, or in any patient with a primary intraventricular hemorrhage. Angiography is almost always negative in chronically hypertensive patients with a hemorrhage in a classic hypertensive location (putamen, thalamus, pons, or cerebellum).

5. **Osmotherapy**

Consider **mannitol (1.0 to 1.5 g/kg IV)** for deepening coma or if clinical signs of brain stem compression are evident (see Chapter 12 for further details). An alternative is 0.5 to 2.0 ml/kg of 23.4% hypertonic saline if the patient is relatively hypotensive or hypovolemic. *Steroids such as dexamethasone have not been shown to be effective in patients with ICH and should not be used.*

6. **Anticonvulsant therapy**

Seizures at onset are unusual but if present should be treated with **phenytoin** or **fosphenytoin 10 to 20 mg/kg IV.** Prophylactic treatment with phenytoin or a similar anticonvulsant for 7 days is an option in patients whose condition is critical enough to require intubation, treatment for increased ICP, or surgery.

Additional guidelines for the management of ICH or SAH are included in Chapter 23 (Cerebrovascular Diseases) and under Management II: General Care in this chapter.

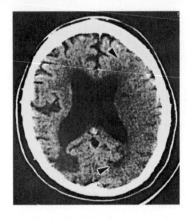

Figure 6–2 Early cerebral infarction, with loss of gray-white definition and sulcal effacement. (*Arrowheads* indicate anterior and posterior borders of the territory of the middle cerebral artery.)

Infarction

Radiographic Assessment

Infarction appears as a lucent (dark) signal on a CT scan but may not be apparent until 12 to 24 hours after onset. Early signs of infarction (Fig. 6–2) are important to recognize and include (1) loss of definition of the gray-white junction, (2) mild sulcal effacement, and (3) subtle, hazy lucency. At many stroke centers, contrast-enhanced *CT perfusion* and *angiography* are increasingly being used as adjuncts to standard CT imaging in the emergency department. Demonstration of an extensive region of hypoperfused brain, or a large-vessel occlusion (Fig. 6–3), can be used to identify good candidates for emergent angiography and possible intra-arterial reperfusion therapy (see below for further discussion).

DWI reveals acute ischemic changes within minutes to hours of onset, long before infarction is present on CT or MR FLAIR images. Accordingly, MRI with DWI is probably the imaging modality of choice for patients with acute stroke. Gadolinium-enhanced perfusion-weighted imaging can also be used to identify regions of "perfusion-diffusion mismatch," much in the way that CT perfusion is used. However, logistical problems often limit the timely performance of MR, which can delay therapy.

AFFECTED VASCULAR TERRITORY

Identification of the affected vascular territory can provide important information regarding the mechanism of the infarction. The topography of the major arterial territories of the brain is shown in Figure 6–4. Examples of the three main patterns of infarction, described below, are shown in Figure 6–5.

1. **Territorial infarction** respects the margins of an entire vascular territory or one of its branches. The cause is usually embo-

Figure 6–3 CT perfusion image demonstrating occlusion of the M1 segment of the left middle cerebral artery *(long arrow)*. Filling of the anterior temporal branches is evident just proximal to the site of occlusion. Posteriorly, there is markedly reduced filling of the sylvian branches of the MCA compared to the contralateral side. (Image provided courtesy of Dr. Michael Lev, Massachusetts General Hospital).

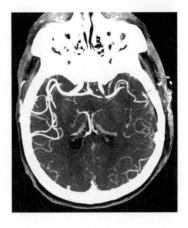

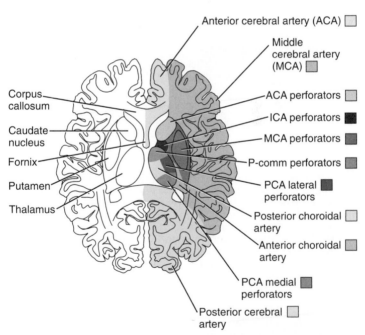

Figure 6–4 Axial section at the level of the thalamus showing the anatomic distribution of the major cerebral vascular territories. P-comm, Posterior communicating artery. (Redrawn from Tatu L, et al: Arterial territories of the human brain: Cerebral hemispheres. Neurology 1998;50:1699-1708.)

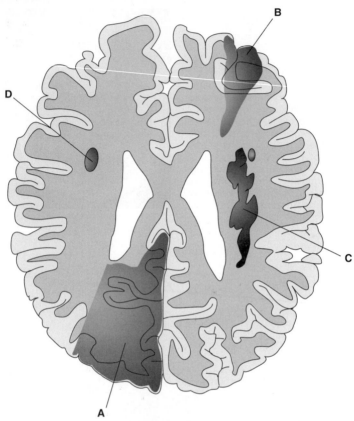

Figure 6–5 Schematic representation of different topographic patterns of cerebral infarction. *A,* Territorial infarction (from posterior cerebral artery occlusion); *B,* watershed border-zone infarction (between the territories of the anterior cerebral artery and the middle cerebral artery); *C,* internal border-zone infarction (deep middle cerebral artery territory); *D,* lacunar infarction (lenticulostriate-penetrating artery occlusion).

lism, with infarction occurring in brain regions immediately distal to the site of occlusion.

2. **Border-zone infarction** may occur either (1) along the boundaries between different vascular territories (watershed infarction) or (2) in the deepest and least well-collateralized regions of a vascular territory (internal border-zone infarction). In either case, the cause is usually distal hemodynamic perfusion failure related to a more proximal stenosis or occlusion.

3. **Lacunar infarction** appears as a small, deep infarction within the territory of a single, small penetrating artery. The mechanism is usually related to occlusion within the course of the small vessel (microatheroma or lipohyalinosis).

Goals of Management

1. **Acute reperfusion to limit or reverse ongoing acute ischemia (6- to 8-hour window)**

   Intravenous thrombolysis with **tissue plasminogen activator (t-PA)** within 3 hours of symptom onset is the only currently approved treatment for reversing ischemia in acute stroke. IV t-PA only rarely results in immediate early neurologic improvement. Rather, it increases the chances of a good recovery at 3 months from approximately 30% to 40%. It carries a 6% risk of symptomatic intracranial bleeding and should not be given if the head CT scan shows subtle early infarct signs involving more than one third of the middle cerebral artery (MCA) territory. Because the risk of hemorrhage increases significantly after 3 hours, this time window must be strictly obeyed.

   If the 3-hour window for IV t-PA is missed, reperfusion for distal ICA, proximal MCA, and basilar artery occlusions can be attempted, because the natural history of these syndromes is uniformly devastating. There is some evidence that intraarterial thrombolysis within 3 to 6 hours (Fig. 6–6), or endovascular mechanical extraction (Merci Concentric clot retrieval device) within 3 to 8 hours, can be effective. The best results

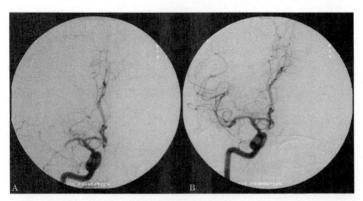

Figure 6–6 Angiogram (anteroposterior view) demonstrating total occlusion of the right M1 middle cerebral artery segment (A) prior to intraarterial thrombolysis, and complete recanalization (B) after the procedure. (Reproduced with permission from Katzan IL, et al. Neurology 1999;52:1081.)

are usually obtained by experienced teams at comprehensive stroke centers.

2. **Preventing neurologic deterioration related to an evolving stroke (72-hour window)**

Stroke progression occurs in 20% to 40% of hospitalized patients with ischemic stroke, with the risk being highest in the first 24 hours. Clinical deterioration can result from one of three mechanisms:

- **Extension of ischemic territory.** This may result from either *progressive thrombosis within an occluded vessel* (e.g., progressive brain stem infarction in a patient with basilar artery thrombosis) or *distal perfusion failure related to a more proximal stenosis or occlusion* (e.g., enlargement of internal border-zone infarction in a patient with internal carotid artery [ICA] occlusion).

  Approach: Full anticoagulation with unfractionated heparin may be used to prevent progressive thrombosis, although there is limited evidence of its efficacy, and its use in general is not recommended. Optimization of volume status and blood pressure may be used to mitigate perfusion failure; the best results occur if the patient has a fluctuating deficit or history of crescendo TIAs, which is suggestive of hemodynamic perfusion failure.

- **Hemorrhagic conversion.** This problem is frequently identified radiographically but seldom results in clinical symptoms. The three main risk factors are increased patient age, large infarct size, and acute hypertension.

  Approach: Defer anticoagulation of high-risk patients; treat severe hypertension.

- **Progressive edema and infarct swelling.** This problem is generally limited to large infarcts. Brain edema generally peaks 3 to 5 days after onset and is rarely a problem within the first 24 hours.

  Approach: Treatment with mannitol is beneficial. Avoid hypotonic fluids. *Steroids are not effective.*

3. **Preventing early recurrent stroke (30-day window)**

Approximately 5% of patients hospitalized for ischemic stroke experience a second stroke within 30 days. This risk is highest (greater than 10%) in patients with severe carotid stenosis and cardioembolism and lowest (1%) in patients with lacunar infarction.

Approach: Early treatment with heparin may reduce the risk of early recurrent stroke in patients with cardioembolism or large-artery stenosis, but has not been proven to do so.

Checklist for Acute Management of Ischemic Stroke

1. **Intravenous thrombolysis (0- to 3-hour window). Give IV t-PA (0.9 mg/kg IV over 1 hour with 10% of the dose given**

TABLE 6–2 **NINDS Exclusion Criteria for IV t-PA Therapy for Acute Ischemic Stroke**

Time of symptom onset unknown or more than 3 hours ago
CT evidence of hemorrhage
Early infarct signs involving >$\frac{1}{3}$ of the MCA territory
Seizure at onset of stroke
Rapidly improving or minor symptoms (e.g., pure sensory, minimal weakness)
Stroke or serious head trauma within preceding 3 months
Gastrointestinal, urinary tract, or other significant bleeding within preceding 21 days
Major surgery or serious trauma within preceding 14 days
Lumbar puncture within preceding 7 days
Arterial puncture at a noncompressible site within preceding 7 days
SBP >185 or DBP >110 despite attempts to control BP
History of coagulopathy or anticoagulant use, documented elevation of INR (>1.7) or aPTT (>1.5 × control) or thrombocytopenia (platelet count <100,000)
Glucose <50 or >400 mg/dl
Pregnancy
Significant MI within past 4 weeks or symptoms of post-MI pericarditis

These contraindications are intended to serve as a guideline. Successful and safe use of IV t-PA has been reported despite the presence of one or more of these complications. Decision making regarding the risks and benefits of t-PA should be individualized.
SBP, systolic blood pressure; *DBP*, diastolic blood pressure.

as an initial bolus; maximum of 90 mg) if onset is definitely within 3 hours and CT shows no signs of widespread early infarction. Exclusion criteria for IV t-PA are shown in Table 6–2. Note that BP must be controlled to ≤180/105 mm Hg prior to giving t-PA, and for at least 24 hours thereafter to minimize the risk of hemorrhagic conversion. Intra-arterial BP monitoring is not recommended because of the risk of hemorrhage. Hyperglycemia is also an important risk factor for hemorrhage after IV t-PA and should be controlled with a regular human insulin infusion of 0.5 to 4.0 U/hr to maintain the serum glucose between 100 to 120 mg/dl for the first 24 hours. In addition to IV t-PA, concomitant application of continuous 2 MHz transcranial Doppler ultrasonography to an occluded MCA for 2 hours was shown to improve recanalization rates and clinical outcome in a phase 2 study, but its use remains experimental.

2. **Intra-arterial reperfusion (3- to 6-hour window).** If an experienced interventional neuroradiologist is available, consider emergent angiography for (1) patients with a large anterior circulation stroke syndrome within 6 hours of onset, or (2) patients with a complete basilar artery territory syndrome within 12 hours of onset. For patients with severe evolving strokes, angiography should be considered even if

BOX 6-3 **Acute Intra-arterial Reperfusion Strategies for Acute Ischemic Stroke**

Thrombolysis. If an emergency angiogram demonstrates a persistent large-vessel occlusion, local intra-arterial thrombolysis with **t-PA (5 to 25 mg) between 3 and 6 hours after onset** can be considered. Depending on the experience and skill of the operator, mechanical clot disruption with a balloon or wire can be combined with IA thrombolysis. This approach was shown to improve outcome in a Phase 2 study (the Pro-ACT trial) but is not approved by the Food and Drug Administration (FDA). The administration of IA t-PA after initial treatment with a full or two thirds dose of IV t-PA (so called "bridging" therapy) has been shown to be feasible, but it remains unclear whether the benefit of this approach outweighs the risk.

Mechanical Thrombectomy. A new FDA-approved alternative to IA thrombolysis for reperfusion is mechanical clot extraction with **the Merci Concentric** retriever device. This corkscrew type can allow the operator to successfully remove an occluding thrombus and recanalize an occluded MCA in approximately 50% of cases. Because the procedure does not involve administration of a thrombolytic, this approach is associated with a smaller risk of hemorrhage and may safely allow reperfusion over a time window extending to 8 hours.

a full dose of IV t-PA has been administered, because the likelihood of complete or partial recanalization for a distal ICA "T-occlusion" or proximal MCA or basilar artery occlusion may be as low as 25% to 50% with IV t-PA alone. The most common approaches for attaining intra-arterial (IA) reperfusion are described in Box 6-3.

3. **Anticoagulation.** Although the use of **IV heparin** (start at **800 U/hr, 20,000 U in 500 ml NS at 20 ml/hr**) for acute ischemic stroke is not generally recommended, it may be a reasonable treatment option to prevent progression or recurrence of stroke in the following situations:
   - Stroke-in-evolution
   - High-grade large-vessel atherostenosis
   - Cardioembolic stroke
   - Arterial dissection
   - Crescendo TIAs
   - Dural sinus thrombosis

   Keep in mind that heparin is relatively contraindicated in patients with large infarcts associated with mass effect or hemorrhagic conversion.

4. Give **aspirin 325 mg PO** within 48 hours of onset. Aspirin is associated with a very small reduction in mortality and the risk of recurrent ischemic stroke.

5. Consider **cardiac rhythm monitoring** for patients with evidence of arrhythmia or myocardial ischemia.
6. **Consider intensive care unit (ICU) observation** in patients with clinical or radiographic signs of massive hemispheric or cerebellar infarction, depressed level of consciousness, respiratory distress, or fluctuating deficits or stroke-in-evolution. In selected cases with a fluctuating deficit and documented large-vessel stenosis or occlusion, a 30-minute trial of induced hypertension with **phenylephrine 2 to 10 μg/kg/min** targeted to raise the systolic BP by 20% can lead to immediate improvement of the neurologic deficit in approximately one third of cases. If no improvement is observed after 30 minutes, the infusion should be stopped. Close clinical, cardiac rhythm, and BP monitoring is essential.
7. **Obtain a neurosurgical evaluation** for possible decompressive surgery in patients with large cerebellar infarction or complete middle cerebral artery territory infarction with midline shift and deteriorating level of consciousness.
8. Consider **MRI** including diffusion-weighted imaging in patients with posterior circulation strokes or if the infarction is not well delineated by CT.
9. **Order a noninvasive neurovascular workup.**

   Proper decisions regarding the treatment of cerebral infarction are based on elucidation of the mechanism of the stroke.

   The following tests should be performed in every patient:
   - *Echocardiography* is an important technique for identifying cardiac sources of emboli. In many patients, transthoracic echocardiography is adequate. *Transesophageal echocardiography* provides more detailed views of the left atrium and aortic arch and is a more sensitive test for detecting mural thrombi and valvular vegetations. An *agitated saline study* ("bubble study") is highly sensitive for detecting right-to-left atrial shunts, consistent with a patent foramen ovale.
   - *Carotid Doppler ultrasonography* is needed to rule out carotid stenosis that is symptomatic and greater than 70%, which is an indication for carotid endarterectomy.

   The following tests should be performed in selected patients:
   - *Transcranial Doppler ultrasonography* can be used to diagnose occlusion or stenosis of the major intracranial arteries. Abnormal intracranial waveforms and collateral flow patterns can also be used to determine whether a stenosis found in the neck is hemodynamically significant.
   - *Magnetic resonance or CT angiography* can be used to diagnose extracranial or intracranial stenosis or occlusion.

- *Holter monitoring* may be useful for detecting intermittent atrial fibrillation.
10. **Consider blood testing** to identify unusual causes of stroke, particularly in young patients.
    - *Blood cultures* if endocarditis is suspected
    - *Procoagulant workup:* protein C activity, protein S activity, antithrombin III activity, lupus anticoagulant, anticardiolipin antibodies, Factor V Leiden mutation, prothrombin gene mutation
        Note: These tests should be obtained before anticoagulation is started.
    - *Vasculitis workup:* antinuclear antibody (ANA), rheumatoid factor (RF), rapid plasma reagin (RPR), hepatitis virus serologies, erythrocyte sedimentation rate (ESR), serum protein electrophoresis (SPEP), cryoglobulins, and herpes simplex virus (HSV) serologies
    - *Coagulation profile* to rule out disseminated intravascular coagulation (DIC)
    - *Beta-human chorionic gonadotropin (β-hCG)* testing to rule out pregnancy in young women with stroke

Refer to **Chapter 23** for further discussion of specific ischemic stroke syndromes, evaluation of TIAs, and the secondary prevention of ischemic stroke.

MANAGEMENT II: GENERAL CARE

Much of the morbidity and mortality associated with stroke is related to nonneurologic complications, which can be minimized by adherence to these guidelines:

1. **Fever**
    Fever exacerbates ischemic brain injury and should be treated aggressively with antipyretics (acetaminophen) or a cooling blanket, if necessary.
2. **Nutrition**
    Stroke patients are at high risk for aspiration. Patients with depressed level of consciousness, brain stem strokes, bilateral strokes, and large hemispheric strokes carry the highest risk. Formal assessment of swallowing ability by a speech pathologist should be completed before patients at risk are fed. Start enteral feeding via a nasoduodenal tube within 24 hours after the stroke if the patient cannot swallow safely.
3. **Intravenous hydration**
    Hypovolemia is common among stroke patients and should be corrected with isotonic crystalloid. Avoiding volume depletion may be particularly important in patients with intracardiac thrombi (dehydration has been linked to progressive thrombus formation) or hemodynamic stroke. Hypotonic

fluids (e.g., D5W and 0.45% saline) can aggravate cerebral edema and should be avoided.

4. **Glucose**

Hyperglycemia and hypoglycemia can lead to exacerbation of ischemic injury. In critically ill stroke patients it seems prudent to prevent hyperglycemia (glucose level higher than 140 mg/dl with intensive insulin infusion (0.5-1.0 U/hr to maintain glucose levels between 90-120 mg/dl).

5. **Pulmonary care**

Chest physical therapy (every 4 hours) should be ordered to prevent atelectasis in immobilized patients.

6. **Head of bed elevation**

Elevate the head of bed 30° to reduce the risk of ventilator associated pneumonia, improve orientation, and minimize ICP.

7. **Activity**

Patients with stroke should be mobilized and engaged in physical therapy as soon as possible. For immobilized patients, order patient turning every 2 hours (to prevent pressure sores) and joint range-of-motion exercises four times a day to prevent contractures. Heel splints to maintain the ankle in dorsiflexion can also prevent shortening of the Achilles tendon. Have the patient taken out of bed to a chair every day as soon as feasible.

8. **Prophylaxis for deep vein thrombosis (DVT)**

Ischemic stroke patients with significant immobility who are not on IV heparin should be treated with Enoxaparin 40 mg once daily or heparin 5000 U every 12 hours to prevent formation of DVT. This treatment can be started safely in patients with ICH after 24 hours.

9. **Bladder care**

Indwelling urinary catheters should be used judiciously; order intermittent catheterization every 6 hours when possible.

Spinal Cord Compression

Spinal cord compression is one of the few true neurologic emergencies. The more severe the syndrome, the more acute the injury is likely to have been. Unlike the brain, which may have remarkable functional recovery, the spinal cord, once damaged, rarely recovers function. Patients with cord compression resulting from neoplastic disease of the spine who cannot walk before the onset of treatment will rarely walk again. Diagnosis of spinal cord injury depends on a clear understanding of the anatomy of the cord and the supportive structures.

PHONE CALL

This chapter will be most useful for patients in whom spinal cord compression is known or suspected. The response to such a call should focus on establishing the diagnosis and assessing the acuteness of the injury.

Questions

1. **What is the patient's general condition?**
2. **What are the vital signs? Is the patient in any respiratory distress?**
3. **Does the patient have back pain?**
4. **Is there history of trauma to the neck or back?**
5. **Does the patient have any known cancer or infection?**
    Back pain in a cancer patient is considered to result from a vertebral metastasis until it is proved otherwise.
6. **How long has the problem been going on?**

Orders

If trauma or an unstable spine is suspected, give the following orders:

1. **Immobilize the neck (back).**
    A Philadelphia collar or a backboard should be used to ensure adequate stability (Fig. 7–1). If such equipment is

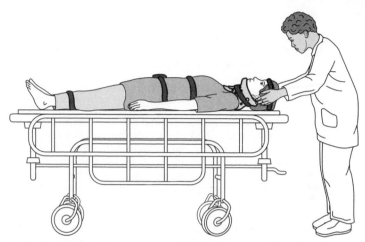

Figure 7–1 Stabilizing the neck and back with a Philadelphia collar and a backboard.

unavailable immediately, the cervical spine can be immobilized by holding the head firmly in a neutral position, using both hands.

2. **Check vital signs.**

Injury above the C5 level may compromise respiratory function. Cervical spinal injury, particularly with complete transection, may result in loss of sympathetic control, causing hypotension and bradycardia. Fever may point to an infectious process.

3. **Obtain plain x-rays of the neck (anteroposterior and lateral).**

Flexion and extension views, if done carefully by an experienced staff, may be helpful. Even if there is no suspicion of trauma, the pattern of bony abnormality may suggest subluxation, unsuspected pathologic fracture from neoplasm, osteomyelitis, or other infection. In most circumstances, plain x-rays can provide quick information that can then be followed up by CT or MRI once an initial assessment is done.

4. **Notify the neurosurgical team or specialized spinal unit, if available.**

Direct trauma to the spinal cord can produce a myelopathy, but it is the secondary effects from bleeding, dislocation, or osseous or articular instability that can be devastating; these secondary effects are preventable if properly identified and addressed.

Inform RN

"Will arrive at the bedside in . . . minutes."

Spinal cord compression is a medical emergency. Delay may cause irreversible neurologic dysfunction.

ELEVATOR THOUGHTS

What is the differential diagnosis of spinal cord compression?

Physical examination and often radiographic evaluation are needed to confirm a compressive myelopathy. You should be thinking first of the three categories of disease that are the most likely to cause spinal cord compression: trauma, infection, and neoplasm. Four other categories complete the differential diagnosis list.

1. **Trauma**

    Trauma is the most acute form of spinal cord compression. A history of a motor vehicle accident or sports-related accident is commonly elicited. Flexion, extension, compression, or rotation injuries in addition to direct blunt or penetrating trauma may produce a compressive myelopathy. Cervical disks tend to herniate centrally, producing an anterior cord syndrome.

2. **Infection**

    Infections of the spine most often occur in the thoracic or lumbar spine. Infections can take the following forms:

    - Epidural abscesses—seen commonly in IV drug users, these are most often bacterial (e.g., *Staphylococcus aureus, Escherichia coli*)
    - Spinal tuberculosis (Pott's disease)—this occurs in debilitated or immunocompromised patients or in those known to have pulmonary tuberculosis
    - Vertebral osteomyelitis—*Staphylococcus* species, *Streptococcus* species, *E. coli*, or *Brucella* species may cause pathologic fractures or produce epidural abscesses

3. **Neoplasm**

    Metastases are the most common neoplasm seen in bony disease of the spine (Fig. 7–2). The thoracic spine is most often affected because of venous drainage of visceral organs through spinal extradural venous plexuses. Meningiomas may appear as extradural tumors, with a predominance in the thoracic region. The female/male ratio is 9:1. Neurofibromas or schwannomas may arise on spinal roots and cause cord compression as they expand. Ependymomas are intrinsic cord tumors that could mimic extra-axial compressive lesions.

4. **Degenerative disease**

    Cervical disks herniate centrally, in contrast to lumbar disks, which herniate laterally and cause radicular symptoms.

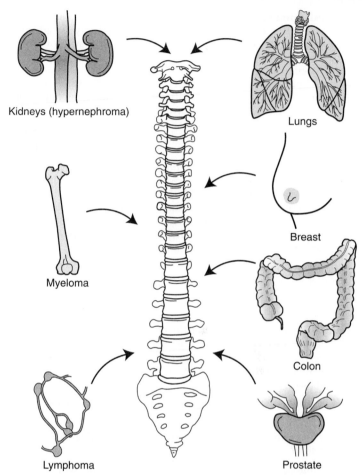

Figure 7–2 Neoplasms that commonly metastasize to or involve the spine: carcinoma of the lung, breast, colon, and prostate; hypernephroma; myeloma; and lymphoma.

Thoracic disk protrusions are rare. An acute cauda equina syndrome may be produced by herniation at L1-L2.

5. **Congenital disease**

Arnold-Chiari malformation, with or without syringomyelia, may produce cervical myelopathy. Congenital defects of the atlantoaxial joint may predispose to subluxation or dislocation. A tethered cord produces a spastic diplegia of the legs. Relatively minor trauma may bring an occult malformation to clinical prominence.

6. **Inflammatory disease**

   Rheumatoid arthritis is the most common disease affecting the stability of the upper cervical spine and may allow atlantoaxial translocations.

7. **Vascular disease**

   Epidural and subdural hematomas of the spine are very rare. They may be seen in patients taking anticoagulant medication. Arteriovenous malformations of the spine are rare.

MAJOR THREAT TO LIFE

- **Respiratory compromise** (cervical lesions) may require immediate intubation. Diaphragm weakness may result in hypoventilation and respiratory acidosis.
- **Autonomic dysregulation may produce hypotension** that does not respond to volume challenge. This phenomenon may be part of spinal shock. The hypotension may respond to pressors (e.g., dopamine).

BEDSIDE

Quick Look Test

What is the general condition of the patient?

Respiratory distress may necessitate immediate intubation. Look for retraction of the supraclavicular muscles as a sign of accessory respiratory muscle use because of diaphragmatic weakness.

Does the patient look cachectic or ill, suggesting cancer or general debilitation?

Is there urinary or bowel incontinence, suggesting sacral cord involvement?

Is there flushing or diaphoresis, suggesting autonomic dysregulation?

Management

If, after a quick look, the patient appears unstable, notify the surgical team, the anesthesiology service, and/or the neurosurgery service and address cardiopulmonary dysfunction. Stability of the neck should be ensured.

1. **Anti-inflammatory treatment**
   a. **Trauma**

      For **acute traumatic spinal cord injury**, the following protocol for methylprednisolone administration should be initiated:

      (1) **Methylprednisolone 30 mg/kg IV bolus over 15 minutes**

(2) 45-minute pause

(3) **Methylprednisolone 5.4 mg/kg/hr continuous IV infusion over the next 23 hours**

b. **Tumor**

For known or suspected **spinal neoplasm**, administer **dexamethasone 100 mg IV bolus** immediately.

2. **Blood tests**

In any patient with suspected spinal cord compression, routine blood tests should be performed in preparation for possible surgical decompression: CBC, chemistry panel, coagulation profile, and blood type and hold.

3. **Imaging**

If the patient is hemodynamically stable and not in respiratory distress, notify the appropriate radiologic personnel. Your patient will require an MRI scan as soon as your examination can provide anatomic localization and a working differential diagnosis. Myelography in combination with CT has nearly uniformly been replaced by MRI. CT may be superior to MRI only in spinal trauma to define subtle bony abnormalities or fractures.

Selective Physical Examination

Do not move the patient with a suspected spine injury until adequate immobilization of the neck or back has been ensured (e.g., with a Philadelphia collar).

The anatomy of the white matter tracts and cell groups in the spinal cord is consistent from patient to patient. Precise localization of the involved level and structure of the cord will, therefore, provide valuable early information about the likely pathogenesis of the injury. An anterior cord syndrome localized to the cervical region, for example, suggests cervical disk herniation. A posterior cord syndrome at the thoracic level suggests bony metastasis. Figure 7–3 shows a representative cross section of the spinal cord. Table 7–1 outlines the features of the main spinal cord syndromes. Note that at each level, lower motor neuron signs result from cell groups exiting the cord at that level, and upper motor neuron signs are present below the level of injury.

General Physical Examination

Vital signs	Evaluate as described earlier; look for any signs of autonomic instability.
HEENT	Trauma to the neck should be suspected when there is trauma to the face and body. Battle's sign (ecchymosis over the mastoid process), raccoon sign (periorbital ecchymosis), hemotympanum, and CSF otorrhea suggest basilar skull fracture.

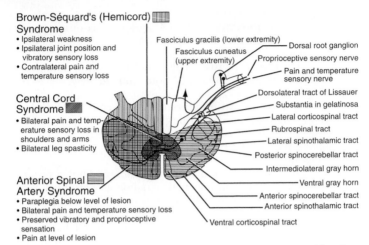

Brown-Séquard's (Hemicord) Syndrome
- Ipsilateral weakness
- Ipsilateral joint position and vibratory sensory loss
- Contralateral pain and temperature sensory loss

Central Cord Syndrome
- Bilateral pain and temperature sensory loss in shoulders and arms
- Bilateral leg spasticity

Anterior Spinal Artery Syndrome
- Paraplegia below level of lesion
- Bilateral pain and temperature sensory loss
- Preserved vibratory and proprioceptive sensation
- Pain at level of lesion

Fasciculus gracilis (lower extremity)
Fasciculus cuneatus (upper extremity)
Dorsal root ganglion
Proprioceptive sensory nerve
Pain and temperature sensory nerve
Dorsolateral tract of Lissauer
Substantia in gelatinosa
Lateral corticospinal tract
Rubrospinal tract
Lateral spinothalamic tract
Posterior spinocerebellar tract
Intermediolateral gray horn
Ventral gray horn
Anterior spinocerebellar tract
Anterior spinothalamic tract
Ventral corticospinal tract

Figure 7–3 Cross section of the spinal cord at the cervical level.

Spine	Percuss the spine with a fist or lightly with a tendon hammer. Tenderness to percussion suggests bony disease and will help localize the lesion for the rest of the examination and for a focal radiographic evaluation. Remember that the spinal cord comes down only to L1 in adults, unless there is a tethered cord. Tenderness in the lower lumbar or sacral spine may cause radicular symptoms but does not suggest cord compression.
Musculoskeletal	Look for signs of rheumatoid arthritis, which can be associated with atlanto-occipital dislocation.

Neurologic Examination

- **Motor**

    Test strength in the legs and the arms. Symmetric loss of lower extremity power with preserved strength in the arms may be the first clue to thoracic cord involvement. If there is bilateral weakness in both the arms and the legs, suggesting cervical involvement, there should be upper motor neuron signs in the legs. Note that if the spinal injury is acute, muscle tone may be decreased below the level of the injury.

- **Sensory**

    Look for a sensory level. Bilateral weakness with a concordant sensory level is pathognomonic for spinal cord injury. Vibra-

TABLE 7–1 **Major Spinal Cord Syndromes**

Syndrome	Common Causes	Features
Hemicord syndrome (Brown-Séquard's paralysis)	Penetrating injury Extrinsic compression	Contralateral spinothalamic loss Ipsilateral paresis Ipsilateral dorsal column loss Preserved light touch *Note:* deficits appear 1 to 2 levels below injury
Anterior cord syndrome	Anterior spinal artery infarct "Watershed" (T4–T6) ischemia Acute cervical disk herniation	Bilateral spinothalamic loss Preserved dorsal column sensation Upper motor neuron paralysis below lesion Lower motor neuron paralysis at lesion Sphincter dysfunction
Central cord syndrome	Syringomyelia Hypotensive spinal cord ischemia Spinal trauma (flexion-extension injury) Spinal cord neoplasm Sphincter dysfunction or urinary retention	Lower motor neuron weakness in arms Variable leg weakness and spasticity Severe pain and hyperpathia Spinothalamic loss in arms
Posterior cord syndrome	Trauma Posterior spinal artery infarct	Dorsal column sensory loss Pain and paresthesias in neck, back, or trunk Mild paresis

tory sense may be the first to go, particularly with a posterior cord syndrome, but the pinprick test (with a previously unused safety pin) is the most precise and reproducible. Remember, pain and temperature sensory neurons entering the cord ascend ipsilaterally for two to three spinal segments in the dorsolateral tract of Lissauer before crossing just anterior to the central canal to join the contralateral spinothalamic tract located in the lateral cord. Therefore, loss of pinprick or temperature sensation at a given level may indicate pathology two to three segments above the level detected on examination. A dermatome chart can be found in Appendix A-5.

Perineal sensory loss (saddle anesthesia) suggests injury to the conus medullaris. Patchy sensory loss in the lower extremities with radicular-type pain and bilateral weakness may suggest involvement of the cauda equina, rather than of the spinal cord.

Mark the borders of a sensory disturbance with a pen for comparison with future examinations.

- **Reflexes**

  Hyporeflexia is often present at the level of the spinal cord injury, with hyperreflexia below the level of injury. If the injury is acute, the only upper motor neuron sign may be a Babinski sign. Loss of the "anal wink" (contraction of the anal sphincter in response to pinprick in the perineum) indicates possible conus medullaris involvement.

- **Cranial nerves and mental status examination**

  These may be done briefly to rule out involvement of CNS structures above the spinal cord. A perisagittal mass lesion, such as a falx meningioma or a CNS lymphoma, may produce bilateral leg weakness and urinary incontinence, mimicking a thoracic cord lesion. Other mental status signs, such as personality change, lethargy, or disinhibition, may be a clue to CNS pathology. Lower brain stem signs may accompany high cervical cord injury, particularly if there is a congenital deformity of the brain or atlantoaxial joint.

Selective History and Chart Review

1. *Reassess the timing, duration, and course of the symptoms.*

   Development over minutes to hours suggests trauma or infarction. Progression over hours to days suggests an infectious etiology. An epidural abscess may be present even in the absence of fever or an elevated white blood cell count. Development of weakness or sensory loss over days to weeks suggests a neoplasm.

2. *Review the presence and character of pain.*

   Radicular pain will help localize and confirm extramedullary spinal involvement. Abrupt onset of radicular or diffuse pain, flaccid weakness, sphincter dysfunction, and a thoracic sensory level suggest spinal cord infarction. Bilateral radicular pain in an unusual distribution (e.g., L2 or L3) may indicate a cauda equina syndrome. Rectal pain may be the first sign of a conus medullaris lesion.

3. *Review the chart for history of illicit drug use* (this predisposes to epidural abscess and osteomyelitis), tuberculosis, or cancer.

4. *Check recent laboratory values* to assess for possible infection or chronic disease.

Surgical Intervention

Fractures, subluxations, and dislocations require reduction into normal alignment. Cervical traction may succeed in reducing a displacement, but it should be performed only by experienced personnel, usually under radiographic guidance. Open stabilization and fusion operations may be required for unstable, complex fractures or dislocations.

Neurosurgical decompressive laminectomy is the operation of choice for epidural abscess. Investigations should proceed without delay when an epidural abscess is suspected to avoid its progression to irreversible spinal cord injury. Patients who are paraplegic at the start of the operation rarely regain function. For pyogenic osteomyelitis, direct ventral spinal canal decompression is often necessary. A second, reconstructive operation may be required after the infection is brought under control with appropriate antibiotics. Decompressive laminectomy may also be needed for acute myelopathy or cauda equina syndrome resulting from disk herniation in the lumbar region. An anterior approach may be necessary to remove a herniated cervical disk. Finally, in the rare case of epidural or subdural hematoma, decompressive laminectomy is again the treatment of choice.

For **neoplastic spinal cord compression,** a combination of high-dose steroids and radiation should be administered. Surgical decompression is generally reserved for spinal instability, progressive neurologic deterioration from bony collapse, intractable pain, and failure of conservative treatment. Once the pressure has been relieved, further treatment usually requires tissue biopsy. If the surgeons have performed a decompression procedure, open biopsy may be possible. An alternative procedure is CT-guided needle biopsy.

Delirium and Amnesia

The term *delirium* is synonymous with the term *acute confusional state*. Delirium is common in hospitalized patients, particularly in the elderly, and refers to an acute, global disorder of thinking and perception, characterized by impaired consciousness and inattention. Restlessness, agitation, and combativeness may be seen, as well as bizarre behavior and delusions. A call to evaluate delirium may therefore be one for "agitation" or "confusion." Delirium may be distinguished from dementia by the fact that with dementia alone, the sensorium remains clear, despite the occurrence of confusion and disorientation. Furthermore, it should be emphasized that although delirium is often defined as a transient condition, it may take days to weeks to clear, and if delirium is left untreated, the mortality rate may be as high as 25% in elderly inpatients. As with other mental status alterations discussed in this book, delirium is a symptom, not a disease. Successful management depends on accurate diagnosis of the underlying condition.

Amnesia is defined as a pure loss of memory without other cognitive dysfunction. Although memory is affected by delirium, amnesia may occur in isolation, with a clear sensorium. **Retrograde amnesia** refers to loss of memory for events before a specific point in time. **Anterograde amnesia** is the inability to lay down new memory. Memory is often categorized into **immediate recall** (seconds), **short-term memory** (minutes to hours), and **long-term memory** (days to years), with short-term memory being the most vulnerable to pathologic processes, both in acute amnestic states and in dementia syndromes. The hippocampi and parahippocampal structures, and dorsomedial thalamus along with the dorsolateral prefrontal cortex, have been implicated in short-term memory function. Verbal memory is mediated predominantly by the left hemisphere, and visuospatial memory is mediated by the right hemisphere. Most of this chapter will focus on diagnosis and management of acute confusional state. Two acute amnestic disorders will be discussed in brief here. Dementia as a disorder of memory along with broader cognitive decline will be discussed in depth is Chapter 27.

PHONE CALL

Questions

1. **Is the patient fully awake and alert? In what way is the patient confused? When did the change occur?**
   Clarify the acuteness and nature of the mental status change. It is important to distinguish between acute and chronic changes and also to distinguish delirium from dementia (see Chapter 27) and stupor (see Chapter 5).
2. **What are the vital signs?**
   Fever suggests infection; tachypnea may suggest hypoxia, metabolic acidosis, or hyperglycemia (Kussmaul's respiration); and irregular heart rhythm may suggest cardioembolic stroke.
3. **Was there any head injury?**
4. **What is the patient's underlying medical condition?**
   Diseases that are likely to cause metabolic disarray, such as renal or liver disease, endocrinopathies, diarrheal illnesses, or malignancy, may alter electrolytes. HIV infection or AIDS opens a wider array of differential diagnoses.
5. **Is the patient diabetic?**
   Both hypoglycemia and hyperglycemia can cause altered mental status.
6. **Is the patient known to be a user of alcohol, nicotine, or other nonprescription drugs?**

Orders

1. Order a finger stick glucose level.
2. If the patient is tachypneic or drowsy, obtain arterial blood gas measurements. A pulse oximeter may be useful for monitoring oxygen saturation.
3. Provide orientation and reassurance to the patient. Make sure the room is well lit. The treatment of the behavioral and emotional manifestations of delirium, to the extent possible, will make the subsequent etiologic evaluation easier.
4. Restrain the patient with a Posey chest restraint if necessary. Significant agitation or combativeness may put the patient or those nearby at risk for physical injury.
5. If possible, do not medicate. Perform the evaluation first. If sedation is given before a good neurologic examination can be obtained, the opportunity for making a diagnosis may be lost.

Inform RN

"Will arrive at the bedside in . . . minutes."

ELEVATOR THOUGHTS

What are the causes of delirium?

V (vascular): stroke (infarct or hemorrhage causing a sensory aphasia), subarachnoid hemorrhage, hypertensive encephalopathy, cholesterol emboli syndrome

I (infectious): herpes simplex encephalitis or other viral encephalitis; bacterial, fungal, or rickettsial meningoencephalitis; neurosyphilis; Lyme disease; parasitic abscess (e.g., toxoplasmosis, cysticercosis), bacterial abscess; HIV encephalitis; systemic infection such as urosepsis or pneumonia

T (traumatic): open or closed head trauma, acute or chronic subdural hematoma

A (autoimmune): systemic lupus erythematosus (SLE), multiple sclerosis

M (metabolic/toxic): hypoglycemia or hyperglycemia, hyponatremia, hypercalcemia, hepatic encephalopathy, uremia, porphyria; drug or alcohol ingestion or withdrawal

I (iatrogenic): drug toxicity (particularly in the elderly)—psychotropic drugs, steroids, digoxin, cimetidine, anticonvulsants, anticholinergics, dopaminergics (see Table 8–1 for common medications with CNS side effects; Table 8–2 lists medications associated with memory impairment), rare-heavy metal poisoning, pellagra, vitamin B_{12} or folate deficiency, Wilson's disease

N (neoplastic): primary brain tumor, metastatic brain disease, paraneoplastic syndrome (limbic encephalitis with small-cell lung cancer)

S (seizure): postictal state, nonconvulsive status epilepticus (rare)

Other (psychiatric): bipolar disorder/mania, psychosis

MAJOR THREAT TO LIFE

- **Expanding mass lesion with impending herniation**

  Although it is rare for a mass lesion to progress to impending herniation without focal neurologic signs, the first changes may be confusion or altered state of consciousness. Progression can be rapid if there is an expanding subdural hematoma or edema from subarachnoid hemorrhage.

- **Bacterial meningitis or encephalitis**

  Bacterial meningitis is a major treatable illness that can be fatal if missed. Other meningitides are likely to be less fulminant yet can also be fatal if left untreated. Herpes simplex encephalitis is the most common sporadic encephalitis. Aside from direct brain damage from infection, encephalitides can produce edema and subsequent herniation.

TABLE 8–1 **Common Medications That Can Cause Delirium**

Dextromethorphan hydrobromide promethazine (Phenergan)
Anticholinergics
   Trihexyphenidyl HCl (Artane)
   Benztropine mesylate (Cogentin)
Anticonvulsants
   Phenytoin (Dilantin)
   Phenobarbital
   Valproic acid (Depakene/Depakote)
Antihistamines
   Diphenhydramine (Benadryl)
   Dextromethorphan hydrobromide promethazine (Phenergan)
   Cimetidine (Tagamet)
Benzodiazepines
   Diazepam (Valium)
   Temazepam (Restoril)
   Triazolam (Halcion)
Corticosteroids
   Prednisone
   Dexamethasone (Decadron)
Dopaminergic drugs
   L-dopa (Sinemet)
   Pergolide (Permax)
   Bromocriptine (Parlodel)
Digoxin
Disulfiram
Indomethacin
Lithium
Opiates

TABLE 8–2 **Medications That May Be Associated with Memory Impairment**

Benzodiazepines
Anticonvulsants (overdose)
Corticosteroids
Isoniazid
Benzodiazepines
Barbiturates
Bromides
Chlorpromazine
Interleukins
Methotrexate
Clioquinol (antifungal)

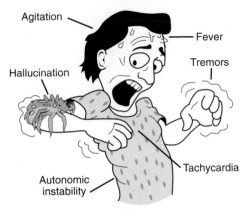

Figure 8–1 Delirium tremens.

- **Delirium tremens**

  Usually occurring more than 48 hours after cessation of alcohol consumption, the autonomic instability of delirium tremens may produce high fevers, tachycardia, and severe fluctuations in blood pressure (Fig. 8–1). The mortality rate is approximately 15%.

BEDSIDE

Quick Look Test

Does the patient look ill or well?

Is the patient in respiratory distress?

What are the vital signs?

If there is a fever, meningitis must be ruled out. An irregular heart rhythm may suggest atrial fibrillation. Markedly elevated blood pressure, particularly diastolic blood pressure greater than 120 mm Hg, may produce hypertensive encephalopathy, which is characterized by headache, confusion, and irritability, with lethargy developing over hours to days.

Selective Physical Examination I

General Physical Examination

Breath	The odor of alcohol or fetor hepaticus may suggest the etiology.
HEENT	Look for external signs of head trauma—scalp lacerations or bruises, Battle's sign, raccoon eyes, papilledema.

Neck	Nuchal rigidity, Kernig's sign, Brudzinski's sign
Cardiopulmonary	Tachypnea can indicate hypoxia or metabolic acidosis. Rales or decreased breath sounds may help diagnose a pneumonia. Listen for irregular heart rhythm and for murmurs to suggest valvular heart disease.
Abdomen	Percuss the liver. Hepatomegaly may be the physical manifestation of hepatic encephalopathy or may direct your management to consideration of alcohol withdrawal. Look for ascites.
Extremities	Look for clubbing as a sign of chronic pulmonary disease, peripheral edema as a sign of cardiac or renal failure, and splinter hemorrhages as a sign of emboli. **Asterixis** is a sign of metabolic disarray, for example, from renal or hepatic failure.

Neurologic Examination

- **Mental status**
  1. Assess the patient's **alertness:** Is the patient fully awake and alert? Assess the patient's **attentiveness.** Does the patient maintain eye contact? Does he or she glance about the room as if having hallucinations? One simple test of sustained attention is to ask the patient to recite the days of the week backward or to count backward from 20 to 1.
  2. Listen for **paraphasias** in spontaneous speech to suggest a sensory aphasia. Test **comprehension.** Ask the patient to follow progressively complex commands (e.g., "Show two fingers," "Point to the ceiling and then to the floor," and "Tap each shoulder twice with your eyes closed").
  3. Assess **thought content.** Tangential or pressured speech, delusions, flight of ideas, hallucinations, perceptual illusions, and disorientation may be seen with psychiatric disease or acute encephalopathies.
- **Cranial nerves**
  1. **Pupils:** Pinpoint pupils may result from opiate overdose. Widely dilated pupils could be a sign of cholinergic overdose (e.g., organophosphate poisoning). Asymmetric pupils can indicate uncal herniation from intracranial mass effect. Argyll Robertson pupils are seen with CNS syphilis (periaqueductal midbrain lesion [see Chapter 21]).

2. **Facial asymmetry** in the form of a flattened nasolabial fold or a wider palpebral fissure may be a subtle sign of an intra-parenchymal mass or stroke.
3. Assess swallowing capacity and gag reflex.

- **Motor**

  Depending on how cooperative your patient is, you may be able to test strength by confrontation. In an inattentive patient, observe limb movements for asymmetry. Lateralizing weakness suggests an intracranial lesion. Tremor may indicate alcohol withdrawal or intoxication.

- **Sensory**

  A detailed sensory examination requires sustained coopera-tion that an inattentive patient often cannot give. Response to a brief noxious stimulus (e.g., a pinch or pulling hair on the arm) is a quick way to assess gross sensory function. If the limb is paretic, the response may be a facial grimace.

- **Gait**

  Ataxia may suggest intoxication.

- **Reflexes**

  Babinski's response or reflex asymmetry suggests lateralized intracranial pathology.

Selective History and Chart Review

1. **Review medications**

   Have any new medications been started recently? Particu-larly in the elderly, drug toxicity is a common cause of change in mental status. See table 8–1 lists common medications that can cause delirium.

2. **Review medical or psychiatric history**

   Known metabolic disorders such as renal or hepatic disease or past episodes of psychosis would be crucial to make a diagnosis.

MANAGEMENT I: CONTROL OF DELIRIUM

1. **Treatment of agitation**

   Treatment of delirium depends on the correct identification of the underlying condition. If agitation or combativeness is likely to interfere with the investigation or if there is physical threat to the patient or to the staff, the best medications to use are butyrophenones (e.g., haloperidol [Haldol]), benzisoxa-zoles (e.g., risperidone), group 3 phenothiazines (e.g., trifluo-perazine), or benzodiazepines. See Table 8–3 for drugs used to control agitation and delirium. **Haldol 2 to 10 mg intra-muscularly (IM)** may be expected to reach peak serum levels in 20 to 40 minutes. Repeating the dose up to 20 mg may be necessary in severe cases. For mild agitation or in the elderly,

TABLE 8–3 **Drugs used in the Treatment of Acute Agitation and Delirium**

Antipsychotics	Starting Dose
Haloperidol (Haldol)	1-2 mg Q 6H PO/IV
Olanzepine (Zyprexa)	5-10 mg QD BID PO/IM
Quetiapine (Seraqual)	25-50 mg PO
Trifluoperazine (Stelazine)	2-5 mg PO/IM PO/IV
Benzodiazepines	
Lorazepam (Ativan)	0.5-2.0 mg IV/IM/PO
Midazolam (Versed)	1-2 mg IV/PO
Diazepam (Valium)	5-10 mg IV/PO

an initial dose of 1 to 2 mg may be sufficient. For moderate agitation, use 4 mg initially. For violent, combative patients, 6 to 10 mg can be used as an initial dose. If an acute dystonic reaction occurs with Haldol, **diphenhydramine 25 to 50 mg IM** may be given, even though the anticholinergic effect may worsen the delirium. Haloperidol should be avoided in alcohol withdrawal, benzodiazepine withdrawal, and hepatic encephalopathy. For acute agitation in these settings, a benzodiazepine such as **lorazepam 1 to 2 mg IM** may be given. (Higher doses may be required if tolerance has developed in the setting of chronic alcohol or benzodiazepine abuse.) **Naloxone (Narcan) 1 to 2 ampoules, given IV, IM, or SC every 5 minutes,** should be reserved for the lethargy of suspected opiate intoxication.

2. **The following blood tests should be ordered immediately:**
   - CBC with differential
   - Electrolyte panel, including stat glucose
   - Full chemistry panel, including liver function tests
   - Urine toxicology screen (if drug intoxication is suspected)
   - Urine and blood cultures (if fever is present)
   - Arterial blood gases
   - Calcium, phosphate
   - Erythrocyte sedimentation rate may be measured, but its specificity is low

3. **A chest x-ray should be obtained if fever or dyspnea is present.**

MANAGEMENT II: TREATMENT OF LIFE-THREATENING DISORDERS

1. **Bacterial meningitis**

   Delirium with fever should be treated as bacterial meningitis until proved otherwise. As a rule, a head CT scan should be ordered before a lumbar puncture is performed. If there is no papilledema on examination, no coagulopathy, and no focal deficit (including gait ataxia), and a head CT is not readily available, a lumbar puncture may almost always be done without risk of herniation. (See Chapter 3 for a discussion of lumbar puncture.) CSF should be sent for cell count, protein and glucose determinations, microbial cultures (bacterial, fungal, mycobacterial), and VDRL test, and for Gram, acid-fast bacillus, and India ink stains. CSF findings in bacterial meningitis are cloudy fluid with 50 to 20,000 white blood cells, predominantly leukocytes, elevated protein level, and decreased glucose level (see Table 21–1). The causative organism may be identified and antibiotic sensitivity may be obtained in more than 80% of the cases. Empirical treatment of bacterial meningitis prior to definitive identification in adults should be **ampicillin 1 g IV every 6 hours** and a third-generation cephalosporin (e.g., **ceftriaxone 2 g IV every 12 hours**). See Chapter 21 for details.

2. **Delirium tremens**

   The autonomic instability of delirium tremens is treated supportively, with acetaminophen (Tylenol) or a cooling blanket for fevers. Continuous cardiac monitoring may be necessary if arrhythmias develop. **Valium 5 to 10 mg IV load, with subsequent doses of 2 to 5 mg IV every 30 to 60 minutes,** should be used. Sedation should be titrated to minimize agitation. Tremulousness may be used as a clinical monitor of the effectiveness of the benzodiazepine. An alternative is **chlordiazepoxide (Librium) 25 to 100 mg every 6 hours PO.** The dose should be tapered as the symptoms subside. **Thiamine 100 mg IV, IM, or PO** should be given daily for 3 days to prevent the development of Wernicke's encephalopathy.

3. **Suspected mass lesion**

   If there is papilledema or a focality on examination, an emergent head CT or MRI scan should be obtained. For mass lesions, refer to the appropriate chapter for treatment of acute stroke (Chapter 6), increased intracranial pressure (Chapter 12), or brain tumor (Chapter 22).

Selective History and Chart Review

Once it is clear that the patient does not have a mass lesion, bacterial meningitis, or delirium tremens, you have time to make a more complete assessment of the situation. If family members are available, try to sort out the acuteness of the change. A chronic or fluctuating course in an elderly person may suggest that the apparent delirium is really a component of dementia. Alzheimer's disease and vascular dementia are the most common causes (see Chapter 27). A subacute course over days, with intermittent fevers, suggests a subacute or chronic encephalomeningitis, such as herpes simplex encephalitis, tubercular meningitis, or cryptococcal meningitis.

Review the chart. What are the patient's medical conditions? What medications is he or she on? Were any medications recently added that are known to have CNS effects (see Table 8–1)? The offending agent should be stopped or substituted. Do the most recent laboratory values suggest metabolic abnormalities? Renal failure and hepatic failure are the most common sources of metabolic encephalopathy (Box 8–1). Is the patient HIV positive? Acute HIV infection may cause a meningoencephalitis. Immunocompromised patients are at risk for a variety of opportunistic infections that can cause encephalomeningitis, particularly cryptococcal and tuberculous meningitis, toxoplasmosis, and CNS syphilis. Malignancy, most notably small-cell lung carcinoma, can cause a paraneoplastic limbic encephalitis, in addition to altering electrolytes with syndrome of inappropriate antidiuretic hormone (SIADH).

BOX 8–1 **Hepatic Encephalopathy**

Hepatic encephalopathy usually appears in a patient with liver function already compromised from alcoholic cirrhosis, chronic hepatitis, or malignancy. An increased protein load, such as from a gastrointestinal bleed, causes ammonia to accumulate in the brain. Whether the high level of ammonia itself or the increase in concentration of its metabolites produces the alterations in consciousness is not known. Examination may reveal abdominal ascites, an enlarged (or shrunken) liver, and asterixis, in addition to changes in mental status, namely inattention, disorientation, and confusion. In the later stages, focal signs such as hemiparesis or dysconjugate gaze may appear. Management is directed at reducing the protein load with dietary protein restrictions and **neomycin 2 to 4 g per day PO,** or **Rifaxamin 200 mg BID,** which reduces the population of ammonia-producing bacteria in the bowel. **Lactulose 15 to 45 ml two to four times per day** to induce diarrhea may also help reduce intestinal bacteria. Ammonia levels should be followed as an indication of the effectiveness of therapy. If acute agitation requires treatment, use benzodiazepines such as **diazepam 5 to 10 mg every 8 hours. Haloperidol should be avoided.** When hepatic encephalopathy is suspected, be sure to obtain a stool guaiac test and a hematocrit.

MANAGEMENT III: TREATMENT OF OTHER DISORDERS

1. **Hypoglycemia and hyperglycemia**

   Hypoglycemia may be rapidly corrected with a bolus of **50 ml D50W IV by direct injection.** Do not forget that **thiamine (100 mg PO or IM)** must be given first to prevent possible induction of Wernicke's encephalopathy. Maintenance with D5W may be necessary if the hypoglycemia is prolonged. Hyperglycemia (diabetic ketoacidosis) requires administration of insulin, repletion of intravascular volume, and often, management of acidosis and potassium. The level of monitoring required is best handled in an intensive care unit (ICU).

2. **Hyponatremia and hypernatremia**

   Management of hyponatremia and hypernatremia usually involves treating the underlying cause (e.g., renal disease, vomiting and diarrhea, hypothalamic or adrenal dysfunction, or SIADH from malignancy or medications). Treatment with IV fluids and electrolytes differs depending on volume status (see Table 21–3). Too rapid a correction of hyponatremia may precipitate central pontine myelinolysis, an acute demyelinating syndrome occurring mostly in patients with poor nutritional status, causing quadriplegia, dysarthria, and pseudobulbar palsy.

3. **Hypocalcemia**

   Severe hypocalcemia (<7.0 mg/dl) may be treated with **10 to 20 ml (1 to 2 g) of 10% calcium gluconate IV in 100 ml D5W over 30 minutes.** If the patient is hyperphosphatemic, correction with glucose and insulin is required before giving calcium IV. Patients on digoxin should have continuous cardiac monitoring, as calcium potentiates digoxin's action.

4. **Uremia with renal failure**

   Symptomatic uremia with renal failure causing delirium may necessitate urgent hemodialysis.

5. **Sepsis**

   Delirium caused by sepsis should clear spontaneously with appropriate treatment of the infection.

6. **Psychiatric causes**

   Psychiatric causes of delirium may generally be treated acutely with **haloperidol 1 to 5 mg PO or IM.** Psychiatric consultation should be obtained for definitive treatment.

7. **Seizures**

   Delirium from a **postictal state** should clear progressively over minutes to hours. An EEG should be ordered within the next few days. **Nonconvulsive status epilepticus** is a neurologic emergency that requires EEG for definitive diagnosis. (See Chapter 4 for further discussion of seizure management.)

8. **Nicotine withdrawal**

In rare instances, delirium can occur in heavy smokers due to nicotine withdrawal. Application of a **transdermal 21-mg nicotine patch** can result in dramatic improvement in some cases.

Other Amnestic Disorders

Transient Global Amnesia (TGA)

Patients with TGA are middle-aged or older, often with hypertension, prior ischemic episodes, or atherosclerotic heart disease, but are otherwise healthy. Typically, they are brought in by a relative or friend because they are "confused." On examination, there are no focal neurologic deficits. Cognitive function and language are intact, except for a profound anterograde amnesia and a retrograde amnesia for the preceding several hours or days. Patients typically appear agitated and will repeat the same question over and over, such as "What am I doing here?" The anterograde amnesia clears gradually after minutes to hours and usually resolves completely within 24 to 48 hours. A residual retrograde amnesia for the hours immediately surrounding the event is often permanent. TGA often appears in the setting of an emotional or physical stress. The pathophysiology is unknown; both epileptic mechanisms and vascular mechanisms have been proposed but have not been proved. The differential diagnosis includes unwitnessed head trauma or seizure, drug intoxication, stroke, dissociative states, and Wernicke-Korsakoff syndrome. The EEG is usually negative, but a positive EEG allows treatment with anticonvulsants to be given. MRI should be obtained to evaluate for a seizure-producing lesion. The condition is self-limiting and there is no specific treatment, although some physicians have advocated using **aspirin 325 mg per day** for secondary prophylaxis. Recurrence occurs in less than one fourth of the patients.

Wernicke-Korsakoff Syndrome

Wernicke-Korsakoff syndrome is a nutritional thiamine deficiency occurring in chronic alcoholics. The acute component (Wernicke's encephalopathy) is characterized by inattentiveness, lethargy, truncal ataxia, and ocular dysmotility (nystagmus—horizontal with or without a vertical or rotary component; and gaze palsy—horizontal or lateral rectus palsy, progressing to complete external ophthalmoplegia). Other signs of nutritional deficiency may be present, such as skin changes or redness of the tongue. If left untreated, the condition is fatal in 10% of patients. Treatment is **thiamine 100 mg IV, IM, or PO daily for 3 days**, along with magnesium and multivitamins. Although the ataxia, inattentiveness, and ocular dysmotility may resolve, the more purely amnestic Korsakoff's syndrome persists in greater than 80% of patients. Korsakoff's syndrome is characterized by moderate to severe anterograde amnesia and patchy long-term memory loss. Unlike patients with TGA, patients with Korsakoff's syndrome are not distressed by their amnesia. Confabulation is often present. Even with good nutrition, the amnesia of Korsakoff's syndrome rarely resolves. Histopathologic examination shows cell loss and degenerative changes in the dorsomedial thalami, the mamillary bodies, the periaqueductal midbrain, and the Purkinje cell layer of the cerebellar vermis.

Head Injury

The initial assessment of head injury in the ER can be frantic, with resuscitation measures, history taking, and examination occurring simultaneously. An organized approach is essential to ensure that vital components of the evaluation are not omitted. **The immediate goal is to judge the severity of the injury as minimal, moderate, or high.** This aspect of the injury can be quickly assessed at the time of arrival.

PHONE CALL

Questions

1. **What are the vital signs?**

    If the patient is in respiratory distress, the spine should be immobilized (this should have been done already) and endotracheal intubation should be performed.

2. **What were the circumstances and the mode of injury?**

    The force and location of head impact should be determined as precisely as possible.

3. **Did the patient experience loss of consciousness?**

    Concussion refers to temporary loss of consciousness that occurs at the time of impact. Because patients are amnestic following concussion, only an eyewitness can accurately gauge the duration of loss of consciousness.

4. **Has the patient's neurologic status deteriorated since the time of impact?**

    Progressive decline in level of consciousness after an injury suggests an expanding *subdural or epidural hematoma.*

5. **What is the patient's level of consciousness now?**

    This should be assessed using the Glasgow Coma Scale (see Table 5–2).

6. **Has the patient recently ingested drugs or alcohol?**

    Intoxication can confound assessments of mental status and may lead to withdrawal symptoms.

7. **Is there significant extracranial trauma?**

    The patient should be quickly examined for external signs of trauma to the neck, chest, abdomen, and limbs.

117

Determination of the Severity of Injury

At this juncture, you should have enough information to classify the injury severity as **minimal, moderate,** or **high.** Subsequent diagnostic testing and management should proceed according to the algorithm in Figure 9–1.

1. **Minimal-risk group**
   - Glasgow Coma Scale score of 15 (alert, attentive, and oriented) and normal neurologic findings on examination
   - No concussion, or concussion in the absence of moderate-risk group criteria
2. **Moderate-risk group**
   - Glasgow Coma Scale score of 9 to 14 (confused, lethargic, or stuporous) or minor focal neurologic deficit (i.e., nystagmus, facial droop)
   - Concussion if age >60 years, headache, or minor external signs of trauma are present
   - Posttraumatic amnesia
   - Vomiting
   - Seizure
   - Major external trauma (Battle's sign, raccoon eyes, etc.)
3. **High-risk group**
   - Glasgow Coma Scale score of 3 to 8 (Table 5–2)
   - Progressive decline in level of consciousness
   - Major focal neurologic deficit (i.e., hemiparesis, aphasia)
   - Penetrating skull injury or palpably depressed skull fracture

Orders

1. **For *all patients*, order cervical spine radiographs (anteroposterior, lateral, and odontoid views).**

   All patients with traumatic injury above the level of the clavicles should have cervical spine films to rule out a fracture. Before a cervical collar can be removed, the cervical spine must be cleared completely from C1 to C7.
2. **For all patients with *moderate or severe injury*, give the following orders:**
   a. **Start an IV line with normal (0.9%) saline or lactated Ringer's solution.**

      Isotonic fluids replace intravascular volume more effectively than do hypotonic fluids, and they do not aggravate cerebral edema.
   b. **Order diagnostic blood tests.**
      (1) Hemoglobin and hematocrit
      (2) CBC and platelet count
      (3) Serum chemistries (glucose, electrolytes, blood urea nitrogen, creatinine)
      (4) PT/PTT

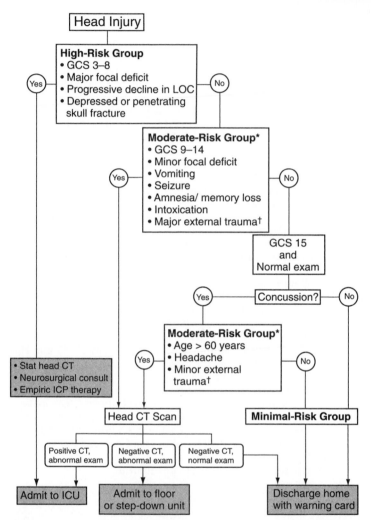

Figure 9–1 Emergency room diagnostic and treatment algorithm for head injury. (Refer to text for details.) CT, computed tomography; GCS, Glasgow Coma Scale score; ICP, intracranial pressure; ICU, intensive care unit; LOC, level of consciousness.
*One or more criteria may be present; †above the level of the clavicles.

    (5) Toxicology screen and serum alcohol level
    (6) Type and hold
  c. **Obtain a head CT scan with bone windows.**
      Skull radiographs are not necessary if a head CT scan is performed, because CT is more sensitive for detecting fractures. Intracranial hemorrhage will be detected in approximately 90% to 100% of high-risk patients, 5% to 10% of moderate-risk patients, and 0% of minimal-risk patients. CT scans should be assessed for the following (Fig. 9–2):
    (1) Epidural and subdural hematoma
    (2) Subarachnoid and intraventricular blood
    (3) Parenchymal contusions and hemorrhages
    (4) Cerebral edema
    (5) Effacement of perimesencephalic cisterns
    (6) Midline shift
    (7) Skull fractures, sinus opacification (air-fluid levels), and pneumocephalus
3. **For** *comatose patients* **(Glasgow Coma Scale score ≤ 8) or in patients with signs of herniation, give the following orders:**
  a. **Elevate head of the bed 30 degrees.**
  b. **Hyperventilate the patient.**
      Intubate the patient. Use intermittent mandatory ventilation (IMV) at a rate of 16 to 20 cycles per minute with tidal volumes set at 10 to 15 ml/kg. Adjust settings to attain a PCO_2 of 28 to 32 mm Hg. Severe hypocapnia (<25 mm Hg) may lead to excessive vasoconstriction and cerebral ischemia and should be avoided.
  c. **Administer mannitol 20% 1.0 to 1.5 g/kg IV.**
      Mannitol should be given "wide open." The patient should be reexamined 30 minutes after mannitol is given to assess for signs of improvement. Additional doses should be guided by an ICP monitor (see Chapter 12).
  d. **Insert a Foley catheter.**
  e. **Obtain a neurosurgical consultation.**

ELEVATOR THOUGHTS

What are the most important sequelae of traumatic head injury?
1. **Concussion**
    Concussion refers to temporary loss of consciousness that occurs at the time of impact. It is usually associated with a short period of amnesia. The majority of patients with concussion have normal CT or MRI scans, reflecting the fact that concussion results from physiologic (rather than structural) injury to the brain. *Approximately 5% of patients who have sustained concussion will have an intracranial hemorrhage.*

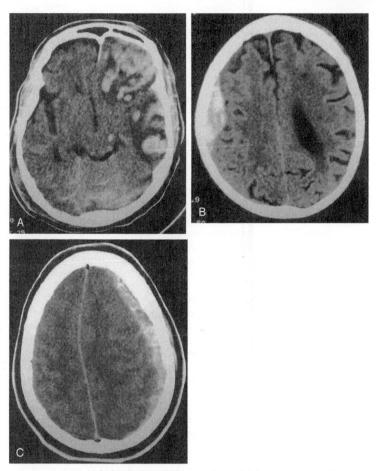

Figure 9–2 *A*, Left frontal and temporal cerebral contusions with surrounding edema. *B*, Small right parietal epidural hematoma *(convex shape)*. *C*, Thin left subdural hematoma *(crescentic, convex shape)*. (Images courtesy of Dr. Robert De La Paz.)

2. **Epidural hematoma**

Epidural bleeding usually results from a tear in the middle meningeal artery. Approximately 75% of such cases are associated with a skull fracture. The classic clinical course (seen in only one third of patients) proceeds from immediate loss of consciousness (concussion) to a lucid interval, which is followed by a secondary depression of consciousness as the epidural hematoma expands. Epidural blood takes on a bulging convex pattern on the CT scan (see Fig. 9–2) because the collection is limited by firm attachments of the dura to the cranial sutures. Progression to herniation and death can occur rapidly because the bleeding is from an artery.

3. **Subdural hematoma**

Subdural bleeding usually arises from a venous source, with blood filling the potential space between the dural and arachnoid membranes. CT usually reveals a crescentic collection of blood across the entire hemispheric convexity (see Fig. 9–2). *Elderly and alcoholic patients are particularly prone to subdural bleeding;* in these patients, large hematomas can result from trivial impact or from acceleration/deceleration injuries (e.g., whiplash injury).

4. **Parenchymal contusion and hematoma**

Cerebral contusions result from "scraping" and "bruising" of the brain as it moves across the inner surface of the skull. The inferior frontal and temporal lobes are the common sites of traumatic contusion (see Fig. 9–2). With lateral forces, contusions can occur just deep to the site of impact (coup lesions) or at the opposite pole as the brain impacts on the inner table of the skull (contrecoup lesions). Contusions frequently evolve into larger lesions over 12 to 24 hours, and in rare instances, contusions can develop de novo 1 or more days after injury ("spät hematoma").

5. **Axonal shearing injury**

Persistent coma occurs frequently in patients with severe head injury with normal CT scans and normal ICP. In these cases, coma results from widespread stretching, shearing, and disruption of axons as a result of rotational forces. Bilateral motor posturing, hyper-reflexia, and dysautonomia are common and result from injury to the corticospinal tracts and autonomic centers in the brain stem. MRI scans show characteristic "shearing lesions" in the dorsolateral midbrain, posterior corpus callosum, and centrum semiovale (Fig. 9–3). Diffuse axonal injury is thought to be the single most important cause of persistent disability in patients with traumatic brain damage.

6. **Skull fracture**

Skull fractures are important markers of potentially serious intracranial injury, but they rarely cause symptoms them-

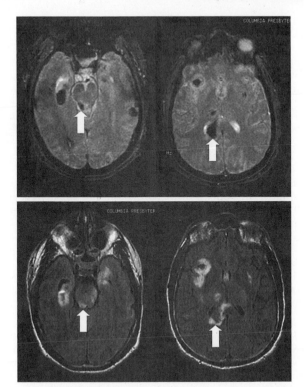

Figure 9–3 Gradient echo (top) and FLAIR (bottom) MR images showing hemorrhagic lesions characteristic of axonal shearing injury involving the right dorsolateral midbrain (right) and right posterior splenium (left). Small contusions of the temporal lobes are also present. (Reproduced with permission from: Mayer SA: Head Injury. In: Rowland LP (ed): *Merritt's Textbook of Neurology*, 11th ed. Baltimore: Lippincott, Williams, and Wilkins, 2005:483-5.)

selves. If the scalp is lacerated over the fracture, it is considered an open, or compound, fracture. *Linear fractures* account for 80% of all skull fractures and can usually be managed conservatively. *Basilar skull fractures* occur with more serious trauma and are frequently missed on routine skull x-ray films. These fractures may be associated with cranial nerve injury or CSF leakage from the nose or ear. *Comminuted and depressed fractures* are often associated with contusions of the underlying brain and usually require surgical debridement.

MAJOR THREAT TO LIFE

- Epidural hematoma
- Subdural hematoma
- Increased ICP

BEDSIDE

Quick Look Test

What is the level of consciousness?

Almost all patients with potentially life-threatening lesions will have depressed level of consciousness (lethargy, stupor, or coma).

Airway and Vital Signs

Is the airway protected? What is the respiratory rate?

Indications for intubation include depressed level of consciousness with inability to protect the airway, respiratory distress (rapid, shallow breathing), or respiratory depression.

What is the heart rate and blood pressure?

If the patient is *hypotensive*, bleeding into the abdomen, thorax, retroperitoneal space, or tissues surrounding a long-bone fracture should be excluded. *Spinal shock* can occur with cord injury and results from acute loss of sympathetic outflow. *Hypertension* associated with a wide pulse pressure and bradycardia (Cushing's reflex) may reflect increased ICP.

Selective Physical Examination

General Physical Examination

Head	The skull should be palpated for fractures, hematomas, and lacerations. *Battle's sign* (ecchymosis over the mastoid process) and *raccoon sign* (periorbital ecchymosis) suggest, but do not confirm, basilar skull fracture.
Ear, nose, and throat	*CSF otorrhea* and *CSF rhinorrhea* result from skull fracture with disruption of the dura. CSF can be differentiated from mucus by its high glucose content on dipstick testing; bloody CSF can be differentiated from frank blood by a positive *halo test* (a "halo" of CSF forms around the blood when CSF is dropped on a cloth sheet). *Hemotympanum* is also

highly suggestive of skull fracture. *Tongue biting* suggests an unwitnessed seizure.

Neck   Do not manipulate the neck until a cervical fracture has been ruled out.

Chest, abdomen, back, pelvis, and extremities   It is essential to rule out important coexisting injuries in patients with head injury. The patient should be thoroughly examined, and x-rays, diagnostic peritoneal lavage, and other interventions should be performed prior to CT scanning as clinically indicated.

Neurologic Examination

Rapid neurologic examination of the patient with head injury should focus on the following:

- **Mental status**
  1. **Level of consciousness**

     Level of consciousness is best documented by using the Glasgow Coma Scale (Table 5–2) and by describing specific stimuli and responses (e.g., "answers with brief confused responses to repeated questioning" or "moans and vocalizes in response to sternal rub").
  2. **Attention and concentration**

     Ask the patient to count from 20 to 1 or recite the months in reverse.
  3. **Orientation**

     Check for orientation to time, place, and situation.
  4. **Memory**

     Document *retrograde amnesia* by asking the patient to recall the last thing he or she remembers prior to the injury. Check for *anterograde amnesia* by asking about the first thing remembered after the injury. Check recall for three objects at 5 minutes.
- **Cranial nerves**
  1. **Pupils**
  2. **Extraocular movements**

     Nystagmus may be found in alert patients with dizziness or vertigo following concussion. An *exodeviated eye with a large pupil* suggests CN 3 compression from uncal herniation.
  3. **Facial nerve**

     The facial nerve is the most commonly injured cranial nerve in patients with closed head injury.
- **Motor**
  1. **Spontaneous movements**

     Preferential movement of the limbs on one side indicates paresis of the unused limbs. If the patient is unresponsive, check for a lateralized localizing response to sternal rub.

2. **Limb tone**

Increased tone may reflect an early stage of decortication (flexor posturing) or decerebration (extensor posturing).

3. **Arm (pronator) drift**

If the patient is unable to follow commands, passively elevate both arms and check to see whether one falls preferentially.

4. **Power**

Check strength against active resistance at the shoulders, wrists, hips, and ankles.

- **Reflexes**
- **Gait**

1. **Normal gait**

2. **Tandem (heel-to-toe) gait**

It is particularly important to check gait in patients with "mild injury" who are treated and released without a CT scan.

MANAGEMENT

Minimal-Risk Group

Patients in this group (see Fig. 9–1) can generally be discharged from the ER **without a head CT scan** as long as the following criteria are met:

- Neurologic examination (especially mental status and gait) is normal.
- Cervical spine radiograph is cleared.
- A responsible person is available to observe the patient over 24 hours, with instructions to return the patient to the ER if late symptoms (listed on a head injury warning card) develop.

Moderate-Risk Group

In patients who have suffered concussion, normal findings on neurologic examination and CT scan eliminate the need for hospital admission. These patients can be discharged home for observation, even in the presence of headache, nausea, vomiting, dizziness, or amnesia, because the risk of development of a significant intracranial lesion thereafter is minimal. Criteria for hospital admission after head injury are shown in Box 9–1.

Severe Head Injury

Following initial assessment and stabilization, the immediate consideration in the patient with severe head injury is whether there is an indication for emergent neurosurgical intervention. If the decision is made to operate, surgery should proceed immediately, because delays can only increase the likelihood of further brain damage during the waiting period.

> BOX 9–1 **Criteria for Hospital Admission Following Head Injury**
>
> • Intracranial blood or fracture identified on head CT scan
> • Confusion, agitation, or depressed level of consciousness
> • Focal neurologic signs or symptoms
> • Alcohol or drug intoxication
> • Significant comorbid medical illness
> • Lack of a reliable environment for subsequent observation

The medical management of patients with severe injury should be carried out in an ICU. Although little can be done about brain damage that occurs on impact, ICU care can play a major role in reducing secondary brain injury from hypoxia, hypotension, or increased ICP.

Checklist for Management of Severe Head Injury in the ICU

1. **Reassess airway and ventilation**

   In general, patients in stupor or coma (those unable to follow commands because of a depressed level of consciousness) should be intubated for airway protection. If there is no evidence of increased ICP, ventilatory parameters should be set to maintain PCO_2 at 40 mm Hg and PO_2 at 90 to 100 mm Hg.

2. **Monitor BP**

   If the patient shows signs of hemodynamic instability (hypo- or hypertension), monitoring is best accomplished with an arterial catheter. Because autoregulation is frequently impaired with acute head injury, mean BP must be carefully maintained to avoid hypotension (mean BP <90 mm Hg), which can lead to cerebral ischemia, or hypertension (mean BP >130 mm Hg), which can exacerbate cerebral edema.

3. **Consult neurosurgery to insert an ICP monitor in patients with a Glasgow Coma Scale score of 8 or less**

   Because severe ICP elevations (Lundberg A waves or plateau waves) occur suddenly and without warning, a monitor should be inserted even if the patient does not currently show signs of increased ICP. Ventricular catheters are advisable if significant intraventricular hemorrhage with hydrocephalus is present. Otherwise, a parenchymal or epidural monitor should be used, because the associated risk of infection is significantly lower (see Chapter 12).

4. **Fluid management**

   Only isotonic fluids (normal saline or lactated Ringer's solution) should be administered to patients with head injury, because the extra free water in half-normal saline or D5W can exacerbate cerebral edema.

5. **Nutrition**

   Severe head injury leads to a generalized hypermetabolic and catabolic response, with caloric requirements that are 50% to 100% higher than normal. Enteral feedings via a nasogastric or a nasoduodenal tube should be instituted as soon as possible (usually by hospital day 2).

6. **Temperature management**

   Fever (temperature >101° F) exacerbates cerebral injury and should be aggressively treated with acetaminophen or cooling blankets.

7. **Anticonvulsants**

   Phenytoin or **fosphenytoin (15 to 20 mg/kg IV loading dose, then 300 mg/day IV)** reduces the frequency of early (i.e., first week) post-traumatic seizures from 14% to 4% in patients with intracranial hemorrhage but does not prevent later seizures. If the patient has not experienced a seizure, phenytoin should be discontinued after 7 to 10 days. Levels should be monitored closely, because subtherapeutic levels frequently result from hypermetabolism of phenytoin.

8. **Steroids**

   Steroids have NOT been shown to favorably alter outcome in patients with head injury and may lead to increased risk of infection, hyperglycemia, and other complications. Large doses of steroids actually increase the risk of death from these complications. For this reason, *steroids such as dexamethasone have no role in the treatment of traumatic brain injury.*

9. **Prophylaxis for DVT**

   Pneumatic compression boots are routinely used in immobilized patients to protect against lower-extremity DVT and the associated risk of pulmonary thromboembolism. **Heparin 5000 U SC every 12 hours or enoxaparin 40 mg SC once a day** should be started 48 hours after injury even in the presence of intracranial hemorrhage.

10. **Prophylaxis for gastric ulcer**

    Patients on mechanical ventilation or with coagulopathy are at increased risk of gastric stress ulceration and should receive **pantoprazole 40 mg IV once daily** or **sucralfate 1 g PO every 6 hours.**

11. **Antibiotics**

    The routine use of prophylactic antibiotics in patients with open skull injuries is controversial. Penicillin may reduce the risk of pneumococcal meningitis in patients with CSF otorrhea, rhinorrhea, or intracranial air but may increase the risk of infection with more virulent organisms.

12. **Follow-up CT scan**

In general, a follow-up head CT scan should be obtained 24 hours after the initial injury in patients with intracranial hemorrhage to assess for delayed or progressive bleeding.

Selected Complications of Severe Head Injury

1. **CSF leaks**

CSF leaks result from disruption of the leptomeninges and occur in 2% to 6% of patients with closed head injury. CSF leakage ceases spontaneously with head elevation alone after a few days in 85% of patients; a lumbar drain may speed this process by limiting flow through the dural fistula in persistent cases. Although patients with CSF leaks are at increased risk for meningitis (usually from pneumococci), administration of prophylactic antibiotics is controversial. Persistent CSF otorrhea or rhinorrhea or recurrent meningitis is an indication for operative repair.

2. **Carotid cavernous fistulae**

Carotid cavernous fistulae, characterized by the triad of *pulsating exophthalmos, chemosis, and orbital bruit,* may develop immediately or several days after injury. Angiography is required to confirm the diagnosis. Endovascular balloon occlusion is the most effective means of repair and can prevent permanent visual loss resulting from retinal venous hypertension.

3. **Diabetes insipidus**

Diabetes insipidus may result from traumatic damage to the pituitary stalk, resulting in cessation of antidiuretic hormone secretion. Patients excrete large volumes of dilute urine, resulting in hypernatremia and volume depletion. **Arginine vasopressin (Pitressin) 5 to 10 U IV, intramuscularly, or SC every 4 to 6 hours** or **desmopressin acetate (DDAVP) SC 2 to 4 µg or IV every 12 hours** is given to control urine output to less than 200 ml/hr, and volume is replaced with hypotonic fluids (D5W or 0.45% saline) depending on the severity of hypernatremia.

4. **Post-traumatic seizures**

Post-traumatic seizures may be **immediate** (occurring within 24 hours), **early** (occurring within the first week), or **late** (occurring after the first week). Immediate seizures do not predispose to late seizures; early seizures, however, indicate an increased risk of late seizures, and these patients should be maintained on anticonvulsants. The overall incidence of late post-traumatic epilepsy (recurrent, unprovoked seizures) after closed head injury is 5%; the risk is as high as 20% in patients with intracranial hemorrhage or depressed skull fractures.

PROGNOSIS

The outcome after head injury is often a matter of great concern, particularly in patients with serious injuries. The admission Glasgow Coma Scale score has substantial prognostic value: patients scoring 3 or 4 have an 85% chance of dying or remaining in a vegetative state, whereas these outcomes occur in only 5% to 10% of patients with a score of 12 or higher. *Postconcussion syndrome* refers to a chronic profile of headache, fatigue, dizziness, inability to concentrate, irritability, and personality changes that develops in many patients following head injury. Often, there is overlap with symptoms of depression.

Ataxia and Gait Failure

True ataxia implies a decomposition of coordinated posture and movement that is normally integrated by the cerebellum. Because almost every component of the nervous system contributes to maintenance of normal movement, gait, and posture, a call for a patient with gait failure requires consideration of a broad differential diagnosis. Successful evaluation begins with assessing the acuteness of the syndrome. Associated signs on examination will help with anatomic localization. Your management may range from emergent neurosurgical decompression of a cerebellar hematoma to a thorough laboratory evaluation to seek a cause for a chronic degenerative disease.

PHONE CALL

Questions

1. **When did the patient last walk normally?**

    This is the key question from which your route of investigation and management will spring. If the patient was known to have been walking normally within the past 24 hours, you must rule out stroke, spinal cord compression (see Chapter 7), or a mass lesion in the posterior fossa. These are medical emergencies. A subacute course (days to weeks) suggests an infectious, inflammatory, or neoplastic process. If the gait deterioration has occurred over weeks to months, your differential diagnosis will be weighted toward degenerative processes, either inherited or acquired.

2. **Has there been any trauma to the head, neck, or back?**

    A traumatic subdural hematoma or injury to the spinal cord or peripheral nerves may alter gait.

3. **What is the patient's level of consciousness?**

    Is the patient alert and awake, agitated, or confused? If a patient has an abnormal mental status in combination with ataxia or gait failure, acute intoxication or significant brain injury is likely.

4. **What are the vital signs?**

    Irregular heart rhythm may suggest cardioembolic stroke; fever may suggest an infectious process.

Orders

1. Maintain the patient at bed rest.
2. Use a chest restraint, if necessary, to prevent the patient from injuring himself or herself.
3. If there has been trauma to the head or neck, stabilize the cervical spine with a cervical collar (see Chapter 7).

ELEVATOR THOUGHTS

What is the differential diagnosis of gait failure?

Gait failure may occur as a result of damage to almost any part of the neural axis. Your initial examination of the patient will help establish whether you are dealing with disturbance of motor, sensory, or cerebellar function. Table 10–1 is an outline of the categories of diseases that cause gait dysfunction and the characteristic features of the gait disturbance. Table 10–2 provides a more detailed differential diagnosis of ataxia.

MAJOR THREAT TO LIFE

- **Cerebellar hemorrhage or infarction**

  Hematoma or infarction in the posterior fossa may progress to herniation and death if the lesion is large. It may require emergent neurosurgical evacuation.
- **Acute intoxication**

  Intoxication with sedatives such as barbiturate or alcohol may present initially as ataxia and may lead to respiratory failure.

BEDSIDE

Quick Look Test

Is the patient awake and alert?

A decreased level of consciousness in the presence of ataxia is more serious than ataxia alone.

Is there any evidence of head or neck trauma?

Head trauma rarely presents as ataxia alone but may require more immediate management. Vertebral artery dissection may result from trauma to the neck.

Has the patient been vomiting?

Nausea, vertigo, and vomiting are common symptoms that accompany posterior fossa disease.

TABLE 10–1 **Clinical Features of Gait Disturbances**

Disease Category	Features of Gait Failure
Focal brain injury (hemiparesis)	Spastically extended leg
	Spastically flexed arm
	Circumduction of paretic foot
Spinal cord injury (paraparesis)	Stiff, effortful movements at knees and hips
	Bilateral circumduction
	Toe-walking or scissoring gait
Peripheral or central deafferentation (sensory ataxia)	Wide-based stance and gait
	High-stepping gait
	Positive Romberg's sign
Cerebellar disease	Titubation (unsteady, oscillating posture) on sitting or standing
	Wide-based stance and gait
	Ataxia: staggering or lurching may be unilateral or bilateral
Normal-pressure hydrocephalus	"Magnetic," shuffling gait
	Many steps taken to turn 180 degrees
Lower motor neuron disease	Distal weakness (e.g., footdrop)
	High-stepping gait
Myopathy	Proximal leg weakness
	Difficulty arising from seated position
	Difficulty climbing stairs
Parkinsonism	Stooped posture
	Shuffling gait
	Retropulsion
	Difficulty initiating and terminating ambulation ("festinating gait")
Congenital/perinatal injury (cerebral palsy)	Spastically extended legs
	Spastically flexed arms
	Scissoring gait
	Adventitial movements (abnormal posturing or movements of one or more limbs)
Movement disorders	Adventitial movements may be present at rest (chorea, athetosis, or dystonia)
	Lurching gait

Selective History and Chart Review

The diagnosis for the etiology of gait failure can often be made on the history alone. If the patient is unable to give a history, get the history from a relative, nurse, or other witness. In the absence of a witness on hand, review the chart.

1. When did the gait disturbance begin?
2. Was the onset sudden or gradual?
3. Why was the patient unable to walk? Was it because of weakness, imbalance, pain, or numbness?
4. Were there any accompanying symptoms?

TABLE 10–2 Differential Diagnosis of Ataxia by
Mode of Onset

Mode of Onset	Disease Process
Acute (minutes to hours)	Cerebellar hemorrhage Cerebellar infarction Acute intoxication Head trauma Basilar migraine Dominant periodic ataxia (in children)
Subacute (hours to days)	Posterior fossa tumor Posterior fossa abscess Multiple sclerosis Toxins/intoxications Hydrocephalus Miller-Fisher variant of Guillain-Barré syndrome Viral cerebellitis (mostly in children)
Chronic (days to weeks)	Alcoholic cerebellar degeneration Paraneoplastic cerebellar syndrome Foramen magnum compression Chronic infection (e.g., Jakob-Creutzfeldt disease, rubella, panencephalitis) Hydrocephalus Vitamin E deficiency Hypothyroidism Inherited ataxias (autosomal recessive or dominant) Idiopathic degenerative ataxias
Episodic	Recurrent intoxications Multiple sclerosis Transient ischemic attacks Dominant periodic ataxia (children)

Modified from Harding AE: Ataxic disorders. In Bradley WG, Daroff RB, Fenichel GM, Marsden CD (eds): Neurology in Clinical Practice. Boston, Butterworth-Heinemann, 1991.

Diplopia, dysarthria, vertigo, or nausea suggests posterior fossa involvement. Unilateral weakness or numbness implies focal hemispheric brain injury (e.g., stroke). Urinary or fecal incontinence suggests spinal cord involvement. Pain radiating into the legs implies nerve root disease.

5. *Is the patient taking any medications that might cause ataxia?*

Most of the effects of medications are dose dependent (Table 10–3).

Selective Physical Examination I

General Physical Examination

Vital signs   Fever may suggest an infectious etiology, such as **abscess, viral cerebellitis, or fungal**

TABLE 10–3 **Medications Known to Cause Ataxia**

Anticonvulsants	Immunosuppressants
Phenytoin	Cyclosporine A
Carbamazepine	Cytosine arabinoside
Primidone	Fluorouracil
Ethosuximide	**Other medications (rarely cause ataxia)**
Methosuximide	Phenothiazines
Sedatives	Monoamine oxidase inhibitors
Barbiturates	Reserpine
Benzodiazepines	Thiothixene
Chloral hydrate	Lithium salts
Paraldehyde	Nitrofurantoin

	infection. Fever may also occur in some of the inherited metabolic ataxias (mostly in children). Irregular heart rhythm may suggest cardioembolic stroke.
HEENT	Look for signs of head trauma. **Subdural or epidural hematoma** may produce hemiparesis.
Abdomen	Look for signs of **chronic alcohol use,** such as hepatomegaly, caput medusae, or ascites. Hepatosplenomegaly may also appear in **Wilson's disease** and in some **inherited metabolic ataxias.**

Neurologic Examination

- **Mental status:** Establish level of alertness and attentiveness by asking the patient to count backward from 20 to 1 or to recite the months of the year backward.
- **Cranial nerves: Gait failure with almost any cranial nerve finding means there is brain stem or cerebellar involvement.**
  1. **Pupils:** Pinpoint pupils may suggest **opiate intoxication;** asymmetric pupils may be a part of Horner's syndrome (miosis, ptosis, and anhidrosis), which, in combination with ataxia and contralateral pain and temperature sensory loss, makes up Wallenberg's (lateral medullary) syndrome. Small, irregular pupils that react to accommodation but not to light (Argyll Robertson pupils) may be a sign of **central nervous system syphilis, brain stem encephalitis, or mass effect on the midbrain.**
  2. **Extraocular movements: Nystagmus, particularly if vertical or dysconjugate, is a sign of injury to the brain stem or cerebellum.** Vertical (upbeat or downbeat) nystagmus is a reliable indicator of cerebellar or brain stem damage (see Chapter 13 for a more detailed discussion of nystagmus).

Horizontal gaze palsies localize disease to a large hemispheric or small pontine lesion. Impaired upgaze, particularly in combination with retraction nystagmus and loss of pupillary accommodation, implies pressure on or damage to the tectum of the midbrain and can be seen in pineal region tumors or in hydrocephalus (Parinaud's phenomenon). CN 6 palsies may be a nonspecific sign of increased ICP. Oculoparesis, in combination with ataxia and areflexia, makes the diagnosis of the **Miller-Fisher variant of Guillain-Barré syndrome.**

3. **CN 7:** Upper motor neuron facial paresis may be part of a hemiparesis or may indicate brain stem involvement if CN 6 is affected on the same side.

4. **CN 8:** Tinnitus or hearing loss with ataxia suggests a **peripheral vestibular neuropathy or labyrinthitis,** particularly if there is a rotational component to the nystagmus.

5. **CN 9 to CN 12:** Dysphagia, nasal speech, dysarthria, or tongue deviation may suggest a **brain stem stroke or mass lesion at the skull base,** producing spastic paraparesis and gait failure in addition to the lower cranial nerve findings.

- **Cerebellar testing:** Rapid, repetitive finger-thumb opposition (rapid alternating movements [RAM]) and finger-nose-finger (FNF) movements are two sensitive screening tests for cerebellar function. Irregular rhythm (dysdiadochokinesis) on finger tapping or ataxia of movements as the finger approaches the target on the FNF test suggests cerebellar dysfunction. The heel-knee-shin (HKS) test is the equivalent of the FNF test for the lower extremities. Figure 10–1 illustrates three common cerebellar tests (the FNF, RAM, and HKS tests). **Unilateral limb ataxia implies ipsilateral cerebellar hemisphere damage** because the cerebellar circuits that coordinate movement cross twice, once while descending in the frontopontocerebellar pathway and a second time while ascending in the dentatothalamic, dentatorubral, and dentatocortical pathways. **Titubation (truncal ataxia) on sitting or standing or gait ataxia in the absence of limb ataxia suggests midline cerebellar damage.**

  If the patient is able to stand, the gait evaluation is a crucial part of the examination for anatomic localization and determination of the underlying pathophysiology. Table 10–1 reviews the features of gait dysfunction that characterize different disease processes. The gait should be tested with the patient walking normally, walking on the toes, walking on the heels, and doing a tandem walk. Observe for symmetry of balance, stride, and arm swing.

- **Motor:** Test for strength by confrontation and look for pronator drift with the arms extended and palms up. (Pronator drift may be the only sign of a subtle hemiparesis.)

Finger-nose-finger test

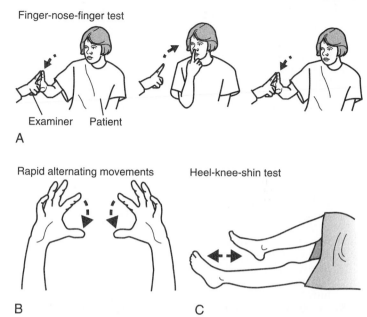

Examiner   Patient

A

Rapid alternating movements   Heel-knee-shin test

B   C

Figure 10–1 Cerebellar function tests. *A,* Finger-nose-finger test. Patient touches the finger of the examiner and his or her own nose sequentially. *B,* Rapid alternating movements. Patient taps the forefinger and thumb together as rapidly as possible. *C,* Heel-knee-shin test. Patient runs the heel up and down the opposite shin as accurately and rapidly as possible.

- **Sensory:** Temperature and vibration are the most sensitive parameters for testing sensory loss. Proprioceptive loss may indicate damaged posterior columns, as occurs in **vitamin B$_{12}$ deficiency** (subacute combined degeneration) or **tabes dorsalis** (a now rare, late complication of syphilis).
- **Reflexes:** Unilateral hyper-reflexia usually accompanies hemiparesis; bilateral hyper-reflexia may indicate myelopathy; and areflexia is seen in peripheral neuropathy and in the **Guillain-Barré syndrome.**

MANAGEMENT I

Acute ataxia, particularly with any accompanying signs or symptoms of posterior fossa disease or increased intracranial pressure, must be treated with utmost urgency.

1. Obtain a noncontrast head CT or MRI scan.

If cerebellar hematoma or infarction is identified, proceed with the next steps.

2. **Admit the patient to an intensive care unit.**
3. **Consult with the neurosurgery service.**

   If there is hematoma near the brain stem or if the hematoma is large, rapid, and irreversible, neurologic deterioration may occur. Delayed deterioration may be the result of a rebleed or reactive edema formation. **Surgical evacuation of cerebellar hematoma greater than 3 cm in diameter has been shown to reduce morbidity and mortality rates for these patients.** Consideration for surgical evacuation is warranted, particularly if the patient is relatively young and is following a deteriorating course. **It may be necessary to place an intraventricular drain if hydrocephalus develops.**

4. **Cerebellar hematomas smaller than 3 cm may be managed medically with reasonably good results.**

   Therapy is largely supportive, with blood pressure control to a target maximum systolic BP (SBP) of 160 to 180 mm Hg and control of coagulopathy with fresh frozen plasma if necessary. Hydrocephalus can develop even with smaller hematomas, necessitating neurosurgical placement of an intraventricular drain.

5. **Cerebellar infarction, if large, may produce the same syndrome of rapid progression to coma as does cerebellar hematoma.**

   As the infarcted territory becomes edematous, compression of the fourth ventricle may produce **obstructive hydrocephalus,** leading to further increase in intracranial pressure. Cerebellar infarction in the posterior inferior cerebellar artery territory carries a worse prognosis than infarction in the anterior inferior cerebellar artery or superior cerebellar artery territories. **Surgical evacuation of a large cerebellar infarction may be lifesaving.** As noted in item 3, placement of an intraventricular drain may become necessary with cerebellar infarction if hydrocephalus develops.

Other causes of gait failure that require immediate management include cord compression or acute myelopathy (see Chapter 7), **subdural or epidural hematoma from head trauma** (see Chapter 9), **acute cerebral infarction** (see Chapter 6), **and acute intoxication** (see Chapter 5).

Selective Physical Examination II

Once posterior fossa lesions have been ruled out by imaging, further examination for systemic signs associated with chronic ataxic disorders should be performed:

Hair	Alopecia may be a sign of **thallium poisoning, hypothyroidism, or adrenoleukomyeloneuropathy.**

Skin	Telangiectases, particularly in the conjunctivae, nose, and ears, or flexures, may be seen in **ataxia-telangiectasia.** Pigmentation may be seen in adrenoleukomyeloneuropathy.
HEENT	Kayser-Fleischer rings appear as a brown border at the edge of the iris in **Wilson's disease.** Retinal angiomas seen on fundoscopic examination may be a part of **von Hippel-Lindau disease** that also includes cerebellar hemangioblastomas. Deafness in combination with short stature is often a sign of **mitochondrial encephalopathy.**
Heart	Cardiomegaly, murmurs, arrhythmias, and heart failure may accompany **Friedreich's ataxia.** Conduction defects on ECG may be present in mitochondrial encephalopathy.
Musculoskeletal	Short stature is characteristic of mitochondrial encephalopathy and ataxia-telangiectasia. Other skeletal deformities may be a part of hereditary ataxias and hereditary motor and sensory neuropathy.

MANAGEMENT II

Diagnostic Testing

Laboratory Investigation

Laboratory investigation should begin with an attempt to diagnose treatable or reversible causes of ataxia or gait failure. Laboratory tests to be performed include the following blood tests:

1. Chemistry panel, including electrolytes, glucose, and liver function tests
2. Urine and serum toxicology screen
3. Vitamin B_{12} and folate levels
4. VDRL test
5. Thyroid function tests
6. Anticonvulsant levels if the patient is taking anticonvulsants
7. Lithium level if the patient is taking lithium
8. Anti-Yo serum antibodies to investigate paraneoplastic cerebellar degeneration from ovarian, lung, or breast carcinoma, or Hodgkin's lymphoma (see Chapter 22)
9. Ceruloplasmin levels (Wilson's disease)

Other Diagnostic Tests

1. **Chest radiograph**
   A chest radiograph may disclose occult neoplasm, raising the possibility of metastatic disease or a paraneoplastic cerebellar degeneration.

2. **Transcranial Doppler ultrasonogram or MR angiogram**
   Vertebrobasilar TIAs or vertebrobasilar insufficiency may be suggested if there is stenosis of the basilar or vertebral arteries.

3. **Visual evoked responses**
   Delayed P100 suggests multiple sclerosis.

4. **Lumbar puncture**
   Oligoclonal bands are present in multiple sclerosis. Abnormal CSF cell count, protein, or glucose may point to an infectious or neoplastic process. Elevated CSF protein without pleocytosis is found in the Miller-Fisher variant of Guillain-Barré syndrome. Cytology may be performed if a CNS- or meninges-based tumor is suspected.

5. **Electromyography (EMG)/nerve conduction studies (NCS)**
   The Miller-Fisher variant of the Guillain-Barré syndrome includes ataxia, oculoparesis, and areflexia. A typical demyelination pattern of slowed conduction velocities and prolonged F waves supports this diagnosis. Gait failure on the basis of neuropathy can also be diagnosed with EMG/NCS.

Treatment of Some of the Reversible Causes of Ataxia

1. **Acute sedative intoxication:** Administer **naloxone (Narcan) 0.4 to 2 mg IV** for opiate overdose; **flumazenil (Romazicon) 0.5 mg IV** for benzodiazepine overdose; admit for observation and supportive therapy.

2. **Anticonvulsant overdose:** Stop administering the anticonvulsant, admit for observation and cardiovascular monitoring, and follow anticonvulsant levels.

3. **Hypothyroidism:** Administer **Synthroid 0.05 to 0.15 mg every day.**

4. **Lithium toxicity:** Admit patient for cardiac monitoring, adjust dose, and follow lithium and electrolyte levels.

5. **Paraneoplastic disorder:** Treating the underlying malignancy may reverse the symptoms in some patients. Immunosuppressive therapy and plasmapheresis have not been proved to be effective.

6. **Vertebrobasilar TIAs:** Admit patient for workup for etiology of TIAs. Anticoagulation may be required (see Chapter 23).

7. **Multiple sclerosis:** Treat with IV methylprednisolone and beta interferon (see Chapter 20).

8. **CNS infections:** Treat with appropriate antimicrobial agents (see Chapter 21).
9. **Miller-Fisher variant of Guillain-Barré syndrome:** A several-day course of plasmapheresis or intravenous immune globulin (IVIG) early in the disease may be effective in halting progression and speeding recovery (see Chapter 15).

11

Acute Visual Disturbances

No symptom may be as disturbing or dramatic to a patient as acute visual loss. Although acute ocular diseases such as glaucoma, uveitis, and retinal detachment may require urgent evaluation by an ophthalmologist, a high percentage of visual disturbances fall within the province of the neurologist. Neurologic visual symptoms may be reported as blurriness, focal obscurations, or positive visual phenomena. Because the visual pathway from the retina to the calcarine cortex is constant from individual to individual, anatomic localization can be made with a high degree of accuracy on physical examination. The progression, associated symptoms and signs, and clinical setting will help you make the correct diagnosis and suggest the proper acute management.

Questions

The following questions will need to be repeated during the selective history and physical examination of the patient. Nonetheless, these questions, asked prior to your arrival at the bedside, will form the starting point for your diagnostic and management algorithm.

1. **Is the visual loss in one or both eyes?**

   This is the first point for anatomic localization. Visual disturbances affecting one eye indicate pathology between the retina and the optic chiasm. Binocular disturbances suggest lesions in the visual pathway between the chiasm and the calcarine cortex.

2. **What is the nature of the visual disturbance?**

   This is an elaboration of question one. Vision can be altered in one of the following ways: monocular visual loss (temporary or permanent), bilateral blindness, a hemifield cut, diplopia, scotomata, or positive phenomena (e.g., flashes or lines). The first description of the disturbance will allow the visual problem to be categorized into specific disease entities.

3. **How old is the patient?**

Certain disorders, such as ischemic optic neuropathy or transient monocular blindness (TMB), are rare in patients under 45 years of age, whereas a first presentation of multiple sclerosis, pseudotumor cerebri, or migraine is much more common in a younger patient.

4. **Is the patient still experiencing the visual symptom?**

Although persistent acute visual loss may require immediate, specific therapy, transient visual loss may be no less ominous as a warning sign for further visual, cerebrovascular, or inflammatory events.

5. **When did the visual disturbance begin?**

Acute monocular blindness is a neuro-ophthalmologic emergency. Ischemia in the retina resulting from a central retinal artery occlusion may be irreversible after 105 minutes. Furthermore, even if the patient presents many hours after the onset of visual loss, efficient and accurate diagnosis may prevent contralateral visual loss due to temporal arteritis or stroke from carotid artery disease.

6. **Was there any trauma or injury to the eyes?**

Eye injury will nearly always require ophthalmologic evaluation. Because a dilated fundoscopic examination by an ophthalmologist will interfere with your ability to get an accurate assessment of pupillary reactivity, you should try to perform your assessment first.

Orders

If there has been eye trauma or if there is a preexisting ophthalmologic condition such as glaucoma, call the ophthalmology service for consultation.

Inform RN

"Will arrive at the bedside in . . . minutes."

ELEVATOR THOUGHTS

What is the differential diagnosis of acute visual disturbance?

The differential diagnosis of acute visual disturbance can be divided into processes affecting one eye or both eyes.

1. **Monocular visual loss**
   - **Retinal ischemia (central [or branch] retinal artery occlusion [CRAO])**

     This occlusion is usually caused by an embolus from the ipsilateral internal carotid artery or from the heart or aortic arch. If the symptoms are transient (TMB or amaurosis fugax), the mechanism may be hemodynamic rather than embolic. Hemodynamic TMB may be caused by perfusion failure in the retinal artery from high-grade carotid stenosis. Patients with vascular causes for retinal ischemia usually have risk factors for cerebrovascular disease, such as hypertension, diabetes, or a history of smoking.

- **Optic nerve head ischemia (anterior ischemic optic neuropathy [AION])**

    Although its pathophysiology is uncertain, this entity is often associated with arteritis. Patients in their 50s or 60s may have systemic lupus erythematosus, polyarteritis nodosa, sickle cell trait, or polycythemia. In patients over 60 years of age, the most common associated arteritis is giant cell (temporal) arteritis, which must be treated emergently.

- **Inflammatory/demyelinating optic neuritis**

    The most common cause for optic neuritis in a patient under 40 years of age is multiple sclerosis, but idiopathic forms and sarcoidosis can be present in older individuals.

- **Retrobulbar mass lesion**

    The lesion may be a **tumor, such as optic glioma, neurofibroma, meningioma, or metastasis, or a giant aneurysm in the cavernous segment of the carotid. Pseudotumor cerebri** (benign intracranial hypertension) can mimic a mass lesion, causing papilledema and visual loss in young women who are often obese and dysmenorrheic. Visual loss may begin unilaterally.

2. **Binocular visual loss**

    Binocular involvement with visual field defects implies pathology at or behind the optic chiasm. Acute binocular visual loss affecting the chiasm, the optic tracts, the thalamus (lateral geniculate body), the optic radiations, or the calcarine cortex is nearly always due to an anatomic lesion such as a **tumor, abscess, or stroke. Migraine** is a notable exception, in which "spreading depression" (a wave of depolarization) is thought to produce neuronal deactivation that moves slowly across the cortex and produces scotomata in one or both visual fields. **Pituitary adenomas** often produce bitemporal visual field defects as pressure from the mass disrupts midline-crossing fibers from both nasal retinae (Fig. 11–1). The farther back along the visual pathway the lesion is located, the more congruous is the visual field defect. Table 11–1 lists unusual visual syndromes associated with occipital cortex lesions.

3. **Diplopia**

    Double vision implies some form of oculoparesis. If diplopia persists when one eye is covered, the etiology is either factitious or an ophthalmologic condition such as retinal detachment, dislocated lens, or keratoconus. For true binocular diplopia, the lesion is almost always in the brain stem or involves CN 3, CN 4, or CN 6. The most common conditions

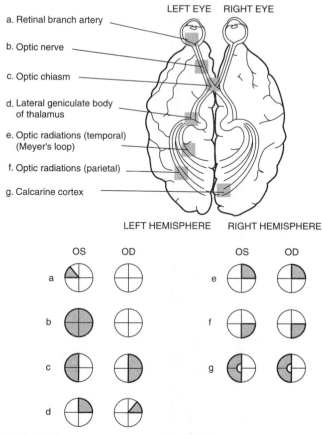

Figure 11–1 Visual field cuts produced by lesions at different points along the visual pathway. a. Monocular segmentanopia produced by a retinal artery branch occlusion in the left eye. b. Monocular blindness produced by a lesion in the left optic nerve. c. Bitemporal hemianopia produced by a mass lesion at the optic chiasm. d. Right segmentanopia produced by a lesion in the lateral geniculate body of the left thalamus. e. Right upper quadrantanopia produced by a lesion in the left temporal optic radiation (Meyer's loop). f. Right lower quadrantanopia produced by a lesion in the left parietal optic radiation. g. Left homonymous hemianopia produced by a lesion in the calcarine cortex of the right occipital lobe. Note that macular vision is sometimes spared because of middle cerebral artery collateral blood flow to the occipital pole. OS, oculus sinister; OD, oculus dexter.

TABLE 11–1 **Unusual Visual Syndromes Associated with Occipital Cortex Lesions**

Syndrome	Localization	Description
Anton's syndrome	Bilateral calcarine	Bilateral loss of vision in which the patient denies blindness
Balint's syndrome	Bilateral occipito-parietal	Simultanagnosia, optic ataxia, and ocular apraxia
Bonnet's syndrome	Unilateral or bilateral calcarine	Lilliputian visual hallucinations in the absence of delirium
Dyschromatopsia	Lingual gyrus	Abnormal color perception contralateral to lesion
Pallinopsia	Incomplete injury or recovery in calcarine cortex	Visual persistence of afterimages
Prosopagnosia	Right or bilateral inferior calcarine (lingual gyrus)	Inability to recognize faces

affecting the brain stem are **stroke** and **multiple sclerosis,** although **brain stem tumors** and **progressive multifocal leukoencephalopathy (PML)** may rarely present with diplopia. The most common systemic condition that affects the ocular cranial nerves is **diabetes mellitus.** A **berry aneurysm** of the posterior communicating artery may also produce diplopia by stretching CN 3 as it passes over the artery on its way forward toward the cavernous sinus. Invasive or metastatic **tumor in the cavernous sinus region** or late **chronic meningitis** may cause oculomotor disturbances. Unilateral or bilateral CN 6 palsies can be a false localizing sign of **increased intracranial pressure** (see Chapter 12). **Hyperthyroidism** may cause diplopia by mechanical limitation of infiltrated, fibrotic ocular muscles. Finally, weakness of the extraocular muscles because of **myasthenia gravis** must be considered in the differential diagnosis of diplopia, particularly if the symptoms fluctuate or appear with fatigue.

Diagnoses for which immediate, specific therapy may arrest loss or restore vision are the following:

- CRAO
- Ischemic optic neuropathy from temporal arteritis
- Pseudotumor cerebri
- Acute glaucoma

Diagnoses for which urgent management may prevent further vision loss or stroke are the following:

- TMB with carotid stenosis
- Retrobulbar mass lesion (aneurysm or tumor)

MAJOR THREAT TO LIFE

Acute visual loss in the absence of other neurologic signs is rarely life threatening.

BEDSIDE

Quick Look Test

Are there any signs of trauma?

Is the patient in any pain or discomfort?

Is one eye affected or are both?

Selective History and Chart Review

Some of the questions asked in the initial telephone interview should be discussed with the patient.

1. **Was one eye affected or were both?**

    It may be difficult for a patient to distinguish between a visual field loss and monocular blindness. A patient will often refer to "the left eye" as being defective when in fact the left hemifield was affected. Ask if the symptoms improve if "the bad eye" is covered.

2. **When and how did the visual disturbance begin?**

    Ask the patient to describe the onset of the symptoms, with particular reference to the location and pattern of the visual disturbance. An obscuration that moves across the visual field "like a shade coming down" is a common description of an arterial occlusion. An altitudinal defect is common with ischemic optic neuropathy. An expanding blind spot may suggest worsening papilledema. Slowly marching lights, particularly the jagged-edged "fortification scotomata," is a common description of migraine, whether or not it is followed by headache. Sudden loss of vision over seconds to minutes suggests a vascular cause. Progression over hours to days may suggest ischemic optic neuropathy, demyelination, mass lesion, or pseudotumor cerebri.

3. **Was there pain?**

    Headache is common in temporal arteritis, pseudotumor cerebri, and migraine. Masticatory claudication and other myalgias may be a tip-off for arteritis. Pain with eye movement is the rule for the inflammatory optic neuritis of multiple sclerosis, but pain is usually absent with retinal embolism and ischemic optic neuropathy. The exception is in carotid artery dissection, which may cause pain in the side of the head or jaw, with radiation into the orbit.

4. **Were there any associated neurologic symptoms?**

Dysarthria, vertigo, nausea, vomiting, and ataxia suggest stroke or mass lesion in the posterior fossa. Urinary incontinence, ataxia, diplopia, and patchy weakness or sensory loss are other presenting symptoms of multiple sclerosis.

Selective Physical Examination

General Physical Examination

Vital signs	Fever may be a feature of temporal arteritis. Cardiac arrhythmia and hypertension are risk factors for cerebrovascular disease.
HEENT	**Palpate the temporal arteries** just anterior and superior to the ear and along the side of the head. Exquisite tenderness strongly suggests temporal arteritis.
	Listen for **carotid bruits.**
	Eye examination. Check for **proptosis** by viewing the orbits from above. A retrobulbar mass lesion may cause the eye to protrude. Gentle palpation of the globe may disclose more resistance to posterior motion. The high pressure of glaucoma may also be detected, if present.

Neurologic Examination

- **Mental status**

    Aphasia or hemineglect may rarely accompany a disruption of optic radiations through the parietal lobe.
- **Cranial nerves**

    Check the following:
    1. **Pupillary reactivity.** Examine each pupil's direct and consensual response to light. Use low ambient light and a bright flashlight for the stimulus. A relative or absolute **afferent pupillary defect (APD).** APD may be detected by swinging the flashlight from one eye to the other. If the pupil enlarges when the flashlight swings to that eye **(Marcus Gunn pupil),** there is pathology in the retina or optic nerve.
    2. **Visual fields.** Test for visual fields by having the patient visually fix on your nose and by holding your hands in two of the four visual quadrants, an arm's length from the patient. Move a finger or briefly display a number of fingers on one or both hands. Test all four quadrants. More subtle visual field loss may be tested by comparing the brightness of a red button or hatpin. Red desaturation may occur without frank blindness. Be sure to check macular vision in the central 6 degrees of vision. Figure 11–1 illustrates the visual field defects expected with lesions at various points along the visual pathway.

TABLE 11–2 **Fundoscopic Features of Some Neuro-ophthalmologic Entities**

Diagnosis	Fundoscopic Appearance
Central retinal artery occlusion	White, ground-glass retina
	"Boxcar segmentation" (clumped red blood cells) in retinal veins (<1 hour)
	Macular cherry-red spot (hours to days)
Branch retinal artery occlusion	Embolic material (bright calcium flecks or lipid yellow Hollenhorst plaques) at arterial branch points
	Arcuate band of retinal infarction
Ischemic optic neuropathy	Disk head pallor, often in the superior or inferior half only
	Papilledema
	Superficial flame hemorrhages
	Optic disk cupping (late)
Optic neuritis	Disk pallor
Pseudotumor cerebri	Papilledema
Foster Kennedy syndrome	Optic atrophy ipsilateral to a retrobulbar mass
	Papilledema in contralateral eye due to increased retrobulbar pressure

3. **Fundoscopic examination.** This can reveal a specific pathology, although an examination adequate to make a definitive diagnosis may require pharmacologic dilation of the pupil. Table 11–2 lists the fundoscopic features of the most important diagnoses of monocular blindness. **Hollenhorst (cholesterol) plaques** in retinal arteries are a sign of cholesterol emboli from atherosclerotic plaque in the aortic arch or carotid arteries.

4. Check **ocular motility** with the following steps:
   A. **Have the patient follow your finger through horizontal and vertical range of motion.** Note oculoparesis if it occurs. Simple observation of the eye movements may be sufficient to diagnose a CN 3 or CN 6 lesion.
   B. **Latent or subtle nonconjugate gaze may be revealed by the cover-uncover test.** Ask the patient to fix on one point such as your finger. Cover one eye, then uncover it. Repeat with the other eye. If the eyes shift when the eyes are uncovered, there is a nonconjugate gaze. Although a positive cover-uncover test may suggest brain stem or cranial nerve pathology, benign, latent phorias in patients with normal vision may cause a positive test.
   C. **Evaluate subtle oculoparesis using a Maddox rod.** If there is preexisting amblyopia or if the patient is suppressing one eye's image, it may be difficult to identify

diplopia without isolating the images from the two eyes. To check for horizontal diplopia, have the patient cover one eye with the Maddox rod, with the slats oriented horizontally, and then have the patient fix on a point light source. Two images should be seen: the point of light will be seen by the uncovered eye and a vertical red line will be seen by the covered eye. If gaze is conjugate, light should bisect the red line. As you move the light laterally, the light and line will move farther apart if there is a paresis of lateral gaze in one eye. This occurs as the image is projected onto the retina, away from the macula in the affected eye. The rules are as follows: (1) the false image is always the one on the outside, and (2) the false image always comes from the affected eye. Figure 11–2 diagrams the use of the Maddox rod. The same procedure can be used to check for a vertical nonconjugate gaze by orienting the slats of the Maddox rod vertically (making the red line horizontal), and moving the light up or down. Again, the image that is on the outside (farther up on upgaze or farther down on downgaze) comes from the affected eye. Impairment of abduction indicates CN 6 or lateral rectus palsy. Impairment of adduction indicates CN 3 or medial rectus palsy. If adduction palsy is accompanied by abduction nystagmus in the opposite eye, this is likely an **internuclear ophthalmoplegia,** suggesting multiple sclerosis in a younger patient or a paramedian midbrain infarct in an older person. *Nystagmus* is discussed in Chapter 13.

- **Coordination and gait**
  Ataxia or dysdiadochokinesis may be a sign of multiple sclerosis or may suggest posterior circulation infarction affecting the cerebellum and the occipital cortex.
- **Sensation**
  Unilateral sensory loss may accompany visual field cuts produced by lesions in the thalamus or parietal lobe.
- **Reflexes**
  Asymmetry may be a subtle sign of brain injury.

MANAGEMENT

Order the following blood tests:
1. ESR
2. CBC with platelet count
3. PT or INR/partial thromboplastin time
4. Chemistry panel including glucose and cholesterol levels

If there is monocular blindness or any suspicion of injury to the eye, have someone call for an ophthalmologic consultation to follow your assessment.

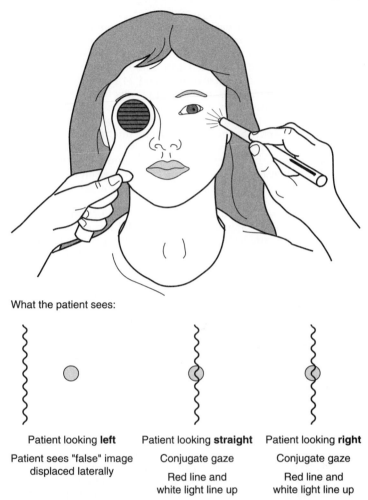

What the patient sees:

Patient looking **left**

Patient looking **straight**

Patient looking **right**

Patient sees "false" image displaced laterally

Conjugate gaze

Red line and white light line up

Conjugate gaze

Red line and white light line up

Figure 11–2 Use of the Maddox rod in a patient with a right CN 3 palsy. Patient sees the red line to the left of the white light on left gaze. This occurs because the red line projects farther laterally onto the retina of the abnormal eye, giving a false image that appears displaced laterally. The gaze is conjugate on primary gaze and on rightward gaze. Right CN 3 palsy would be confirmed by holding the Maddox rod so that the red line is oriented horizontally and asking the patient to look upward. The red line would then appear above the white light.

1. **CRAO**

   Restoration of vision is usually possible only within the first 90 to 120 minutes after the occlusive event, although reversal of blindness has been reported up to 12 hours after embolus. Local intra-arterial thrombolysis with t-PA may be possible. Treatment between 12 and 24 hours would be considered heroic. Standard treatment in the hyperacute phase is aimed at dislodging the embolic particle and lowering the intraocular pressure. This is accomplished by laying the patient flat and applying **ocular massage** (intermittently, pressing firmly on the globe every 4 seconds). If segmentation can still be seen in the retinal veins, you should consult an ophthalmologist to perform an anterior oculocentesis. The presence of a cherry-red spot suggests that the retina has been infarcted.

   Apart from treating the eye itself, CRAO requires a search for an embolic source. **Duplex Doppler ultrasonography** of the carotid arteries and echocardiography seeking a cardioembolic source should be performed urgently. **Intravenous (IV) heparin at 800 U/hr (no bolus), aiming for a PTT of 1.5 to 2.0 times the control value,** may be given as a bridge to oral anticoagulation if a cardioembolic source is known, provided there are no contraindications to anticoagulation therapy. **Patients with ipsilateral carotid stenosis greater than 70% should be referred for carotid endarterectomy** or **carotid angioplasty** and stenting to reduce the risk of stroke. Long-term anticoagulation with warfarin (Coumadin) is indicated if a cardioembolic source such as atrial fibrillation or an intracardiac thrombus is identified or if the patient has a hypercoagulable state such as anticardiolipin antibody syndrome.

2. **Arteritic ischemic optic neuropathy**

   Identifying temporal arteritis is of utmost importance. Because the prognosis for recovery of vision is less than 15% for the first eye, and because contralateral blindness may occur in up to 40% of patients, early recognition is important. Realistically, if visual loss is the presenting symptom, therapy is aimed at preventing involvement of the contralateral eye. Anorexia, fever, myalgias, and jaw claudication accompanying visual loss and headache in a patient over 65 years of age firmly establish the diagnosis clinically. Less typical presentations are possible. Sedimentation rate, C-reactive protein, and fibrinogen levels are usually markedly elevated. **Prednisone 100 mg by mouth (PO)** once a day should be started immediately, then tapered slowly after several weeks. **IV methylprednisolone 1 g per day** may also be used in the acute phase. Temporal artery biopsy should be arranged within a week. Corticosteroids generally have to be continued for 1 to 2 years. The ESR can be used as a marker of disease activity.

3. **Transient monocular blindness**

   Patients with painless transient monocular visual loss, particularly those with risk factors for cerebrovascular disease, should be evaluated for risk of stroke. TMB is a classic warning sign for high-grade carotid stenosis. As in CRAO, the patient should be referred for duplex Doppler ultrasonography, echocardiography, and usually magnetic resonance (MR) angiography. Maintaining the patient on an antithrombotic agent, either **acetylsalicylic acid (aspirin) (ASA) 81 or 325 mg once a day** or **IV heparin at 800 U/hr** if he or she is awaiting imminent endarterectomy, will reduce the risk of stroke or recurrent TIA (see Chapter 23). Most interventional neuroradiologists favor a combination of 81 mg ASA and 75 mg clopidogrel in preparation for carotid stenting.

4. **Retrobulbar mass lesion**

   In a patient with a suspected retro-orbital mass, high-quality imaging is the key to accurate diagnosis. **MRI with gadolinium contrast enhancement** will help define soft-tissue masses. **Computed tomography (CT) scan with thin cuts through the orbits** can help define any bony erosion. Appropriate **surgical referral** to an ophthalmologist or neurosurgeon should be made.

5. **Inflammatory optic neuritis**

   Optic neuritis is the presenting symptom for multiple sclerosis in approximately 15% of patients. Optic neuritis occurs at some point in the course of the disease in approximately 50% of patients with multiple sclerosis. As with treatment of other flares of multiple sclerosis, treatment of optic neuritis is **IV methylprednisolone 1 g for 7 to 10 days**, followed by a tapering dose of oral prednisone. Beta interferon or other immunomodulatory drugs may be indicated. (see Chapter 20) Oral prednisone as a first line of treatment for acute optic neuritis has been shown to be ineffective. Patients older than 45 years of age may have idiopathic optic neuritis that is steroid responsive.

6. **Pseudotumor cerebri**

   Visual loss is the most significant and dreaded complication of pseudotumor cerebri. Papilledema may occur with or without decreased acuity, but once visual loss begins, urgent therapy is imperative to prevent progression to blindness. Visual disturbance usually begins with an expanding blind spot or with constriction of the peripheral fields. Formal visual field testing may help evaluate the extent of loss. For mild visual loss, give **acetazolamide 500 mg PO two times a day.** This treatment is aimed at relieving increased intracranial pressure. For severe visual loss, the addition of **methylprednisolone 250 mg IV four times a day** (with an appropriate gastrointestinal protective medication such as ranitidine) may be vision saving. For patients whose visual loss is unresponsive to medical therapy, consult an ophthalmologist for **optic nerve sheath fenestration.** Periodic lumbar punctures or lumboperitoneal shunting has been advocated by some physicians, but the results of these treatments are inconsistent (see also Chapter 14).

Increased Intracranial Pressure

Increased ICP is not a symptom. Rather, intracranial hypertension is a pathologic state common to a variety of serious neurologic illnesses (Table 12–1). All conditions that result in increased ICP are characterized by an increase in intracranial volume. Accordingly, all therapies for ICP (hyperventilation, mannitol, etc.) are directed toward reducing intracranial volume.

Normal ICP is less than 20 cm H_2O, or 15 mm Hg. Because elevations beyond these levels can rapidly lead to brain damage and death, prompt recognition and treatment are essential. This chapter will be most useful in cases in which the pathology is known, and increased ICP is the suspected cause of clinical deterioration.

PHONE CALL

Questions

1. What is the patient's underlying neurologic problem?
2. Why is increased ICP suspected?
3. What is the patient's current level of consciousness?

BEDSIDE

Quick Look Test

Does the patient have clinical signs of increased ICP?

Increased ICP should be suspected in patients with known or suspected intracranial pathology (e.g., stroke, trauma, or neoplasm) who exhibit the following symptoms and signs:

Signs that are almost always present:
- Depressed level of consciousness (lethargy, stupor, coma)
- Hypertension, with or without bradycardia

Symptoms and signs that are sometimes present:
- Headache
- Vomiting

TABLE 12–1 **Conditions Associated with Increased ICP**

Intracranial mass lesions
Subdural hematoma
Epidural hematoma
Intracerebral hemorrhage
Brain tumor
Cerebral abscess

Increased CSF volume (or resistance to outflow)
Hydrocephalus
Benign intracranial hypertension (pseudotumor cerebri)

Increased brain volume (cytotoxic cerebral edema)
Cerebral infarction
Global hypoxia-ischemia
Reye's syndrome
Acute hyponatremia

Increased brain and blood volume (vasogenic cerebral edema)
Head trauma
Meningitis
Encephalitis
Lead encephalopathy
Eclampsia
Hypertensive encephalopathy
Dural sinus thrombosis
Subarachnoid Hemorrhage

CSF, cerebrospinal fluid; ICP, intracranial pressure.

- Papilledema
- CN 6 palsies

Remember, however, that these signs may be nonspecific. For this reason, the only way to confirm the diagnosis and properly treat increased ICP is to measure it.

Does the patient have clinical signs of herniation?

Clinical signs of herniation, listed here, result from *brain stem compression:*

- Loss of pupillary reactivity
- Impairment of eye movements
- Hyperventilation
- Motor posturing (flexion or extension)

When ICP is differentially increased across the tentorium (as is usually the case with hemispheric mass lesions), pressure gradients lead to downward displacement of brain tissue into the posterior fossa. Herniation is often rapidly fatal but can be reversed in some cases by treatments that reduce intracranial volume and ICP.

MANAGEMENT I

Emergency Measures for Reduction of ICP

If the clinical signs described under **Bedside** are identified in a comatose patient, the emergency measures listed in Box 12–1 can "buy time" prior to CT scan and a definitive neurosurgical procedure (craniotomy, ventriculostomy, or placement of an ICP monitor).

Placement of an ICP Monitor

Most clinicians would not treat a patient with suspected high blood pressure without measuring it. However, empirical therapy for increased ICP (i.e., repeated doses of mannitol) without monitoring is used all the time, to the great disadvantage of the patient. This approach is unsatisfactory because most ICP treatments are effective for a short time only, lose their efficacy with prolonged use, and have side effects. Optimally, therapy should be given when ICP is high and should be withheld when it is normal. Only use of an ICP monitor can make this possible.

Indications for ICP monitoring (all three conditions should be met):
1. **The patient is in a coma (Glasgow Coma Scale score of <8).**
2. **Brain imaging shows intracranial mass effect or global brain edma.**
3. **The prognosis is such that aggressive treatment in the ICU is indicated.**

ICP Monitors

If the decision has been made to treat the patient for suspected ICP, and surgical reduction of intracranial volume (i.e., ventriculostomy or craniotomy) is not feasible, an ICP monitor should be placed. There are three main types of monitors shown in Fig. 12–1.

BOX 12–1 Emergency Treatment for Elevated ICP in an Unmonitored Patient

1. Elevate head of bed 30 to 45 degrees.
2. Intubate and hyperventilate (target partial pressure of carbon dioxide [P_{CO_2}] is 28 to 32 mm Hg).
3. Insert a Foley catheter.
4. Administer **mannitol (20%) 1 to 1.5 g/kg intravenous (IV) rapid infusion.**
5. Administer **normal saline (0.9%) at 100 ml/hr (avoid hypotonic fluids).**
6. Consult the neurosurgery service.

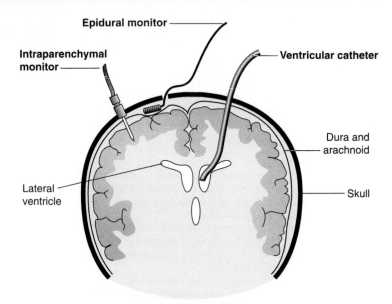

Figure 12–1 ICP monitoring devices.

1. **Ventricular catheter**
   Once inserted, a ventricular catheter is connected to both a pressure transducer and an external drainage system via a three-way stopcock. The major advantage to ventricular catheters is that they allow treatment of increased ICP via drainage of CSF. The main disadvantage is the high infection rate (10% to 20%), which increases dramatically after 5 days.
2. **Intraparenchymal probe (Camino, Codman)**
   These devices are easy to insert and very accurate, and the infection rate is exceedingly low (approximately 1%).
3. **Epidural transducer (Gaeltec)**
   These devices are inserted deep to the inner table of the skull and superficial to the dura. They are associated with a minimal infection rate but have a tendency to malfunction and to have a baseline drift (>5 to 10 mm Hg) after more than a few days of use.

ELEVATOR THOUGHTS

What are the physiologic principles of ICP?
   If you are caring for a patient with increased ICP, a firm understanding of intracranial physiology is essential.

Intracranial Anatomy

There are three principal components of volume within the cranium of the normal adult: brain (1400 ml), blood (150 ml), and CSF (150 ml). CSF is produced by the choroid plexus within the ventricles at a rate of approximately 20 ml/hr, resulting in the formation of almost 500 ml/day. Normal ICP ranges from 50 to 200 mm H_2O (4 to 15 mm Hg). CSF is reabsorbed across the convexity of the meninges into the venous circulation via arachnoid granulations. These pathways normally offer little resistance to CSF outflow. For this reason, jugular venous pressure is normally the principal determinant of ICP.

Intracranial Compliance

Because the cranial vault is a rigid, fixed container, any increase in intracranial volume can lead to increased ICP. In clinical practice, the most common mechanisms of increased intracranial volume are **extrinsic mass lesions, hydrocephalus, and cerebral edema (brain swelling).** Initially, as volume is added to the intracranial space, increases in pressure are minimal because of the highly compliant nature of the intracranial contents; as intracranial volume increases, CSF is displaced through the foramen magnum into the paraspinal space, and blood is displaced from compressed brain tissue. When these mechanisms are exhausted, however, intracranial compliance decreases, and further increases in intracranial volume lead to dramatic elevations of ICP (Fig. 12–2).

Cerebral Perfusion Pressure

Cerebral perfusion pressure (CPP) is routinely monitored in conjunction with the ICP because it is an important determinant of cerebral blood flow (CBF). CPP is defined by the equation

$$CPP = MABP \text{ (mean arterial blood pressure)} - ICP$$

When autoregulation is intact, CBF is maintained at a constant level across a wide range of CPPs (50 to 150 mm Hg). However, in injured brain with impaired autoregulation, CBF approximates a straight-line relationship with CPP; that is, reductions of CBF are more severe at any given level of reduced CPP (Fig. 12–3). **CPP must be closely regulated within 70 to 120 mm Hg in patients with increased ICP,** because reductions below this level can lead to secondary hypoxic-ischemic damage, whereas excessive increases can lead to "breakthrough" hyperperfusion and aggravation of cerebral edema.

ICP Waveforms

The normal ICP waveform (see Fig. 12–2) reflects a transient surge in cerebral blood volume that occurs with each heartbeat. As ICP rises and intracranial compliance decreases, the amplitude of the ICP

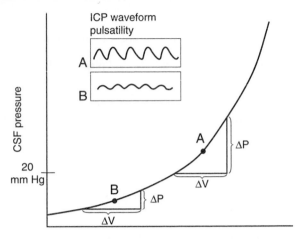

Figure 12–2 Intracranial pressure (ICP)-volume curve. At low pressures (point B) the intracranial compartment is compliant, meaning that large increases in volume (ΔV) lead to small increments in pressure (ΔP). At higher pressures (point A) the intracranial space becomes less compliant. As a result, the amplitude and pulsatility of the arterial reflection in the ICP waveform increases *(inset).* CSF, cerebrospinal fluid.

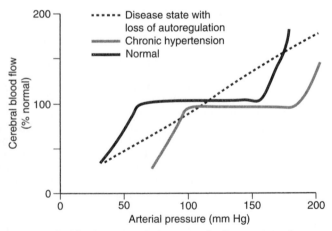

Figure 12–3 Cerebral autoregulation curve. In disease states (e.g., vasospasm or ischemia), cerebral blood flow becomes pressure passive *(dotted line).* With chronic hypertension, the autoregulatory curve shifts to the right.

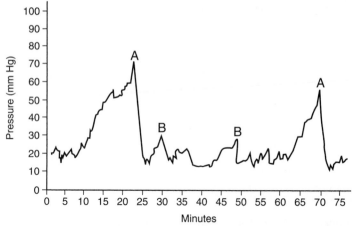

Figure 12–4 Pathologic intracranial pressure elevations. A = Lundberg A (plateau) waves; B = Lundberg B waves. (Redrawn from Chestnut RM, Marshall LF: Treatment of abnormal intracranial pressure. Neurosurg Clin North Am 1991;2:267-284.)

waveform increases, and superimposed pathologic ICP elevations can occur. Two types of pathologic ICP waves have been described (Fig. 12–4):

1. **Lundberg A waves (plateau waves).** Plateau waves are dangerous elevations of ICP; they can reach levels of 20 to 80 mm Hg and are generally from 5 minutes to 1 hour in duration. When severe, they are associated with reduced CPP (less than 60 mm Hg) and CBF and with global hypoxic-ischemic injury.

2. **Lundberg B waves.** These waves are of lesser amplitude (10 to 20 mm Hg) and duration (1 to 5 minutes) than plateau waves and thus are less dangerous. Clinically, they are a useful marker of abnormal autoregulation and reduced intracranial compliance.

MANAGEMENT II

General Measures for Treating Patients with Increased ICP

1. **Elevate head of bed by 30 to 45 degrees and maintain a straight head position.**

   Head elevation reduces ICP by reducing jugular venous pressure and by enhancing venous outflow. Sharp head angulation should be avoided, because it may cause jugular venous compression, increased venous backpressure, and increased ICP.

2. **Prevent seizures.**

   Seizures can lead to profound elevations of CBF, intracranial blood volume, and ICP, even in patients who are paralyzed. **Fosphenytoin (10 to 20 mg/kg loading dose; then 3 to 5 mg/kg per day)** is the preferred agent for seizure prophylaxis.

3. **Treat fever aggressively.**

   Fever can exacerbate ICP, and it lowers the threshold for neuronal death. Treatment with **acetaminophen (650 mg every 4 hours), indomethacin (25 mg every 6 hours),** or a **cooling blanket** can be effective.

Steps for Treating an "ICP Crisis" in an Intubated, Monitored Patient

Proper treatment of increased ICP requires an organized, stepwise approach (Box 12–2). Brief elevations of ICP (lasting only 1 to 5 minutes) occur frequently with suctioning, coughing, and repositioning and do not require aggressive treatment. **In general, the following measures should be instituted only when the ICP is elevated above 20 mm Hg for a period of 10 or more minutes.**

1. **Removal of intracranial mass or drainage of CSF**

   Remember that reduction of intracranial volume is the only definitive treatment for increased ICP. Consider a repeat CT scan in a patient with increasing ICP. If a ventricular catheter is in place, the system should be opened for drainage, and 5 to 10 ml of CSF should be removed. Emergent Craniotomy or hemicraniectomy is the ultimate intervention for an ICP crisis.

2. **Sedation and paralysis**

   In patients with reduced intracranial compliance, physical agitation or fighting the ventilator can lead to elevated ICP because of increased intrathoracic, jugular venous, and arterial

---

BOX 12–2 **Stepwise Treatment Protocol for Elevated ICP in a Monitored Patient (ICP >20 mm Hg for >10 Minutes)**

1. Consider repeat CT scanning or definitive neurosurgical intervention (e.g., craniotomy or ventriculostomy)
2. Sedate patient to attain a quiet, motionless state
3. Optimize CPP with vasopressors to maintain >70 mm Hg, or with blood pressure-lowering agents maintain <120 mm Hg
4. Mannitol 0.25 to 1.5 g/kg IV every 1 to 6 hours
5. Hyperventilate to maintain P_{CO_2} between 28 and 32 mm Hg
6. Pentobarbital infusion

pressures. *Before further measures are instituted, agitated patients with increased ICP should be sedated to the point at which they are motionless and quiet.*

Note: Intravenous sedatives cause apnea and hypotension and thus require intubation and intravascular blood pressure monitoring. The following agents can be used:

- **Morphine IV** is an opioid with sedative-hypnotic and analgesic effects. The dose is **2 to 5 mg IVP every hour.**
- **Fentanyl IV** (supplied as 50 μg/ml) is also an opioid and is 100 times more potent than morphine. For rapid control of agitation, give **25 to 100 μg IVP.** For sustained sedation, give **fentanyl IV infusion 4 mg/250 ml normal saline (NS).** Start at 5 ml/hr (1.33 μg/min); the range is 8 to 23 ml/hr (2 to 6 μg/min).
- **Propofol IV (10 mg/ml)** is a powerful sedative-hypnotic drug whose effect is more rapidly reversible than that of fentanyl. The typical maintenance dose is **5 to 50 μg/kg/min (0.3 to 3 mg/kg/hr);** this translates into 2 to 20 ml/hr for a 70 kg person.

3. **CPP optimization**

   If ICP remains elevated in a sedated patient, optimization of CPP should be attempted using vasoactive agents *before* mannitol and hyperventilation are administered.

   - If CPP is >120 mm Hg and ICP is >20 mm Hg, BP should be lowered. *However, CPP should not be allowed to fall to <70 mm Hg.* Agents for controlling hypertension include the following:
     1. **Labetalol IV (5 mg/ml)** is a combined alpha-1 and beta-1 blocker. For immediate control of BP, **push 20 to 80 mg every 10 to 20 minutes.** Once the desired BP is attained, start **200 mg/200 ml NS (1 mg/ml) at 2 mg/min (120 ml/hr) and titrate.**
     2. **Nicardipine IV** is a rapidly titratable calcium channel blocker. Start with **25 mg/250 ml NS at 5 ml/hr (8 μg/min) and titrate.**
   - If CPP is <70 mm Hg and ICP is >20 mm Hg, BP should be elevated and CPP raised to >70 mm Hg; this can lead to a reflex reduction of ICP by reducing the cerebral vasodilatation that occurs in response to inadequate perfusion. Pressor agents for raising CPP include
     1. **Norepinephrine (4 mg/250 ml N5NS)** infusion starting at a dose of 8 μg/min (30 ml/hr), adjusted to maintain desired target CPP (range 2-12 μg/min).
     2. **Phenylephrine (10 mg/250 ml)** is a pure alpha agonist. Start at **15 ml/hr (10 μg/min)** and titrate upward to a maximum of 200 μg/min.

4. **Mannitol**

Mannitol, an osmotic diuretic, lowers ICP via its cerebral dehydrating effects. The effects of mannitol are biphasic. Rapid infusion immediately creates an osmotic gradient across the blood-brain barrier, resulting in movement of water from brain to the intravascular compartment. The result is decreased brain tissue volume and, hence, reduced ICP. The secondary effect of mannitol results from its action as an osmotic diuretic. As mannitol is cleared by the kidneys, it leads to free water clearance and increased serum osmolality. As a result, even after the mannitol is gone, an intracellular dehydrating effect is maintained as water flows down the osmotic gradient, from the intracellular to the extracellular space.

- **The initial dose of mannitol 20% solution is 1 to 1.5 g/kg, followed every 1 to 6 hours with doses of 0.25 to 1.5 g/kg as needed.** The effect on ICP is maximal when mannitol is given rapidly (over 10 minutes).
- The effect of mannitol on ICP begins in 10 to 20 minutes, reaches its peak between 20 and 60 minutes, and lasts for 3 to 6 hours.
- Adverse effects of mannitol therapy include exacerbation of congestive heart failure (because of the initial intravascular volume load); volume contraction, hypokalemia, and profound hyperosmolality (after prolonged use); acute tubular necrosis (because of excessive hyperosmolality); and rebound increases in ICP.
- Patients treated repeatedly with mannitol require measurements of serum electrolytes and osmolality every 6 hours, and careful measurement of intake and output. Volume lost through urine should be replaced with NS (0.9%) to avoid volume depletion.

5. **Hyperventilation**

By acutely lowering the P_{CO_2} level to 28 to 32 mm Hg, *hyperventilation can lower ICP within minutes.* The alkylosis caused by hypocarbia leads to cerebral vasoconstriction, reduced cerebral blood volume, and decreased ICP.

- Hyperventilation is best accomplished by increasing the ventilatory rate (16 to 20 cycles/min) in mechanically ventilated patients, or by using a face mask with an Ambu bag in nonintubated patients.
- *The peak effect of hyperventilation on ICP is generally reached within 30 minutes.* Over the next 1 to 3 hours, the effect may gradually diminish as compensatory acid-base buffering mechanisms correct the alkylosis, but exceptions can occur.
- Once ICP is stabilized, hyperventilation should be tapered slowly over 6 to 12 hours, because abrupt

cessation can lead to vasodilatation and rebound increases in ICP.

Note: Beware that prolonged severe hyperventilation (PCO_2 less than 25 mm Hg) may actually exacerbate cerebral ischemia by causing excessive vasoconstriction.

6. **Pentobarbital**

High-dose barbiturate therapy, given in doses equivalent to those inducing general anesthesia, can effectively lower ICP in most patients refractory to the steps outlined above. The effect of pentobarbital is multifactorial but most likely stems from coupled decreases in cerebral metabolism, blood flow, and blood volume. In addition, pentobarbital causes profound hypotension and usually requires the use of vasopressors to maintain CPP at or higher than 70 mm Hg.

- **Pentobarbital typically requires a loading dose of 10 to 20 mg/kg, given in repeated 5 mg/kg boluses,** until a state of flaccid coma with preserved pupillary reactivity is attained. IV pressors (dopamine, phenylephrine) should be ready at the bedside to maintain BP and CPP.
- **Maintenance doses are usually 1 to 4 mg/kg/hr (order as 500 mg/250 ml NS, starting at 35 ml/hr).** Continuous or intermittent EEG monitoring should be used, with the infusion rate titrated to a burst-suppression pattern.
- If ICP is adequately controlled with pentobarbital, it is generally maintained for 24 to 48 hours. It can then be discontinued abruptly, with a washout period lasting from 24 to 96 hours.
- Failure of ICP to respond to pentobarbital is an ominous sign. If ICP remains markedly elevated (higher than 30 mm Hg), discontinuation of all aggressive measures should be considered.

7. **Hypothermia**

Lowering body temperature to 33°C can reduce ICP elevations that are refractory to CPP optimization, osmotherapy, hyperventilation, and pentobarbital anesthesia. In general this technique should be applied by experienced intensivists.

Dizziness and Vertigo

Dizziness and vertigo are among the most common neurologic complaints. The etiology of these conditions may range from benign labyrinthitis to serious cardiac syncope to life-threatening cerebellar hemorrhage. Vertigo may be defined specifically as a sensation of movement—either of the environment or of the patient. A spinning sensation is most commonly described, but feelings of acceleration or other movement may also be reported. Dizziness, on the other hand, may be used to mean vertigo, but it may also mean lightheadedness, fatigue, or a general sense of illness.

PHONE CALL

Questions

1. **Does the patient have a normal level of consciousness?**
   Vertigo followed by a decreased level of consciousness may be a sign of impending herniation, a neurologic emergency.
2. **When did the dizziness or vertigo begin?**
   In general, a more acute onset requires a greater urgency in making a diagnosis.
3. **What are the vital signs?**
   Rapid, slowed, or irregular heart rhythm may suggest cardiac syncope or cardioembolic stroke. Fever may suggest infection. Tachypnea may be a sign of heart failure or an anxiety attack.

Orders

1. Obtain a finger stick glucose.
2. Obtain orthostatic blood pressure.
3. Obtain an ECG.

Inform RN

"Will arrive at the bedside in . . . minutes."

ELEVATOR THOUGHTS

What is the differential diagnosis of dizziness and vertigo?

The most common causes of dizziness and vertigo are **orthostatic hypotension, medication side effect, benign positional vertigo,** and **labyrinthitis.** A more complete differential diagnosis follows.

V (vascular): brain stem stroke (most often pontine, brachium pontis, or cerebellar), cerebellar hemorrhage, AVM (rare), brain stem TIAs resulting from vertebrobasilar stenosis ("insufficiency") or embolism, vasodepressor syncope, postural hypotension, cardiac arrhythmia

I (infectious): syphilis, viral or bacterial meningitis, otitis media with labyrinthitis, Lyme disease involving the vestibular cranial nerve, viral cerebellitis (mostly in children)

T (traumatic): head trauma or postconcussional syndrome

A (autoimmune): multiple sclerosis

M (metabolic/toxic): diabetes with hypoglycemia, dehydration, drug toxicity (Table 13–1)

I (idiopathic/iatrogenic): benign positional vertigo, Meniere's disease

N (neoplastic): neurofibroma, schwannoma, or meningioma of the acoustic nerve; brain stem glioma; posterior fossa metastasis

S (seizure/psychiatric)

MAJOR THREAT TO LIFE

Cerebellar infarction or hemorrhage

TABLE 13–1 **Common Medications That Cause Vertigo and Dizziness***

Anticonvulsants: carbamazepine, phenytoin, primidone, ethosuximide, methsuximide
Antidepressants: nortriptyline and other tricyclic antidepressants
Antihypertensives: enalapril
Antihistamines: ranitidine, cimetidine
Antiarrhythmics: flecainide
Antibiotics: streptomycin, tobramycin, gentamicin
Analgesics: propoxyphene (Darvocet), naproxen, indomethacin
Neuroleptics: phenothiazines
Tranquilizers: diazepam, chlordiazepoxide, meprobamate
Aspirin
Digoxin

*Many medications have dizziness as a side effect. This is a partial list.

BEDSIDE

Quick Look Test

Is the patient awake and alert?

Lethargy may indicate a brain stem or cerebellar stroke with potential for herniation or progression to coma.

Selective History and Chart Review

1. **Is the dizziness lightheadedness or true vertigo?**

   Lightheadedness, a swimming sensation, faintness, or other similar symptoms point to a systemic disorder such as cardiac syncope, postural hypotension, or systemic infection. True **vertigo,** on the other hand, suggests neurologic dysfunction. The physical examination will help clarify the differential diagnosis, which will focus on distinguishing a peripheral cause from a central nervous system cause for vertigo.

2. **What is the time course of the symptoms?**

   As already noted, an acute onset of vertigo may indicate posterior fossa stroke or hemorrhage. Rapid onset of lightheadedness can occur with cardiac disease. A more gradual onset may suggest medication toxicity, infection, tumor, or demyelinating disease. If this is an episode in a series of recurrences, Meniere's disease or benign positional vertigo may be the cause.

3. **Do the symptoms change with changes in head position?**

   Dizziness on standing may indicate orthostatic hypotension; dizziness or vertigo with head turning may be a sign of benign positional vertigo or labyrinthitis.

4. **Has the patient begun any new medications recently?**

   Table 13–1 shows common medications that cause vertigo. Dizziness without true vertigo is one of the most common side effects of medication. Refer to the *Physician's Desk Reference* for medications not listed in the table.

5. **Are there any accompanying symptoms?**

   Ask about symptoms specific to the brain stem, including diplopia, dysarthria, and ataxia. Tinnitus may localize the problem to the inner ear. If there is posterior neck or head pain, consider vertebral artery dissection and stroke.

Selective Physical Examination

General Physical Examination

HEENT	Be sure to look into the external auditory canal for vesicles of herpes zoster. Unilateral hearing loss and tinnitus are reliable signs of injury outside the brain stem.

Abdomen   Hepatomegaly, ascites, and caput medusae are signs of chronic alcohol abuse.

Neurologic Examination

1. **Mental status**

   Ensure that the patient is awake, alert, and attentive. Decreased attentiveness may suggest drug toxicity or metabolic disarray. If there is vertigo with decreased alertness, see Chapter 5 for further management.

2. **Cranial nerves**

   Any cranial nerve abnormality in combination with dizziness or vertigo should be considered a sign of brain injury until it is proved otherwise.

   a. Nystagmus

   When vestibular input to the brain stem is disrupted (e.g., damage to the vestibular nerve or inner ear apparatus), the eyes will drift toward the affected side. Repeated corrective saccades result in nystagmus, with the fast phase away from the lesion. The sensation of movement experienced with vertigo is the illusion of environmental drift as the eyes move through the slow phase of nystagmus in the other direction. Corrective saccades are suppressed by visual tracking systems so that there is a sensation of continued field shift in one direction. Oscillopsia—the illusion of the environment's jumping or oscillating—is actually quite rare. Nystagmus subtypes are listed in Table 13–2. A common and crucial differential diagnosis that arises in almost every case of vertigo is whether the process is peripheral, and often benign, or whether it represents a lesion in the brain stem or cerebellum. Certain characteristics of nystagmus can help identify the site of pathology (Table 13–3).

   (1) Look for nystagmus in the primary gaze by having the patient fix on your finger. More subtle nystagmus can be seen by looking for oscillations of the fundus on indirect ophthalmoscopy.

   (2) Have the patient follow your finger through the full range of horizontal and vertical gaze. The hand should be kept at a distance of 2 to 3 feet to minimize convergence, which should be tested separately.

   (3) Provocative tests may be helpful in distinguishing peripheral from central injury.

   (a) Nystagmus should be looked for with the patient in different positions, particularly if the patient notes a positional component to the vertigo. The Bárány maneuver is useful in helping to distinguish the positional vertigo of a benign vestibular disorder from a brain stem lesion (Fig. 13–1).

TABLE 13–2 **Subtypes of Nystagmus**

Physiologic nystagmus
Fine nystagmus at ends of gaze, extinguishes after a few beats
Significance: none, if symmetric

Asymmetric horizontal nystagmus
Horizontal or rotational
Fast phase always in one direction
Worse with gaze in one direction than in the other
Often made worse with change in head position
Significance: most often labyrinthine or vestibular disease (benign
positional vertigo, labyrinthitis, Meniere's disease), but may be due
to cerebellar or brain stem lesions

Vertical nystagmus
Upbeat or downbeat nystagmus
May be present with sedative or anticonvulsant medication
Significance: if no drug toxicity is present, vertical nystagmus almost
always means brain stem disease at the midbrain or craniocervical
junction

Dissociated or abduction nystagmus
Unilateral horizontal fast component in direction of gaze in the
abducted eye
Significance: internuclear ophthalmoplegia (e.g., in multiple sclerosis)

Convergence-retraction nystagmus
Part of Parinaud's syndrome of impaired upgaze, impaired pupillary
reaction, convergence insufficiency
Fast component is convergence and retraction of both globes
Significance: mass lesion compression of the tectum of the midbrain,
for example, by pineal tumor, or a midbrain stroke in the region of
the aqueduct of Sylvius

Pendular nystagmus
Usually horizontal
Sinusoidal waveform (oscillation, equal velocity in either direction)
Significance: congenital; if acquired, most commonly multiple
sclerosis; also cerebrovascular disease of the cerebellum or brain
stem

Periodic alternating nystagmus
Horizontal, with fast phase alternating directions in cycles of 1 to 3
minutes
May coexist with downbeat nystagmus
Significance: congenital or acquired lesions at the craniocervical
junction

Ocular dysmetria
Overshooting on attempt to refix on an eccentric target (e.g., moving
from the examiner's nose to a finger held to the side)
Overshooting may be followed by ever-shortening saccadic corrections
Significance: cerebellar disease

Ocular bobbing
Repetitive rapid conjugate downward movement followed by slow
drift back to primary position
Found in comatose patients
Significance: severe central pontine destruction

TABLE 13–3 **Characteristics of Nystagmus Arising from Peripheral or Central Causes**

Nystagmus from peripheral causes
    Extinguishes with repetitive provocative maneuvers
    Exhibits latency of several seconds with provocative maneuvers
    Rotational nystagmus
    Hearing loss or tinnitus
    No accompanying brain stem signs
Nystagmus from central causes
    Any vertical nystagmus
    Accompanying brain stem signs
    Does not extinguish with provocative maneuvers
    No latency with provocative maneuvers

A rotational component, a latency of a few seconds in onset of the nystagmus, and a lessening of the magnitude of the response with subsequent trials all suggest peripheral lesions.

(b) Injecting cold water into the ear on the side of an intact vestibular pathway (see Fig. 5–3) will result in nystagmus, with the fast component beating away from the stimulus. If the patient is comatose, cold water will induce the ipsiversive gaze with no contralateral corrective saccades. Be sure you view an intact tympanic membrane before attempting this test. Also be warned that the stimulus may produce nausea in an awake patient.

b. Diplopia, dysarthria, facial motor or sensory asymmetry, decreased gag response, or asymmetry of tongue protrusion

Any of these should alert you to the possibility of a CNS lesion.

3. **Cerebellar**

Evaluate for limb ataxia and gait ataxia.

MANAGEMENT

1. **Rule out a posterior fossa mass lesion.**

Because the consequences of missing a cerebellar hematoma or posterior fossa tumor can be serious, a **noncontrast CT scan** should be obtained in all cases of first-time vertigo, particularly in the elderly, and certainly if there is any hint of brain stem involvement. CT is poor at identifying smaller lesions and infarcts in the posterior fossa because of the substantial bony artifact. If a brain stem lesion is suspected but not identified on CT, an **MRI scan** should be obtained.

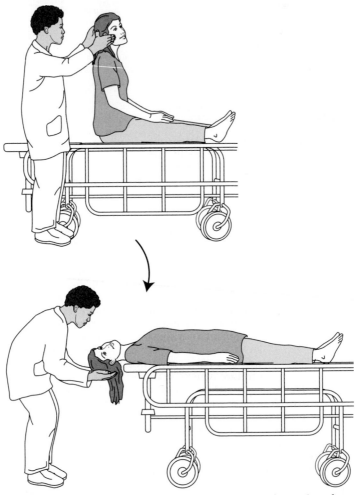

Figure 13–1 Bárány maneuver. The physician moves the patient from a sitting to a supine position, with the head rotated to one side and hyperextended 30 degrees. The test is positive if vertigo is recreated. Nystagmus should be seen with the onset of symptomatic vertigo.

2. **Correct any obvious metabolic disorder,** or discontinue, taper, or substitute any toxic medication. Treat cardiac syncope if present.
3. **Identify a possible peripheral cause.**

    If no posterior fossa lesion and no metabolic abnormality are identified, a peripheral cause for vertigo may be present.

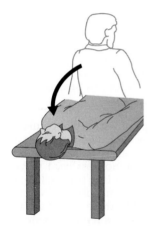

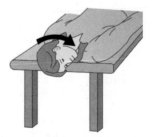

Step 1: Move from sitting to reclining position with the head extended 45 degrees over the end of the table, turned with the "bad" ear down (e.g., left)

Step 2: Turn the head to the right slowly over 1 minute

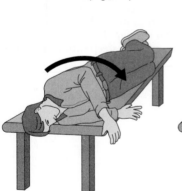

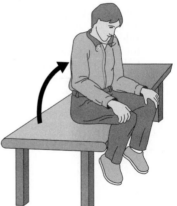

Step 3: Roll over onto the right side, with the head looking down at the floor

Step 4: Slowly return to sitting position with the chin tilted down

Figure 13–2 Four-step canalith repositioning procedure for benign positional vertigo (modified Epley maneuver). The clinician should support and rotate the patient's head in steps 1 and 2.

Such causes include labyrinthitis (postinfectious congestion or inflammation of the labyrinths), Meniere's disease (recurrent attacks of severe vertigo, nausea and vomiting, tinnitus, and hearing loss), and benign positional vertigo. An **electronystagmogram** may be useful in making a diagnosis of peripheral vestibulopathy. An audiogram may be useful in diagnosing Meniere's disease.

4. **Treat benign positional vertigo empirically.**

Benign positional vertigo is a type of vertigo that occurs in adults over 50 years of age. This type of vertigo is thought to arise when particulate debris accumulates in the posterior semicircular canal. Particular head positions or head movement may cause the particles to stimulate hair cells and produce the sensation of movement. Benign positional vertigo may respond to **meclizine 25 mg PO three times a day.** Central causes of dizziness generally do not respond to meclizine. Nonmedicational treatment of benign positional vertigo has been successful in many cases. The two approaches are desensitization exercises, in which the patient moves through a series of repetitive head and body positions twice daily, and canalith repositioning procedures, such as the modified Epley maneuver, in which the head is rotated slowly from the bad side to the good side in an effort to move the particles out of the posterior semicircular canal (see Fig. 13–2). Following the Epley maneuver, the patient is asked to sleep sitting up for two nights.

Headache

Headache is one of the most common complaints presenting to neurologists. In general, headaches can be grouped into two broad diagnostic categories. One group comprises the **primary headache** disorders, for example, migraine, tension-type, and cluster headaches. The second category comprises **secondary headaches** resulting from intracranial lesions, systemic diseases, or local diseases of the eye or nasopharynx. The goal in evaluating headache is to establish the diagnosis and initiate effective treatment.

PHONE CALL

Questions

1. **How severe is the headache?**

    Remember that severity is subjective and you should ask how the attacks disable the patient.

2. **Does the headache reach full intensity instantly or gradually?**

    Sudden onset of extremely severe headache is suggestive of subarachnoid hemorrhage, meningitis, or dural sinus thrombosis. Benign headaches can occasionally have a "thunderclap" presentation, but the more ominous causes need to be excluded. When patients describe a new attack as, "the worst headache of my life," consider a secondary headache. However, the "worst headache of my life" is usually their worst migraine. A subarachnoid hemorrhage must be considered when the headache reaches full intensity in an instant.

3. **How long does the headache last?**

    Migraines typically last 4 to 72 hours. Cluster typically lasts 30 to 180 minutes. Chronic migraine and chronic tension-type headaches are often continuous.

4. **When did the headaches begin and have they been continuous or progressive?**

    Headaches with a recent onset that have become continuous for several days or progressively worse over time suggest

175

a symptomatic etiology such as subarachnoid hemorrhage, subdural hematoma, brain abscess, or brain tumor. A stable headache pattern over years is almost always indicative of a primary headache. Remember, having a primary headache such as migraine or tension does not grant an individual immunity to developing tumors or infections. Worsening of a preexisting headache type should raise concern over the development of a secondary headache.

5. **What are the vital signs?**

    Significant hypertension can cause headache or trigger a migraine. Fever generally suggests an infection or inflammatory disorder.

6. **Has there been a change in level of consciousness?**

    This always suggests an ominous headache. Never assume a primary headache syndrome in a person with an impaired sensorium. Basilar migraine can present with an impaired sensorium, but all such individuals require a careful evaluation before that diagnosis can be made.

7. **Is the patient experiencing nausea or vomiting?**

    Nausea and vomiting most often occur with severe migraine but can also accompany conditions associated with increased ICP.

Orders

1. Place the patient in a quiet, darkened room.
2. Start D5NS IV at 80 ml/hr if nausea and vomiting are severe.
3. Obtain a body temperature
4. Order an ESR and a CBC, particularly if the patient is older than 50 years of age.
5. If you are confident that the headache represents a chronic, recurrent, and previously diagnosed primary headache, the patient can be treated with an agent that has previously relieved the headache or with injectable **sumatriptan,** intravenous **dihydroergotamine (DHE),** intravenous **prochlorperazine,** or **ketorolac** (see dosages in Table 14–1).

ELEVATOR THOUGHTS

What causes headache?

Primary Headache Disorders

1. Tension-type headache
2. Migraine headache
3. Cluster headache
4. Paroxysmal hemicranias
5. Trigeminal neuralgia

TABLE 14–1 **Selected Medications Used for Acute Therapy of Migraine**

Serotonin (5-HT1B/1D) Receptor Agonists (Triptans)

Sumatriptan (Imitrex)	6 mg SQ, may repeat after 1h, max 12 mg qd; 25-100 mg PO, repeat q2h PRN, max 200 mg qd (25-, 50-mg tabs); 20 mg nasal spray, repeat q2h PRN, max 40 mg qd (spray 5, 20 mg)
Naratriptan (Amerge)	2.5 mg PO may repeat after 4h, max 5 mg qd (1-, 2.5-mg tabs)
Rizatriptan (Maxalt)	5-10 mg PO may repeat after 2h, max 30 mg qd (5-, 10-mg tabs)
Zolmitriptan (Zomig)	2.5-5 mg PO STAT, can repeat once after 2 hours, max 10 mg qd; nasal spray 5 mg, may repeat once after 2 hours
Frovatriptan (Frova)	2.5-mg tablets, may repeat once after 4 hours if needed
Almotriptan (Axert)	6.25- and 12.5-mg tablets, may repeat after 2 hours, (max 25 mg daily)
Eletriptan (Relpax)	40-mg tablets, may repeat once if needed

Nonsteroidal Anti-inflammatory Agents (NSAIDs)

Acetaminophen (Tylenol)	650-975 mg PO q4h PRN (325-mg tabs)
Aspirin	650-975 mg PO q4h PRN (325-mg tabs)
Diclofenac (Cataflam)	100 mg PO STAT, 50 mg PO q8h PRN (50-mg tabs)
Indomethacin (Indocin)	25-50 mg PO/PRN q8h PRN (25-, 50-mg caps, 50-mg supp)
Ibuprofen (Motrin, Advil)	400-800 mg q6h PRN (200-, 400-, 600-, 800-mg tabs)
Ketorolac (Toradol)	10 mg q4h PRN, up to 5 days total duration (10-mg tabs)
Naproxen (Naprosyn)	500-1000 mg at onset, 250-375 mg q4h PRN (250-, 375-, 500-mg tabs)
Piroxicam (Feldene)	20 mg PO qd (10-, 20-mg tabs)
Sulindac (Clinoril)	150-200 mg PO qd (150-, 200-mg tabs)

Non-narcotic Analgesic Combinations

Acetaminophen/butalbital/ caffeine (Fioricet, Esgic)	1-2 tabs q4h PRN, max 6 per day, 325/50/40 mg, Should not be used more than twice weekly
Aspirin/butalbital/caffeine (Fiorinal)	1-2 tabs q4h PRN, max 6 per day; 325/50/40 mg, should not be used more than twice weekly
Isometheptene/ acetaminophen/ dichloralphenazone (Midrin)	2 capsules at onset, repeat 1 q1h PRN, 65/325/100 mg, maximum of 5 per day, 10 per week

TABLE 14–1 **Selected Medications Used for Acute Therapy of Migraine—cont'd**

Ergot Medications

Ergotamine/caffeine (Cafergot, Ercaf, Wigraine)	1-2 tabs PO at onset 1/100 mg repeat q30 min PRN, max 6 tabs/attack; suppositories 2/100 mg PRN, up to 2 per attack; should not be used more than twice weekly
Dihydroergotamine (DHE-45, Migranal nasal spray)	1 mg IV/IM/SC, repeat q1h PRN, max 2 mg IV or 3 mg SC/IM qd; nasal spray 1 in each nostril, repeat q15 min PRN, max 6 sprays/day (0.5 mg per spray)

Symptomatic Headache Disorders

1. Vascular
   - Subarachnoid hemorrhage
   - Intracerebral hemorrhage
   - Cerebral infarction
2. Infectious
   - Meningitis
   - Sinusitis
   - Infections remote from the nervous system
3. Post-traumatic headache
4. Increased intracranial pressure
   - Intracranial mass lesions (brain tumor, hemorrhage, abscess, etc.)
   - Malignant hypertension
   - Idiopathic intracranial hypertension (pseudotumor cerebri)
5. Decreased intracranial pressure
   - Spontaneous intracranial hypotension
   - Postlumbar puncture headache
6. Giant cell arteritis
7. Drug exposure or withdrawal
   - Nitrate exposure
   - Selective serotonin reuptake inhibitors; trazodone
   - Calcium channel blockers
   - Caffeine withdrawal
   - The overuse of any analgesics used to treat headache attacks

MAJOR THREAT TO LIFE

- **Subarachnoid hemorrhage**
  Aneurysmal subarachnoid hemorrhage, if not properly diagnosed, can lead to fatal rebleeding.
- **Bacterial meningitis**
  Bacterial meningitis must be recognized early if antibiotic treatment is to be successful.
- **Herniation from intracranial mass lesions**
  Herniation may occur as a result of a tumor, subdural or epidural hematoma, brain abscess, or any other mass lesion.

BEDSIDE

Quick Look Test

Does the patient look well (comfortable), sick (uncomfortable), or critical (about to die)?
Most patients with chronic headache look well, whereas those with severe migraines, subarachnoid hemorrhage, or meningitis look sick.

Airway and Vital Signs

What is the body temperature?
Fever associated with headache suggests meningitis. However, headache can also represent a nonspecific reaction to a systemic febrile illness.

What is the BP?
Contrary to popular belief, headache is rarely caused by hypertension, unless the hypertension is acute and severe (diastolic pressure greater than 120 mm Hg). Hypertension may also reflect subarachnoid hemorrhage, acute stroke, or increased ICP from an intracranial mass lesion.

Selective History and Chart Review

A detailed, well-focused history is the most important tool in diagnosing the cause of headache. The following questions are important:

1. **What is the quality of the pain?**
   Tension-type headache is frequently described as tight, aching, and band like. Migraine and headaches caused by infection often have a throbbing quality, although 40% of the time migraine is nonthrobbing.

2. **Where is the pain located?**
   Tension-type headache is usually generalized and most prominent in the neck, occiput, and forehead. Alternating

unilateral headaches suggest migraine. Cluster headaches are periorbital, maxillary, or supraorbital and always unilateral.

3. **What time of day do the headaches occur?**

Tension-type headaches typically develop in the late morning or the early afternoon and resolve with sleep. Cluster headaches often strike after the patient has gone to sleep and tend to occur at the same time every day.

4. **Do warning symptoms occur before the headaches begin?**

Migraine is often preceded by prodromal symptoms of hunger, restlessness, yawning, depression, or euphoria. "Classic migraine," now referred to as "migraine with aura," is preceded by a transient neurologic symptom that is usually visual (i.e., scintillating scotomas) but can involve lateralized numbness, weakness, or aphasia. Neurologic symptoms that persist once the headache has started can occur in migraine but also suggest a structural lesion (i.e., neoplasm or arterio-venous malformation, or cerebral infarction).

5. **Do any factors precipitate the headaches?**

Migraine is frequently precipitated by emotional stress or relaxation following stress, fatigue, alcohol, hunger, or menstruation.

6. **Are any symptoms associated with the headache?**

Nausea, vomiting, photophobia, and phonophobia are highly characteristic of migraine. Ipsilateral tearing or nasal congestion occurs with cluster headache or migraine.

7. **Is there a history of chronic or recurring headaches?**

The longer a headache has lasted in its present form, the more likely it is to be benign. Headaches that are qualitatively different from previous headaches should raise suspicion for a symptomatic etiology.

8. **Do headaches run in the family?**

Migraine is familial in approximately 80% of cases. Cluster is only rarely seen in multiple family members.

Selective Physical Examination

In most patients with headache, the neurologic and physical examinations are normal. The primary purpose of the initial screening examination is to check for signs of meningismus, increased intra-cranial pressure, or neurologic focality. The main focus should be on examination of the head, ears, nose and throat, and neck.

HEENT   Sinus tenderness (sinusitis)

Temporal artery tenderness (temporal arteritis or migraine)

Conjunctival injection (cluster headache)

Eye: Corneal clouding, scleral injection, conjunctival injection (a red eye), or decreased visual acuity suggests an ocular cause of head pain. Note that most head pain is referred to the eye and temple; if the eye is "white" and the pain is in the eye, it is unlikely that the pain is ocular in origin.

Cranial bruit: (arteriovenous malformation)

Neck   Check for nuchal rigidity, Kernig's, or Brudzinski's signs (Fig. 14–1) (subarachnoid hemorrhage or meningitis), and cervical muscle spasm (tension-type headache or migraine).

Selective Neurologic Examination

1. Level of consciousness
2. Confusion or disorientation
3. Pupillary symmetry
4. Papilledema and spontaneous venous pulsations
5. Retinal hemorrhages (flame or subhyaloid)
6. Pronator drift

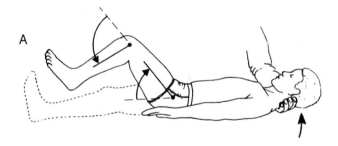

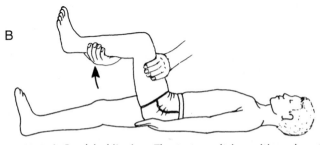

Figure 14–1 *A*, Brudzinski's sign. The test result is positive when the patient actively flexes the hips and knees in response to passive neck flexion by the examiner. *B*, Kernig's sign. The test result is positive when pain or resistance prevents full extension of the knee from the 90-degree hip/knee flexion position. (From Marshall SA, Ruedy J: On Call: Principles and Protocols, 4th ed. Philadelphia, Elsevier, 2004.)

7. Deep tendon and plantar reflexes
8. Gait: hemiparetic, ataxic, observe arm swing at the same time

RADIOLOGIC EVALUATION

Radiologic testing is not necessary if the patient has a long history of characteristic primary headaches (migraine, tension-type, or cluster), a normal neurologic examination, and no fever or meningismus.

1. **Obtain a CT scan in patients with the following:**
   - Extremely severe headache reaching full intensity instantly (thunderclap headache)
   - Headache with progressive onset over days to weeks that is not similar to previous headaches
   - Altered mental status (even if intoxicated)
   - Focal neurologic signs
   - Papilledema, subhyaloid hemorrhages
2. **If subarachnoid hemorrhage or meningitis is suspected and the CT scan is negative, a follow-up LP is mandatory.**

   Fifteen percent of patients with aneurysmal subarachnoid hemorrhage have a negative CT scan. In these instances, the diagnosis can be made only by CSF examination (increased numbers of red blood cells and xanthochromia are present).

   When bacterial meningitis is suspected, it is a good idea to obtain a CT scan before performing an LP, as long as administration of antibiotics is not delayed. CT scanning prior to LP is mandatory in those with a depressed level of consciousness, neurologic focality, papilledema, or AIDS, because of the increased likelihood of detecting a mass lesion. As long as the patient does not look terribly ill, antibiotics should be held until after the LP, as long as both the CT and LP can be performed within 1 hour. Otherwise, treat first, keeping in mind that the CSF culture results may be negative. Empirical treatment of suspected meningitis in healthy adults consists of **ceftriaxone 1 g IV every 12 hours** and **vancomycin IV 1 g every 12 hours.**

MANAGEMENT: SPECIFIC DISORDERS AND THEIR TREATMENT

Migraine Headache

The term, "migraine" is often used erroneously to describe any severe headache. However, migraine is a specific clinical syndrome with a distinct pathophysiology. The diagnosis of migraine is based not only on the quality and location of the pain (i.e., often throbbing

TABLE 14–2 **Checklist of Common Migraine Triggers**

Alcohol (e.g., red wine)
Environmental factors (e.g., weather, altitude, time zone changes)
Caffeine (e.g., coffee, chocolate)
Monosodium glutamate (MSG; found in Chinese food)
Nitrates (e.g., processed foods, hot dogs)
Bright lights and glare
Hormonal changes in women (e.g., menstrual cycle)
Hunger
Sleep deprivation
Medications (over-the-counter and prescription)
Emotional stress

and unilateral) but on the characteristic symptoms associated with the headache, a recurrent pattern to the attacks, the headache duration, and the triggers of the attack (Table 14–2).

Migraine without Aura (Common Migraine)

Migraine without aura is defined by the following criteria:
1. **Recurrent headaches of 4 to 72 hours' duration with at least two of the following characteristics:**
   - Unilateral location
   - Pulsating quality
   - Severe enough in intensity to limit daily activity
   - Aggravated by physical activity
2. **In addition, at least one of the following characteristics must be present:**
   - Nausea or vomiting
   - Photophobia and phonophobia
        Eighty percent of migraines have no aura. Migraine pain does not have to be unilateral and, in fact, is bilateral in 40% of cases. Neck pain is commonly seen with migraine and does not mean that the diagnosis is tension-type headache. The pain of migraine is not always pulsatile.

Migraine with Aura (Classic Migraine)

This condition consists of typical migraine headache pain associated with, and generally preceded by, an aura—a fully reversible symptom indicative of focal cerebral dysfunction. Auras have their onset over at least 4 minutes and last less than an hour. Therefore the focal symptoms do not reach full intensity immediately. In the typical patient experiencing migraine with aura, the aura precedes the headache by 10 to 20 minutes, and the headache follows within an hour. In some patients, aura may persist into the headache phase, or the aura may occur without the subsequent development of headache (accompanied migraine). These rules are important because one third of patients with TIAs or strokes get headache, and it is necessary to differentiate these from migraines with aura.

Common types of aura include the following:

- **Homonymous visual disturbance.** Often occurs with scintillating (i.e., sparkling) objects and blind spots, or zigzag lines enlarging in the periphery
- **Unilateral paresthesias or numbness.** The paresthesias often are seen in the beginning and are replaced by numbness as the attack progresses
- **Unilateral weakness**
- **Aphasia or other language disorder**

Migraine with Prolonged Aura or Migrainous Infarction (Complicated Migraine)

This refers to a migraine headache with particularly prolonged or persistent neurologic deficits, suggestive of cerebral infarction. In these patients, all vasoconstrictors such as ergots or triptans should be avoided because they may precipitate cerebral infarction. In patients with documented infarction, antiphospholipid antibodies or other hypercoagulable conditions should be ruled out.

Status Migrainosus

This refers to a state of prolonged severe migraine, generally exceeding 3 days in duration. In some cases, treatment for status migrainosus may require hospitalization for IV hydration and intravenous therapy.

Opthalmoplegic Migraine

This unusual variant of migraine begins with periorbital headache and is accompanied by vomiting. As the headache progresses, ptosis and opthalmoplegia may develop.

Treatment

Start by identifying and eliminating triggers. Many women experience fewer migraines after discontinuing oral contraceptives. Alcohol, excessive caffeine use, stress or relaxation following stress, over- or undersleeping, hunger, and menstruation commonly precipitate attacks in a migrainous patient.

Most patients presenting to the physician with migraines have disabling attacks, whereas those who suffer mild migraines commonly self-treat with success and do not seek medical attention. Moderate-to-severe migraine headaches require acute therapy, usually with a triptan, which should be taken as soon as possible after the start of the headache in an attempt to cut it short *(abortive therapy)*. Triptans and ergots are contraindicated in patients with cardiovascular, cerebrovascular, and peripheral vascular disease. In attacks that are historically disabling, it is important to avoid "step care," because this approach causes a delay in using the most effective treatments. The goal of therapy is to be free of all migraine symptoms within 2 hours. The overriding principle of acute migraine therapy is to treat early in the attack and with a sufficiently high dose of medication.

The response to a triptan, or any migraine medication, should not be considered a diagnostic test of migraine. Seven triptans are available in the United States, all in tablet form. **Sumatriptan** is also available in injectable and nasal spray formulations, which have an advantage over tablets when nausea or vomiting is prominent. **Zolmitriptan** is also available as an intranasal formulation. Agents used for acute therapy of migraine, including the triptans, are listed in Table 14–1. Adjunctive therapy with antiemetics (**metoclopramide 10 to 20 mg orally every 6 hours,** or **prochlorperazine suppositories 25 mg every 8 hours**) may be added to reduce nausea and vomiting.

Mild migraine headaches may respond to symptomatic treatment with nonsteroidal anti-inflammatory drugs (NSAIDs) such as **ibuprofen** or **naproxen,** or occasionally combination medications (**Fioricet, Esgic, Midrin,** etc.). **Butalbital**-containing medications, in particular, if used more than twice a week, have a high likelihood of triggering drug-induced headaches (rebound headaches).

Those with frequent disabling attacks of migraine (more than one or two per week) or who fail to respond to acute therapy alone are candidates for preventive therapy. Agents used for migraine prevention are listed in Table 14–3. Beta blockers, tricyclic antidepressants, and antiepileptics such as **valproic acid** and **topiramate** are the usual first-line agents. Preventive medications in migraine may have a latency period of several weeks before they become effective. Side effects are often most prominent during this period when the agents are ineffective, and patients should be encouraged to give these agents an adequate trial.

Protocols for the *emergency room treatment of severe migraine* are shown in Table 14–4. In most cases, those seeking care in the emergency room have prolonged attacks, and the usual oral therapies are not likely to be effective. Intravenous hydration is important for those with intractable vomiting. If injectable sumatriptan is unsuccessful, "cocktail" treatment with prochlorperazine, DHE, and dexamethasone can break the cycle of intractable migraine in most patients. The use of DHE is contraindicated within 24 hours of the use of a triptan (and vice versa). Opioids are less effective in the treatment of migraine than they are for visceral pain syndromes. In some cases, the migraine headache can last for days (*status migrainosus*). In these cases the addition of a corticosteroid such as dexamethasone 2 to 6 mg every 6 hours to any acute therapy will reduce the likelihood of symptom recurrence.

TABLE 14–3 **Drugs Used for Preventive Therapy of Migraine**

Beta Blockers	
Propranolol (Inderal, Inderal LA)	40-320 mg daily (10-, 20-, 40-, 60-, 80-mg tabs qid; 60-, 80-, 120-, 160-mg long-acting tabs bid)
Nadolol (Corgard)	20-120 mg qd (20-, 40-, 80-, 120-mg tabs)
Atenolol (Tenormin)	25-100 mg qd (25-, 50-, 100-mg tabs)
Tricyclic Antidepressants	
Amitriptyline (Elavil)	25-200 mg qhs (10-, 25-, 50-, 75-mg tabs)
Nortriptyline (Pamelor)	25-200 mg qhs (10-, 25-, 50-, 75-mg tabs)
Doxepin (Sinequan)	25-200 mg qhs (25-, 50-, 75-, 100- and 150-mg tabs)
Anticonvulsants	
Valproic acid (Depakote, Depakene)	250-1500 mg PO daily (125, 250, 500 mg tid)
Topiramate (Topamax)	50-200 mg daily (25-, 100-mg tabs)
Calcium Channel Blockers	
Verapamil (Calan, Calan SR)	80-160 mg daily (40-, 80-, 120-mg tabs q8h; sustained release 120-, 180-, 240-mg qd)
Antiserotonin Drugs	
Cyproheptadine (Periactin)	2-4 mg qid (4-mg tabs)
MAO Inhibitor	
Phenelzine (Nardil)	15-30 mg PO tid (15-mg tabs); careful training of both practitioner and patient is essential when these are used

Tension-Type Headache

Tension-type headaches were previously known as "muscle contraction headaches," although muscle contraction and psychologic tension have little to do with the pathogenesis. Most people experience tension-type headaches to some degree, and the pain is usually mild and successfully treated with over-the-counter medications. Although tension-type headaches are the most common headache type, only 3% of those presenting for a medical evaluation of their recurring headaches have tension-type headaches. Most patients describing tension-type headache have multiple headache types, and

TABLE 14–4 **Protocol for the Emergency Room Treatment of Migraine**

Mild-to-moderate migraine
Administer sumatriptan 6 mg SC.
Prolonged, refractory, or severe migraine
1. Insert IV line or Heparin-lock. Hydrate with D5NS 80-100 ml/hr for persistent vomiting.
2. **Prochlorperazine (Compazine) 10 mg IV over 5 minutes;** repeat every 20 minutes to max of 30 mg. Observe for orthostatic hypotension and dyskinesias.
3. If no response, administer dihydroergotamine **(DHE 45 1 mg IV push over 2 minutes);** do not use if a triptan has been administered in the last 24 hours.
4. Follow with **dexamethasone (Decadron) 4 to 12 mg IV.**
5. Repeat 1 mg DHE 45 every 1 to 2 hours as needed (maximum 3 mg/day).
6. Consider **IV valproic acid (1000 mg in 50 cc of normal saline, administered over 5 minutes).**
7. Consider **magnesium sulfate 1-2 g intravenously.**

---

their tension-type headache is part of the spectrum of their migraines. Headaches that never go away or that grow worse as the day progresses suggest tension-type headache. The pain is usually bilateral, most prominent in the occiput and frontal regions, and described as tight, pressing, or band like. Associated neck and scalp muscle tightness is common, but no prominent sensory or autonomic symptoms are seen, such as photophobia, phonophobia, and nausea or vomiting. *Chronic daily headache* usually refers to chronic tension-type headaches or migraines that are often, but not invariably, associated with overuse of acute drugs.

Treatment

Most patients respond to relaxation techniques and NSAIDs such as ibuprofen or naproxen (see Table 14–1). An antidepressant may be helpful, although the success of tricyclic antidepressants in headache treatment is independent of their antidepressant effect. Muscle relaxants are of little value in the treatment of these headaches.

Medication Overuse Headache

Those suffering from episodic headaches, upon taking excessive drugs in the attempt to obtain relief, can transform their episodic attacks into chronic daily headaches. Most of these individuals are migraineurs. Over a period of weeks to months, they develop a generalized, pervasive headache with superimposed paroxysms of the original headache type. If the patient has chronic daily headache caused by medication overuse, it is necessary to taper and discontinue the analgesics. There is little possibility of a spontaneous remission, and these individuals need to stop the offending agent. Prescribing additional analgesics only prolongs the problem. While the patient is suffering from these attacks, preventive medications should be initiated, even though they will not be immediately effective. Acute medications should be significantly limited in frequency. Caffeine use should also be limited in these patients because of the ability of caffeine to cause rebound headaches. Patients with medication-induced headache never improve while they are overusing these agents.

Cluster Headache

Cluster headache is characterized by excruciating unilateral head pain, is often localized to the orbit, temple, and cheek, and is associated with ipsilateral tearing, conjunctival injection, and nasal congestion. Men are affected three times more often than are women. The pain is described as sharp, boring, and piercing and occurs in brief episodes (15 minutes to 3 hours) without prodrome or aura. The pain develops to full intensity over a few minutes (shorter time than a migraine, longer time than a subarachnoid hemorrhage), and ipsilateral facial flushing, Horner's syndrome, and exacerbation of symptoms by alcohol are often noted. Although migraineurs prefer to lie in bed in a dark room with attacks, cluster patients pace relentlessly and often exhibit manic behavior. The headaches occur in "clusters," during which time sufferers develop one or more attacks daily for a period of 2 weeks to 3 months, interspersed by headache-free intervals lasting from months to years. Cluster headaches occur most commonly in the early morning or late at night, often awakening the person out of sleep ("alarm clock headaches"), and they frequently occur with regularity at a particular time of day.

Treatment

Cluster headaches are not a variant of migraine and require different treatment.

1. **Sumatriptan 6 mg SC** is the only form of sumatriptan and the only triptan appropriate for the treatment of cluster.

2. **Oxygen 100% at 8 to 12 L/min** using a non-rebreathing mask should be initiated as soon as the attack begins and continued for 5 minutes after the attack is terminated. Patients should be instructed to inhale deeply but not hyperventilate. Many cluster patients are smokers and need to be advised of the dangers of smoking while using oxygen.

4. **DHE 1 mg IV** can be used by the emergency room but cannot be self-administered at home. An intravenous antiemetic must be administered prior to the use of intravenous DHE to avoid vomiting.

5. **Lidocaine 4% 1 ml intranasally** for attacks centering in the cheek or upper teeth: For those experiencing the predomi-

nance of pain in the eye and temple, this will not be very effective. Patients are instructed to lie on a bed and extend their head 30 degrees and laterally rotate their head 30 degrees to the side of the attack. The lidocaine is dispensed in a dropper bottle and released far into the nose, and the head position is maintained for 5 minutes.

Analgesics, including opioids, are notoriously ineffective in the treatment of cluster. In almost all cluster headache patients, prophylactic medications are required. Commonly used preventive agents include the following:

1. **Prednisone 60 to 80 mg per day,** slowly tapered
2. **Verapamil 240 to 720 mg daily**
3. **Lithium 300 mg three to four times a day**
4. **Valproate 500 to 1500 mg daily**
5. **Topiramate 75 to 200 mg daily**

Individuals experiencing a cluster are generally started on prednisone and concomitantly placed on verapamil with lithium, valproate, or topiramate. Frequently the verapamil needs to be increased to 720 mg in order to be effective. The prednisone is tapered over 2 to 3 weeks, during which time the other prophylactic agents are increased into a therapeutic range. Acute therapies need to be made available to these sufferers throughout their cluster period. After several weeks, when the patient appears to be free from attacks, the prophylactic medications are slowly withdrawn.

Postconcussion Headache

After concussion, patients may complain of headache, dizziness, poor concentration, and irritability (postconcussional syndrome). Brain imaging is normal, as is the neurologic examination, except for the occasional finding of nystagmus. In many cases, there is coexisting depression, anxiety, or potential for secondary gain, such as a disability claim or litigation.

Treatment

Begin with NSAIDs (see Table 14–1) and provide reassurance; in most cases, the symptoms remit over a period of weeks to months. In protracted cases with depressive symptoms, a tricyclic antidepressant or centrally acting muscle relaxant (**tizanidine 4 mg tid** or **baclofen 10 mg tid**) might be used. Headaches following head injury can be multifactorial, and evaluations of the facet joints and brain (ruling out a chronic subdural hematoma or hydrocephalus) are appropriate even if the initial evaluation was nonrevealing.

Idiopathic Intracranial Hypertension (Pseudotumor Cerebri)

Also known as "benign intracranial hypertension," this illness is characterized by the triad of headache, papilledema, and increased ICP in the absence of an intracranial mass lesion or hydrocephalus.

The disease occurs most commonly in young obese women; however, this patient profile is not invariable. The key to establishing the diagnosis is excluding other causes of increased ICP, including a mass lesion, dural sinus thrombosis, chronic meningitis, hypervitaminosis A, and tetracycline or corticosteroid exposure. Depressed level of consciousness and focal neurologic deficits do not occur, except for occasional CN6 palsies, which represent a nonspecific sign of increased intracranial pressure. The main hazard in idiopathic intracranial hypertension is visual loss that results from optic nerve damage and can be permanent.

Whenever idiopathic intracranial hypertension is suspected, MRI of the brain and magnetic resonance venography should be performed to rule out a mass lesion, hydrocephalus, or dural sinus thrombosis. If the MRI is normal, LP establishes the diagnosis by the finding of normal CSF under increased pressure (greater than 20 cm H_2O).

Treatment

Approximately one third of patients have spontaneous remission of headache after the first LP. Many patients will respond to repeated LPs and removal of CSF performed every few days to every few weeks. However, medication therapy is generally recommended. In the extremely obese, weight reduction is recommended. Acetazolamide 250 to 500 mg three times a day or furosamide 40 to 80 mg daily can reduce CSF production and ICP. **Topiramate 50 to 300 mg bid,** a carbonic anhydrase inhibitor that often causes weight loss, can also be used. All of these patients need to have baseline visual field and acuity testing and serial visual field testing to evaluate their blind spots. Fundus photography can be helpful, because the resolution of the headache and the visual problems do not necessary parallel each other. If visual loss progresses despite medical therapy, a lumboperitoneal shunt or optic nerve sheath fenestration may be necessary.

Temporal (Giant Cell) Arteritis

Temporal arteritis, a systemic illness of elderly patients, is characterized by inflammatory infiltrates of lymphocytes and giant cells in extradural and cranial arteries. It occurs almost exclusively in patients over 50 years of age. Most patients have systemic symptoms of low-grade fever, diffuse myalgias, weight loss, weakness, and malaise (polymyalgia rheumatica). The ESR is elevated in almost all patients, usually to high levels (60 to 120 mm/hr). Jaw claudication or tongue claudication is an uncommon, but useful, diagnostic clue.

Treatment

The most feared complication of temporal arteritis is visual loss (ischemic optic neuropathy; see Chapter 11), which occurs in 10%

to 30% of untreated patients because of involvement of the ophthalmic artery. If the diagnosis is suspected, immediately start prednisone 100 mg daily and schedule the patient for a temporal artery biopsy. False-negative biopsy results can occur, particularly if thin sections of a long artery section are not studied. In most patients, prednisone will abolish all symptoms very rapidly and normalize the ESR in 2 to 4 weeks. Because the illness is self-limited, maintenance steroids (10 to 20 mg per day) can usually be discontinued within 6 months to 2 years.

Trigeminal Neuralgia

Also known as "tic douloureux," this illness is characterized by brief, sharp, lancinating paroxysms of pain in the distribution of the trigeminal nerve. As in all neuralgias, the pain has an abrupt onset, and jabs may be repetitive and follow the distribution of a particular nerve. In the case of trigeminal neuralgia, the maxillary (V2) and mandibular (V3) divisions are most frequently affected, and involvement of the ophthalmic division (V1) alone is exceedingly rare. Trigger points can often be found on the face, usually in the same region as the pain. For this reason, the pain is often related to activities such as tooth brushing, shaving, or eating. More than 90% of patients present after age 40, and women are more often affected than men. If trigeminal neuralgia is associated with trigeminal sensory loss, other cranial nerve deficits, or onset before age 40, MRI should be performed to rule out neoplasm or multiple sclerosis. Vascular compression of the trigeminal nerve near the pons underlies most cases of trigeminal neuralgia but may not be appreciated on MRI scan. *Glossopharyngeal neuralgia,* a rare disorder similar to trigeminal neuralgia, is characterized by lancinating pains in the oropharynx that radiate to the ear. The pain is triggered by swallowing, yawning, sneezing, or coughing. Serious intracranial pathology is more likely to be seen in glossopharyngeal neuralgia. Treatment is the same as for trigeminal neuralgia but is more likely to be refractory to medical therapy.

Treatment

The most effective treatment is **carbamazepine 200 to 600 mg tid** or **oxcarbazepine 300 to 900 mg bid.** The initial dose of carbamazepine is 200 mg two times a day and is gradually increased to the minimal effective and tolerated dosage. **Phenytoin 300 to 400 mg daily** is an alternative to carbamazepine but is less effective. **Baclofen 10 to 20 mg four times a day, gabapentin 100 to 800 mg three times a day, valproate 250 to 500 mg tid,** or **topiramate 50 to 300 mg bid** may also be effective in some patients. In refractory cases, microvascular decompression of the trigeminal nerve, radiofrequency rhizotomy, glycerol rhizotomy, or gamma knife of the trigeminal nerve may be required.

SPONTANEOUS INTRACRANIAL HYPOTENSION

This unusual disorder, which resembles post-LP headache, is characterized by headache that worsens after standing. Associated symptoms include nausea, vomiting, tinnitus, and vertigo. The pathogenesis is related to spontaneous leakage of CSF along the craniospinal axis. By definition, CSF pressure is low (less than 6 cm H_2O), and the diagnosis is confirmed by meningeal enhancement on MRI (seen early on).

Treatment

If prolonged bed rest fails to relieve the symptoms, most patients will respond to autologous epidural blood patch at the level of CSF leakage. At times this site may be difficult to ascertain, and CT of brain and paranasal sinuses, CT myelography, and radionuclide cisternography may be necessary.

Neuromuscular Respiratory Failure

Generalized weakness is the primary problem in patients with severe neuromuscular disease. Weakness of the bulbar or respiratory muscles leads to life-threatening respiratory compromise by two mechanisms: (1) lack of upper airway protection and (2) hypoventilation because of respiratory muscle weakness. The most common diseases presenting as acute paralysis and ventilatory failure are **myasthenia gravis** and **Guillain-Barré syndrome** (acute inflammatory demyelinating polyneuropathy). Your management should be directed toward stabilizing the patient, assessing the need to intubate and ventilate, and establishing a diagnosis. Because patients with neuromuscular disease can deteriorate rapidly, close observation and meticulous airway and ventilatory management in the early stages are critical.

PHONE CALL

Questions

1. **What are the vital signs?**
2. **Is the patient in respiratory distress?**
   Rapid, shallow breathing is a danger sign of impending ventilatory failure. Patients with acute weakness who are in obvious respiratory distress should be intubated immediately.
3. **Over what time period has the weakness developed?**
   Fluctuating weakness that has been present for weeks or months is characteristic of myasthenia gravis. Progressive ascending paralysis over hours to days is suggestive of Guillain-Barré syndrome.
4. **Has the patient had difficulty swallowing?**
   Dysphagia (coughing or choking after swallowing) is a symptom of bulbar muscle weakness. Affected patients are at risk for aspiration and should be given NPO.

Orders

1. **Administer oxygen.**

   For mild to moderate respiratory distress, order 40% oxygen via face mask and reassess oxygen requirements on arrival at the bedside.

2. **Perform bedside pulmonary function tests.**
   - *Vital capacity* is the maximal exhaled volume after full inspiration and is normally 60 ml/kg (approximately 4 L in a 70-kg person). Patients generally require intubation when vital capacity falls below 15 ml/kg (approximately 1 L).
   - *Peak inspiratory pressure* (normally greater than 50 cm H_2O) measures the force of inhalation generated by contraction of the diaphragm and is an index of the ability to maintain lung expansion and avoid atelectasis.
   - *Peak expiratory pressure* (normally greater than 60 cm H_2O) correlates with the strength of cough and the ability to clear secretions from the airway.

3. **Measure arterial blood gas levels on room air.**

   Hypercarbia (PCO_2 greater than 45 mm Hg) results from alveolar hypoventilation. *Hypoxia* (PO_2 less than 75 mm Hg) is indicative of impaired ventilation-perfusion matching and in this setting is usually related to atelectasis or pneumonia.

4. **Obtain a chest radiograph.**
5. **Keep the patient NPO.**
6. **Insert an intravenous line.**

   IV access should be established in the event of an acute deterioration. Dehydration resulting from recent dysphagia is also common.

ELEVATOR THOUGHTS

What can cause generalized weakness leading to respiratory failure?

An anatomic approach is the most useful way to classify causes of generalized weakness. Further discussion of many of the entities listed here can be found later in this chapter.

1. **Spinal cord lesion**
   - Cervical cord compression
   - Transverse myelitis
2. **Motor neuron lesion**
   - Amyotrophic lateral sclerosis
   - Polio
3. **Peripheral nerve lesion**
   - Guillain-Barré syndrome (acute inflammatory polyneuropathy)
   - Chronic inflammatory demyelinating polyneuropathy
   - Diphtheritic polyneuropathy
   - AIDS-related

- Demyelinating polyneuropathy
- Toxic neuropathy (lead, arsenic, hexacarbons, dapsone, nitrofurantoin)
- Lyme disease
- Tick paralysis
- Critical illness polyneuropathy
- Acute intermittent porphyria

4. **Neuromuscular junction lesion**
   - Myasthenia gravis
   - Lambert-Eaton syndrome
   - Botulism
   - Organophosphate poisoning

5. **Muscle lesion**
   - Polymyositis or dermatomyositis
   - Critical illness myopathy
   - Hyperthyroid myopathy
   - Mitochondrial myopathy
   - Acid maltase deficiency (Pompe's disease)
   - Periodic paralysis (hyperkalemic or hypokalemic)
   - Congenital myopathy (muscular dystrophy)

MAJOR THREAT TO LIFE

- **Hypoxia**

  Inadequate oxygenation is the most worrisome end result of any process leading to shortness of breath. Hence, your initial assessment should be directed toward ascertaining whether significant hypoxia is present.

BEDSIDE

Quick Look Test

Does the patient look well (comfortable), sick (uncomfortable), or critical (about to die)?

Agitation, diaphoresis, difficulty finishing sentences, accessory respiratory muscle contraction, and rapid or labored breathing may signal impending respiratory failure.

Airway and Vital Signs

Is the upper airway clear?

Weakness of the tongue and oropharyngeal muscles can lead to upper airway obstruction, which increases resistance to airflow and the work of breathing. *Stridor* is indicative of potentially life-threatening upper airway obstruction.

Weakness of the laryngeal and glottic muscles can lead to impaired swallowing and aspiration of secretions. A *wet, gurgled voice* and *pooled oropharyngeal secretions* are the best clinical signs of significant dysphagia.

What is the respiratory rate?

Check for *paradoxical respirations* (Fig. 15–1), inward movement of the abdomen on inspiration, which is indicative of diaphragmatic paralysis.

What is the heart rate and blood pressure?

Sinus tachycardia, hypertension, or BP lability can result from dysautonomia in Guillain-Barré syndrome.

What is the temperature?

Fever should raise suspicion for aspiration pneumonia.

Selective History

To make the diagnosis, it is important to establish the time course and distribution of weakness. Key questions to keep in mind when obtaining a history in patients with generalized weakness include the following: (1) Is a spinal cord lesion a possibility? (2) Is the process purely motor or is sensation involved? (3) Is the patient at risk for sudden respiratory failure?

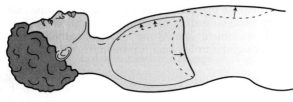

Normal inspiration

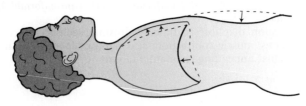

Paradoxical respiration

Figure 15–1 Paradoxical respirations. With normal inspiration *(top)*, contraction and downward movement of the diaphragm cause the abdomen to move outward. With paradoxical respiration *(bottom)*, outward expansion of the chest leads to passive upward movement of the diaphragm and inward movement of the abdomen.

1. **When did the weakness develop?**

   Early symptoms of weakness can be subtle. Ask about difficulty arising from a chair, climbing stairs, lifting packages, combing or brushing hair, or turning keys or doorknobs.

2. **Was there an antecedent illness?**

   Approximately 70% of cases of Guillain-Barré syndrome are triggered by an antecedent viral illness or *Campylobacter jejuni* gastroenteritis. Respiratory crisis in myasthenia gravis is triggered by infection in approximately 40% of patients.

3. **Does the weakness fluctuate?**

   Fluctuating weakness (on an hourly basis) is almost pathognomonic for myasthenia gravis.

4. **Has there been any blurred or double vision?**

   Blurred vision occurs with botulism.

5. **Has there been any neck or back pain?**

   Neck pain should raise suspicion for a cervical cord lesion. Low backache occurs frequently with Guillain-Barré syndrome.

6. **Has there been any numbness or tingling?**

   Distal paresthesias are common in Guillain-Barré syndrome.

7. **Have there been any muscle aches, cramps, or tenderness?**

   Aching and tenderness generally occur with myopathy. Cramps can occur with motor neuron disease or with severe electrolyte derangements.

8. **Has there been any exposure to toxins or insecticides?**

   Organophosphate is the most common toxin that can lead to respiratory failure.

Selective Physical Examination

Once the patient has been stabilized, the goal is to identify signs of airway or respiratory compromise and to search for clues to the diagnosis.

General Physical Examination

HEENT	Oropharynx: Check for *pooled secretions,* which are diagnostic of impaired swallowing and ability to handle secretions. *Exudative pharyngitis* occurs with diphtheria.
	Swallow test: Give the patient a small amount (3 oz) of water to drink. Coughing after swallowing is diagnostic of aspiration.
	Speech: Check for *dysphonia.* A nasal voice results from palatal paralysis. A soft, strangulated voice results from vocal cord paralysis. Evaluate *dysarthria* by checking the buccal (ma, ma), lingual (la, la), and pharyngeal (ga, ga) components of articulation.
Respiratory	Lungs: Auscultate for wheezes, rales, rhonchi, or consolidation.

Diaphragm: Palpate for normal, outward abdominal movement during inspiration.

Cough: Check the strength of the patient's cough.

Ventilatory reserve: Ask the patient to inhale fully and count from 1 to 25. A patient with adequate ventilatory reserve should be able to do this in a single breath.

Skin   Rashes: Check for a rash (Lyme disease, dermatomyositis).

Neurologic Examination

- **Pupils:** Pupillary reactivity may be lost with botulism or in the Miller-Fisher variant of Guillain-Barré syndrome (triad of ophthalmoplegia, ataxia, and areflexia).
- **Extraocular muscles:** *Ptosis and ocular muscle weakness* is characteristic of myasthenia gravis but can occur with the Miller-Fisher variant of Guillain-Barré syndrome, botulism, diphtheria, polymyositis, Graves' disease, mitochondrial myopathy, or critical illness myopathy.
- **Face, palate, tongue, and neck strength**
- **Limb strength**
- **Fasciculations:** Fasciculations are seen with motor neuron disease or organophosphate poisoning.
- **Reflexes:** *Areflexia* is **always** seen with Guillain-Barré syndrome.
- **Coordination:** Ataxia occurs with the Miller-Fisher variant of Guillain-Barré syndrome.
- **Sensation:** A cervical or upper thoracic *sensory level* associated with quadriparesis suggests a cervical cord lesion. Mild sensory loss in the distal extremities is common in Guillain-Barré syndrome.

MANAGEMENT

Airway Management and Mechanical Ventilation

Criteria for Intubation

A number of factors must be considered when deciding when to intubate and ventilate. The most important factor, perhaps, is the overall comfort level of the patient. Decisions must be individualized, but the following criteria may be helpful:

- Reduction of vital capacity to 15 ml/kg (approximately 1 L in a 70-kg person)
- PO_2 less than 70 mm Hg on room air
- PCO_2 greater than 50 mm Hg associated with acidosis (pH less than 7.35)
- Severe oropharyngeal paresis with inability to protect the airway

Remember that conservative, early intubation and institution of positive-pressure ventilation can minimize the development of atelectasis and pneumonia and may lead to earlier extubation.

Initial Ventilator Management

The initial goals of ventilator management immediately after intubation are (1) to provide rest and (2) to promote lung expansion. These goals are best accomplished using intravenous sedation and *continuous mandatory ventilation (CMV)* at a rate of 6 to 8 breaths per minute, using tidal volumes of 10 to 15 ml/kg. *Positive end-expiratory pressure (PEEP)* aids in the expansion of collapsed alveoli and should be used in all patients at levels of 5 to 15 cm H_2O. Use of higher tidal volumes and generous application of PEEP is acceptable as long as peak airway pressures are <30 cm H_2O, and may be beneficial for promoting lung expansion.

Patients with long-standing weakness and CO_2 retention should be intentionally hypoventilated (PCO_2 at or higher than 45 mm Hg). Overventilating to normal or reduced PCO_2 levels will result in alkalosis and renal serum bicarbonate wasting, which in turn will make it more difficult to successfully wean the patient.

Bronchoscopy

Fiberoptic bronchoscopy for pulmonary toilet should be performed aggressively in patients with hypoxia, severe atelectasis, or lobar collapse because of mucus plugging.

Tracheostomy

After the patient has been on mechanical ventilation for approximately 2 weeks, tracheostomy should be performed. Compared with prolonged (more than 2 weeks) endotracheal intubation, tracheostomy (1) is more comfortable, (2) poses less risk of permanent laryngeal or tracheal injury, (3) facilitates weaning from mechanical ventilation by reducing dead space and airway resistance, and (4) makes it easier to clear airway secretions by cough or suctioning. Early tracheostomy within the first week of intubation is reasonable in patients who have severe weakness and clear risk factors for a prolonged course of mechanical ventilation (Table 15–1).

TABLE 15–1 **Risk Factors for Prolonged (>2 Weeks) Ventilator Dependence in Patients with Neuromuscular Respiratory Failure**

- Age >50 years
- Failure to tolerate >12 hours of CPAP with pressure support ≤5 cm H_2O
- Vital capacity fails to exceed 25 ml/kg within 6 days of intubation
- Preintubation serum bicarbonate ≥30 mg/dl (chronic respiratory acidosis)
- Preexisting lung disease

BOX 15–1 **Criteria for Initiating Ventilator Weaning**

1. Vital capacity greater than 15 ml/kg
2. Peak inspiratory pressure greater than 25 cm H_2O
3. PO_2 greater than 80 mm Hg on 40% inspired oxygen with PEEP <10 cm H_2O.
4. No adverse medical conditions: severe infection, hypotension, anemia, gastric distention, volume overload, or cardiac arrhythmias

---

Weaning to Extubation

Criteria to be met before daily spontaneous breathing trials are initiated are listed in Box 15–1. Barring a clear contraindication, spontaneous breathing trials should begin approximately 3 days after intubation.

Continuous positive airway pressure (CPAP) with pressure support is the preferred initial mode for weaning patients with respiratory muscle weakness. Each time the patient inhales, "pressure support" delivers additional inspiratory volume until a preset level of pressure is reached. The amount of inspiratory pressure support given (range, 5 to 15 cm H_2O) should be initially adjusted to attain tidal volumes of approximately 300 to 500 ml in an adult. We advocate daytime spontaneous breathing trials and "resting" the patient on CMV overnight (Box 15–2).

Extubation can be performed once the patient has demonstrated the ability to tolerate long periods (e.g., overnight) on CPAP with pressure support equal to 5 cm H_2O without fatigue. Fluctuating pulmonary function tests, excessive secretions, or concurrent medical problems (i.e., infection or cardiovascular instability) are relative contraindications to extubation. Extubation should always be performed early in the day.

General Care of the Patient with Neuromuscular Respiratory Failure

1. **Elevate the head of the bed**
   With diaphragmatic weakness, lung volumes become diminished and work of breathing increases in the supine position. Head elevation also reduces the risk of ventilator-associated pneumonia.
2. **Chest physical therapy**
   Chest percussion and airway suctioning are essential for preventing mucus plugs and aiding in the clearing of secretions. Prescribe *incentive spirometry* every 6 hours if the patient is not intubated.

> BOX 15–2 **Spontaneous Breathing (Weaning) Trial Protocol**
>
> 1. Begin the trial by switching the ventilator mode from synchronized intermittent mandatory ventilation (SIMV) or continuous mandatory ventilation (CMV) to *continuous positive airway pressure (CPAP) with pressure support (PS) of 5 cm H_2O.*
> 2. After 5 minutes, record the respiratory rate and mean tidal volume, and increase the level of PS as needed to attain a respiratory rate (RR) <30 per minute and tidal volume (TV) >300 ml.
> 3. Obtain a baseline arterial blood gas (ABG) and record the RR and TV hourly.
> 4. Write an order to "call MD to bedside if RR >30, TV <300 ml, O_2 saturation <95%, or obvious for agitation or respiratory distress." *An increasing respiratory rate combined with falling tidal volumes is the most reliable indicator of respiratory fatigue.* If this call is made, perform a clinical assessment, obtain a follow-up ABG, and return the patient to SIMV or CMV.
> 5. The level of pressure support may be decreased by 1 to 2 cm H_2O every 2 to 4 hours if the patient remains comfortable.
> 6. If the patient appears comfortable after 12 hours with PS = 5 cm H_2O, try to have the patient continue on CPAP overnight. If they have tolerated the spontaneous breathing trial for 24 hours, consider extubation or converting to trach collar.

3. **Serial measurements of vital capacity**

   Vital capacity should be checked every 4 to 6 hours in nonintubated patients and every 12 to 24 hours in intubated patients.

4. **Prophylaxis for DVT**

   In addition to dynamic compression stockings, order enoxaparin 40 mg SC once daily or heparin 5000 U SQ every 12 hours.

5. **Nutrition**

   Patients with bulbar weakness should be made NPO and fed via a *small-bore nasoduodenal tube.* When attempting to wean a CO_2 retainer, use a nutritional supplement with a high ratio of carbohydrate to lipid (e.g., Pulmocare) to minimize CO_2 production.

6. **Fluids and electrolytes**

   Hypokalemia and *hypophosphatemia* can exacerbate muscle weakness and should be periodically checked for and treated.

7. **Bowel and bladder care**

   Paralysis predisposes to constipation and can be prevented with **docusate sodium (Colace) 100 mg three times a day and milk of magnesia 30 ml every night.** Intermittent straight catheterization carries a lower risk of infection than an indwelling Foley catheter.

SPECIFIC DISORDERS

Guillain-Barré Syndrome

Guillain-Barré syndrome is a monophasic, acute inflammatory demyelinating polyneuropathy. The etiology is related to an autoimmune attack directed against surface antigens on peripheral nerves, resulting in focal segmental demyelination.

Onset

In approximately 70% of cases, the syndrome follows a respiratory or gastrointestinal infection by 5 days to 3 weeks. Viral upper respiratory infection and *Campylobacter jejuni* gastroenteritis are the most common precipitating infections. Other causes include HIV infection, immunization, pregnancy, Hodgkin's disease, and surgery.

Clinical Features

The syndrome usually begins with rapidly progressive ascending paralysis, associated with cranial nerve and respiratory muscle weakness, loss of deep tendon reflexes, and distal paresthesias and sensory loss. Unlike other neuropathies, proximal muscles are often affected more than distal muscles. The weakness progresses over 7 to 21 days; the median duration from onset to maximal weakness is 12 days. Respiratory failure requiring intubation occurs in 20% of patients. Papilledema, autonomic disturbances (e.g., hypertension, hypotension, urinary retention, sinus tachycardia, cardiac arrhythmias), and SIADH are seen in some patients.

Laboratory Data

The CSF classically shows dissociation between albumin levels and cytologic findings, with elevated protein levels and normal white blood cell counts (5 cells/μl or fewer). The elevation in the protein level can sometimes take up to 2 weeks to develop. A mild lymphocytic or monocytic pleocytosis is sometimes seen (10 to 100 cells/mm^3) and should raise suspicion for an infectious polyradiculopathy (e.g., HIV, CMV, West Nile virus, or Lyme disease) or poliomyelitis. Nerve conduction studies show loss of F waves and reduced conduction velocities. Reduced motor fiber amplitudes reflect secondary axonal damage and imply a worse prognosis for recovery.

Treatment

Patients with signs of respiratory muscle weakness should be admitted to an ICU for observation until it is clear that the illness has stabilized. **Plasmapheresis,** when initiated within 10 days of the onset of symptoms, can speed the onset of recovery. A total of five treatments are performed every 1 to 2 days, with a total of 2 to 4 L

BOX 15–3 **Checklist for the Management of Guillain-Barré Syndrome**

1. *Diagnostic workup:* Lumbar puncture, electromyography/nerve conduction studies, hepatitis and Lyme disease serologies, CMV, EBV, HSV, and HIV titers, urine porphyrin levels, urine heavy metal screen, stool analysis for *Campylobacter*
2. *Pain management:* Pain can be severe and may result from meningeal inflammation or neuropathic mechanisms. **NSAIDs (ketorolac 30 mg IM every 6 hours)**, opioids **(morphine 2-10 mg every 2 to 4 hours as needed)**, or a fentanyl (duragesic patch) 25 µg/hr are most effective.
3. *Dysautonomia:* The most frequent cardiovascular manifestation of dysautonomia is sustained hypertension and tachycardia. Treatment with beta blockers (propranolol **PO 10 to 40 mg every 6 hours** or **labetolol infusion**) may be desirable in older patients with coronary artery disease.

---

of plasma exchanged for 5% albumin during each treatment. High-dose **IVIG, 0.4 g/kg per day for 5 consecutive days,** has been shown to be as effective as plasmapheresis and may be slightly superior. Rebound deterioration after completing a course of IVIG can sometimes occur. The management of pain and dysautonomia is discussed in Box 15–3.

Prognosis

Features shown to have a poor prognosis in Guillain-Barré syndrome include (1) advanced age, (2) very low distal motor amplitudes, (3) rapidly progressive weakness occurring over the first week, and (4) respiratory failure requiring intubation.

Myasthenia Gravis

Myasthenia gravis is caused by an antibody-mediated attack on nicotinic acetylcholine receptors, resulting in a defect in neuromuscular transmission. This phenomenon manifests clinically as *fluctuating weakness* and *muscle fatigability*, the hallmarks of myasthenia gravis.

Clinical Features

Fluctuating weakness is typical of myasthenia gravis; it tends to involve the eyes (in 90% of patients), face, neck, and oropharynx (in 80% of patients), and limbs (in 60% of patients). The age distribution at onset is bimodal, with an early peak between ages 20 and 40 (primarily in women) and a later peak between ages 50 and 80 (in both sexes). The limbs are almost never affected in isolation. Sensation is always normal, and reflexes are preserved unless the muscle is plegic. Most patients reach the maximum severity of their disease within the first 1 to 2 years; thereafter, spontaneous remission is common (in approximately 30% of patients), and the disease process tends to become less severe. *Malignant thymoma* is present in approximately 15% of patients with myasthenia and is associated with more severe disease.

Myasthenic crisis is defined by respiratory failure requiring intubation and mechanical ventilation. Crisis is most often provoked by infection (in 40% of patients) but can also occur spontaneously (in 30% of patients) or result from aspiration, surgery, pregnancy, medications (Table 15–2), or emotional upset. Approximately 25% of patients can be extubated within 1 week, 50% within 2 weeks, and 75% within 1 month. One third of patients intubated for crisis will proceed to experience a second crisis. Although a crisis is by definition life-threatening, with modern ICU management, death (approximately 5% mortality rate) results only from overwhelming medical complications (e.g., myocardial infarction, sepsis).

Laboratory Data

The diagnosis of myasthenia gravis can be established with the following tests:

1. *Edrophonium (Tensilon) testing* reveals transient improvement in patients with ocular and facial weakness. **Edrophonium 10 mg** is used in adults; infuse 2 mg initially and observe for severe cholinergic muscarinic effects such as nausea, bradycardia, and hypotension. **Atropine 0.4 mg** should be kept at the

TABLE 15–2 **Drugs That Can Exacerbate Weakness in Myasthenia Gravis**

Antibiotics
Aminoglycosides (gentamicin, streptomycin, others)
Peptide antibodies (polymyxin B, colistin)
Tetracyclines (tetracycline, doxycycline, others)
Erythromycin
Clindamycin
Ciprofloxacin
Ampicillin
Antiarrhythmics
Quinidine
Procainamide
Lidocaine
Neuromuscular junction blockers (vecuronium, pancuronium, others)
Quinine
Steroids
Lithium
Magnesium toxicity
Verapamil
Thyroid hormones (thyroxine, levothyroxine, others)
Beta blockers (propranolol, timolol, others)
Chloroquine
Phenytoin
Penicillamine (induces autoimmune myasthenia gravis)

bedside and can be used to reverse these symptoms. If there are no severe effects, inject the remaining 8 mg and observe for improvement, which generally occurs within 2 to 10 minutes.

2. *Repetitive nerve stimulation* at 2 to 3 Hz characteristically produces a greater than 10% decrement in amplitude between the first and fifth compound muscle action potential. Sensitivity and specificity are 90% when weak, proximal muscles are tested; however, sensitivity falls to less than 50% in myasthenic patients without limb weakness.

3. *Single-fiber EMG* reveals "jitter," variation in the time interval between firing of muscle fibers in the same motor unit. Single-fiber EMG is highly sensitive (sensitivity greater than 95%) for myasthenia gravis but is not specific.

4. *Acetylcholine receptor antibodies* are present in approximately 80% of patients with generalized myasthenia but in only 50% of patients with ocular myasthenia. Titers do not correlate with the severity of illness.

5. *Anti-MuSK (muscle-specific tyrosine kinase) antibodies* are present in half of patients who lack acetylcholine-receptor antibodies. Anti-MuSK-positive patients tend to be female, with predominant neck and orophayryngeal weakness. They respond variably to acetylcholinesterase inhibitors and do not tend to respond to thymectomy, but usually improve after plasmapheresis.

Treatment

Therapeutic options for treating myasthenia gravis (see Box 15–4) can be divided into three categories: *symptomatic therapy* (with acetylcholinesterase inhibitors), *short-term disease suppression* (with plasmapheresis and IVIG), and *long-term immunosuppression* (with thymectomy, steroids, or chemotherapy).

BOX 15–4 **Checklist for the Management of Myasthenic Crisis**

1. Eliminate and avoid all contraindicated medications (see Table 15–1).
2. *Diagnostic workup:* Edrophonium test, acetylcholine receptor antibody level, repetitive nerve stimulation, single-fiber EMG, thyroid function tests, chest CT scan.
3. *Treatment:* Anticholinesterase medications should be *discontinued* while patients are mechanically ventilated because they lead to excessive stimulation of secretions (see Table 15–2). A course of plasmapheresis or IVIG is indicated in all patients.

Symptomatic therapy. Acetylcholinesterase inhibitors (Table 15–3) improve myasthenic weakness by allowing acetylcholine to accumulate at the neuromuscular junction. **Pyridostigmine (Mestinon) is started at 30 mg PO three times a day, increased to 60 to 120 mg every 4 to 6 hours as a maintenance dose, and increased to 120 mg every 3 hours as a maximal dose.** A long-acting 180-mg tablet (Mestinon Timespan) can be given at bedtime for patients with nocturnal or morning weakness. Excessive muscarinic side effects (e.g., pulmonary secretions, diarrhea) can be controlled by concurrently giving an antimuscarinic agent such as **glycopyrrolate (Robinul) 1 to 2 mg PO three times a day** or **propantheline bromide (Pro-Banthine) 15 mg PO four times a day.**

Short-term disease suppression. This is indicated to hasten clini-cal improvement in hospitalized patients. **Plasmapheresis (five exchanges of 2 to 4 L every 1 to 2 days)** can lead to improvement within days, but the effect is short-lived, lasting only 2 to 4 weeks. Similar benefits have been reported in 70% of patients treated with **IVIG (0.4 g/kg daily for 5 days),** but experience with this therapy remains limited.

Long-term immunosuppression. This treatment is indicated when weakness is inadequately controlled with anticholinesterase medications. **Prednisone** is most commonly prescribed; to use the lowest dose possible, start with **15 to 20 mg per day** and gradually increase to **40 to 100 mg per day over 4 to 8 weeks** until an adequate response is achieved. Temporary worsening of symptoms within the first 2 weeks of starting steroids can be expected in up to 40% of patients. **Azathioprine 1 to 2 mg/kg PO per day** can also be used for long-term immunosuppression in patients who cannot tolerate the side effects of steroids. **Thymectomy** leads to disease remission in 40% of patients and clinical improvement in another 40%, but these benefits can take months or years to occur. Thymectomy is indicated in any patient between the ages of 15 and 60 with thymoma or with generalized myasthenia.

Uncommon Causes of Paralysis and Respiratory Failure

Botulism

Botulism is caused by an exotoxin produced by *Clostridium botulinum,* an anaerobic, gram-positive, spore-forming rod that contaminates food. Weakness occurs because the toxin is a potent inhibitor of presynaptic acetylcholine release. Clinical symptoms begin within 12 to 24 hours of ingestion and are characterized by gastrointestinal complaints, dilated and nonreactive pupils, blurred vision, and weakness that begins with the extraocular and oropharyngeal muscles before becoming generalized. Urinary retention, dry mouth, and anhidrosis may also occur. **Botulism trivalent antitoxin (one vial**

TABLE 15–3 Anticholinesterase Drugs Used for Myasthenia Gravis

	Route	Equivalent Dosage	Onset	Maximal Response	Dosage Range
Pyridostigmine bromide (Mestinon)	PO*	60 mg	30 to 60 minutes	1 to 2 hours	30 to 120 mg every 3 to 8 hours
Pyridostigmine long-acting (Mestinon Timespan)	IM, IV†	2 mg	5 to 10 minutes	20 to 30 minutes	—
	PO	—	3 to 5 hours	3 to 5 hours	180 mg per day at night
Neostigmine bromide (Prostigmin)	PO	15 mg	30 minutes	1 hour	15 to 30 mg every 2 to 3 hours
Neostigmine methylsulfate (Prostigmin injectable)	IV†	0.5 mg	1 to 2 minutes	20 minutes	0.5 to 1 mg every 2 hours
	IM	1.5 mg	30 minutes	1 hour	1.5 to 3 mg every 2 to 3 hours

*Can be given as a tablet or as a liquid.
†Equivalent IV dose of pyridostigmine or neostigmine is one thirtieth of the oral dose.

IV and one vial IM every 2 to 4 hours) should be given as soon as possible. **Guanidine hydrochloride (40 mg PO every 4 hours)** is an acetylcholine agonist that can counteract the presynaptic blockade caused by the toxin.

Poliomyelitis

Poliovirus is an enterovirus that can cause selective destruction of motor neurons in the spinal cord and brain stem, resulting in flaccid, areflexic paralysis. Modern vaccination has made the disease a clinical rarity. Acute paralysis from poliomyelitis is differentiated from that caused by Guillain-Barré syndrome by the presence of headache, high fever, mental status changes, asymmetric weakness, and neutrophils in the CSF.

Tetanus

Tetanus results from an exotoxin produced by *Clostridium tetani,* an anaerobic gram-positive coccus that can infect soft-tissue wounds. The toxin results in neuronal hyperexcitability; the result is seizures, autonomic instability, and sustained "tetanic" muscle contractions involving the jaw ("lockjaw"), neck, back, and respiratory muscles. Treatment is directed toward (1) assisting ventilation, which may require intubation and administration of neuromuscular blocking agents; (2) neutralizing the toxin with intramuscular or intrathecal **tetanus immune globulin 250 U (single dose);** and (3) eradicating the soft-tissue infection with **procaine penicillin 1.2 million U every 6 hours for 10 days.**

Syncope

Syncope is brief loss of consciousness caused by a sudden reduction of cerebral blood flow. *Presyncope* refers to the situation in which there is reduction of cerebral blood flow and a sensation of impending loss of consciousness, although the patient does not actually pass out. Presyncope and syncope represent degrees of the same disorder and should be addressed as manifestations of the same underlying problem. Your task is to discover the cause of the syncopal attack.

PHONE CALL

Questions

1. **Did the patient actually lose consciousness?**
   Ask if the patient was aware and remembers the entire event.
2. **Is the patient still unconscious?**
   If so, this is coma (see Chapter 5) until proven otherwise.
3. **What are the vital signs?**
   Bradycardia suggests a vasovagal event.
4. **Was the patient standing, sitting, or lying down when the attack occurred?**
   Syncope in the recumbent position is almost always cardiac in origin. Syncope that occurs immediately after standing up suggests orthostatic hypotension.
5. **Was any seizure-like activity witnessed?**
   Brief minor seizure activity is a common consequence of syncope. As opposed to a primary seizure, it occurs after a presyncopal prodrome of dizziness, diaphoresis, and graying of vision.
6. **Did the patient sustain any injury from the fall?**
   Serious injury is more characteristic of cardiac syncope.

Orders

If the patient is still unconscious, give the following orders:
1. Administer IV D5W to keep the vein open (KVO) if IV is not already in place.

209

2. Turn the patient onto the left side (this maneuver minimizes the risk of upper airway obstruction and aspiration).
3. Order a stat 12-lead ECG and rhythm strip.
4. Obtain a finger stick glucose level.

If the patient has regained consciousness, if there is no evidence of head or neck injury, and if the vital signs are stable, do the following:

1. Instruct the RN to keep the patient supine for at least 10 to 15 minutes, until the patient feels comfortable. To return the patient to bed, slowly raise the patient to the sitting position, and then to a standing position.
2. Have the RN check orthostatic vital signs (BP and heart rate with the patient lying down and standing).
3. Order an ECG and rhythm strip.
4. Have vital signs taken every 15 minutes until you arrive at the bedside. Instruct the RN to call you back immediately if the patient becomes unstable before you are able to perform your assessment.

ELEVATOR THOUGHTS

What causes syncope?

A comprehensive list of the differential diagnoses for syncope and the approximate relative frequency of each of the main categories in an ER population are given here. **Note that neurologic and psychiatric causes are at the bottom of the list and in combination account for only 5% of all patients presenting with syncope.** In the majority of patients (90%), syncope results from a transient drop in systemic BP and can be explained on the basis of reflex vasodilation, cardiac disease, orthostatic hypotension, or medications. *Accordingly, your initial evaluation should focus on excluding these conditions before a neurologic diagnosis is seriously considered.* Symptoms or precipitants that suggest a particular cause of syncope are listed in Table 16–1.

1. **Reflex vasodilation (60% of ER patients)**
   a. Vasodepressor (vasovagal, neurocardiogenic) syncope
   b. Carotid sinus syncope
   c. Situational syncope
      (1) Micturition syncope
      (2) Defecation syncope
      (3) Cough syncope
2. **Cardiac causes (25% of ER patients)**
   a. Arrhythmias
      (1) Tachycardias
         (a) Ventricular tachycardia/fibrillation
         (b) Supraventricular tachycardia
      (2) Bradycardias

TABLE 16–1 Symptoms That are Characteristic of a Specific Cause of Syncope or Loss of Consciousness

Symptoms	Diagnosis
Episodes occur with a sudden, unexpected or unpleasant stimulus, and are associated with a prodrome	Vasovagal syncope
Episodes occur with micturition, defecation, coughing, or swallowing	Situational syncope
Episodes occur with head turning or use of a tight collar	Carotid sinus syncope
Episodes occur immediately upon standing	Orthostatic hypotension
Vertigo is associated with dysarthria, diplopia, or vertigo	Vertebrobasilar insufficiency
Episodes occur with arm exercise	Subclavian steal syndrome
Patient is confused after episode, or loss of consciousness lasts longer than 5 minutes	Seizure
Differences are found in blood pressure or pulse between the two arms	Subclavian steal or aortic dissection
Syncope and murmur occur with changes in position (i.e., getting out of bed)	Atrial myxoma
Patient has sudden loss of consciousness with no prodrome	Arrhythmia
Patient has a family history of sudden death	Long QT syndrome

Adapted from Kapoor WN. Syncope. N Engl J Med 2000;343:1856.

        (a) Sick sinus syndrome
        (b) Second- and third-degree heart block
        (c) Pacemaker malfunction
    b. Flow failure
      (1) Obstruction to left ventricular outflow
        (a) Aortic or mitral stenosis
        (b) Hypertrophic obstructive cardiomyopathy
        (c) Aortic dissection
      (2) Obstruction to pulmonary outflow
        (a) Pulmonary stenosis
        (b) Pulmonary embolism
        (c) Atrial myxoma
      (3) Pump failure
        (a) Myocardial infarction
        (b) Cardiac tamponade
3. Orthostatic (postural) hypotension (10% of ER patients)
    a. Volume depletion (anemia, dehydration)
    b. Drug-induced (Table 16–2)
    c. Autonomic dysfunction
      (1) Central: Shy-Drager syndrome
      (2) Peripheral: autonomic neuropathy

TABLE 16–2 **Drugs and Medications That Can Cause Syncope**

Antihypertensive agents
Nitrates
Calcium channel blockers
Diuretics
Angiotensin-converting enzyme inhibitors
Beta blockers
Others (hydralazine, prazosin)
Antiarrhythmic agents (long QT syndrome, torsades de pointes)
Quinidine
Procainamide
Disopyramide
Sotalol
Amiodarone
Tricyclic antidepressants
Monoamine oxidase inhibitors
Phenothiazines
Levodopa
Digoxin
Ethanol
Marijuana

4. **Neurologic causes (5% of ER patients)**
    a. Seizure (technically not syncope, but mimics syncope)
        (1) Unwitnessed tonic-clonic seizure
        (2) Atonic seizure (drop attack)
    b. TIA
        (1) Brain stem ischemia
            (a) Vertebrobasilar stenosis/occlusion
            (b) Subclavian steal syndrome
        (2) Bilateral hemispheric ischemia from carotid artery stenosis or occlusion
    c. ICP
        (1) SAH
        (2) Space-occupying lesion (e.g., brain tumor)
5. **Psychiatric causes (less than 1% of ER patients)**
    a. Hyperventilation
    b. Conversion disorder (technically not syncope but mimics syncope)

MAJOR THREAT TO LIFE

- *Aspiration* is the main threat if the patient is still unconscious.

    Remember that syncope generally lasts only a few minutes. If the patient remains persistently unconscious (longer than 15 minutes), the diagnosis is coma, and your evaluation should proceed as outlined in Chapter 5.

- *Fatal cardiac arrhythmia* is the main hazard once the patient has regained consciousness.

If a cardiac rhythm disturbance is suspected, the patient should be attached to an ECG monitor, and consideration should be given to observing the patient in an ICU. Other potentially life-threatening illnesses that can present with syncope include subarachnoid hemorrhage, gastrointestinal bleeding, pulmonary embolism, aortic dissection, and myocardial infarction.

BEDSIDE

Quick Look Test

Does the patient look well (comfortable), sick (uncomfortable), or critical (about to die)?
Most cases of syncope are brief (loss of consciousness less than 5 minutes), and many patients look well shortly after regaining consciousness. Others may appear nauseated, pallid, and diaphoretic; these signs represent the systemic autonomic response to hypotension and should resolve rapidly.

Are there any external signs of head or neck trauma?
Significant head injury is unusual after syncope but should be checked for. In most cases, a period of presyncope warns the patient that something is amiss and allows him or her to avoid a hard fall. **Cardiac syncope often occurs without warning and is more likely to lead to traumatic injury.**

Airway and Vital Signs

Abnormal vital signs can help make your diagnosis of the specific cause of syncope much easier.

Is the airway clear?
If the patient is still unconscious, ensure that he or she is lying on the left side and that respirations are adequate.

What is the heart rate?
Supraventricular or ventricular tachycardia should be documented on ECG tracings. If the patient is hypotensive, call for a cardiac arrest team and treat immediately with electrical cardioversion.

Sinus bradycardia implicates vagally mediated vasodepressor syncope. In this case, both the heart rate and the BP should normalize quickly as the patient remains supine.

What is the BP?
Persistently low BP or significant orthostatic hypotension combined with normal sinus rhythm or sinus tachycardia implicates volume

depletion. Begin IV volume resuscitation with D5NS and order a stat hematocrit. Rule out gastrointestinal (GI) bleeding and ruptured aortic aneurysm, which rarely present with syncope.

Hypertension, if found in association with headache, stiff neck, or altered level of consciousness, may indicate subarachnoid hemorrhage.

What is the temperature?

Patients with syncope are rarely febrile. If *fever* is present, it is usually due to a concomitant illness not related to the syncopal attack. If the syncopal attack was unwitnessed, be careful to exclude meningitis or encephalitis associated with a seizure.

Selective History

History should be obtained from the patient as well as from witnesses, if available. Focus on events immediately preceding and following the attack.

1. **Has this ever happened before?**

   If it has, ask the patient if a diagnosis was made after the previous attack.

2. **What do the patient or witnesses recall from the period immediately before the syncope?**
   - Syncope occurring while changing from the supine or the sitting position to the standing position suggests *orthostatic hypotension.*
   - Palpitations or the complete absence of prodromal symptoms suggest *cardiac arrhythmia.*
   - A prodrome of dizziness, lightheadedness, pallor, diaphoresis, and dimming of vision (i.e., presyncope) is highly characteristic of *reflex vasodepressor syncope.*
   - Syncope after turning the head to one side, especially if the patient is wearing a tight collar, may represent *carotid sinus syncope.*
   - Syncope during or immediately following Valsalva's maneuver (coughing, micturition, defecation) can result from mechanical disruption of venous return and is termed *situational syncope.*
   - One or more episodes of vertigo, diplopia, dysarthria, numbness, weakness, or ataxia preceding the attack, alone or in combination, are suggestive of *vertebrobasilar insufficiency.*
   - An aura (unusual smell or taste, abdominal sensations, visual or sensory hallucinations) may point to a *seizure* as the cause of an unwitnessed attack.

3. **How does the patient feel upon waking from the syncopal attack?**

   Headache suggests *subarachnoid hemorrhage.* Persistent lethargy and confusion are atypical for true syncope and suggest an unwitnessed *seizure* or *subarachnoid hemorrhage.*

4. **Were any shaking movements observed?**

   Loss of consciousness associated with simultaneous generalized tonic-clonic activity is diagnostic of seizure. *Caution:* Be aware that minor twitching, myoclonic activity, or a single convulsion that **follows** loss of consciousness is common and reflects a *secondary* consequence of cerebral ischemia.

5. **Was the patient incontinent of stool or urine?**

   If the attack was unwitnessed, incontinence is highly suggestive of a seizure. Be aware that incontinence can also occur with true syncope.

6. **Is there any history of cardiac disease, seizure, stroke, or TIA?**

   These may point to an obvious cause of syncope.

7. **Has the patient been feeling ill recently?**

   Ask about symptoms of infection, diarrhea, peptic ulcer, chest pain, palpitations, or neurologic dysfunction, which may point to a predisposing illness.

8. **What are the medications?**

   Refer to Table 16–2 for a list of medications that can cause syncope.

Selective Physical Examination

Your physical examination is directed toward finding a cause for the syncope. However, a search for evidence of injuries sustained by a fall is equally important at this time.

General Physical Examination

Vital signs	• Repeat now, including *orthostatic* tests if not performed yet
HEENT	• Fundoscopy: look for SAH
	• Tongue lacerations, especially at lateral borders (seizure)
	• Ecchymoses, abrasions, lacerations
Neck	• Neck stiffness (SAH)
Cardiac	• Heart murmur (mitral, pulmonic, or aortic stenosis)
	• Pericardial rub (cardiac tamponade)
GU	• Urinary incontinence (seizure)
Rectal	• Heme-positive stool (GI bleeding)
Extremities	• Palpate for evidence of fracture

Neurologic Examination

- Lethargy, confusion, or disorientation (seizure, SAH)
- Hemianopia or aphasia (stroke, CNS mass lesion)

- Diplopia, nystagmus, facial weakness or numbness, dysarthria, or dysphonia (vertebrobasilar ischemia)
- Hemiparesis/pronator drift (Todd's paralysis, stroke, CNS mass lesion)
- Cogwheel rigidity (Shy-Drager syndrome)
- Stocking-glove sensory loss and areflexia (peripheral and autonomic neuropathy)
- Appendicular or gait ataxia (vertebrobasilar ischemia)

DIAGNOSTIC TESTING

Apart from an ECG, there are no laboratory tests that are routinely indicated for the evaluation of syncope. In approximately 50% of cases, a careful history, examination (including orthostatic BP), and ECG are all that are needed to establish a diagnosis (for instance, a clear-cut case of vasovagal syncope in a patient having blood drawn).

If the cause of syncope is unexplained and the history and examination are not suggestive of a neurologic cause, further workup should be directed toward ruling out a cardiac cause of syncope. The reason for this is that untreated cardiac syncope carries a substantial risk of subsequent sudden death (approximately 30% over the next 12 months). Tests to rule out a cardiac cause of syncope may include the following:
- Echocardiography
- Cardiac telemetry
- Holter monitoring
- Head-up tilt table testing
- Signal-averaged electrocardiography (SAECG)
- Electrophysiologic (EP) studies
- Cardiac stress testing
- Coronary angiography
- Chest CT angiogram or ventilation-perfusion scan

If a neurologic cause of syncope is suggested by history or examination, specific testing may include the following (refer to the next section on specific neurologic causes of syncope to guide your selection):
- 3-minute trial of hyperventilation
- EEG (with and without sleep)
- Head CT or MRI
- Transcranial Doppler ultrasonography (intracranial vertebral and basilar arteries)
- Duplex Doppler ultrasonography (extracranial carotid and vertebral arteries)
- Magnetic resonance or CT angiography
- Cerebral angiography
- EMG/NCS

MANAGEMENT

Approach to Syncope: A Neurologist's Perspective

Step 1: Rule out medical causes of syncope. As stated previously, neurologic causes of syncope are unusual. When called in consultation to evaluate for a possible neurologic etiology, the first step is to verify that the more common and easy-to-identify medical causes have been excluded. Important tests to rule out a medical cause of syncope in the ER include the following:

- Orthostatic BP
- ECG
- Cardiac auscultation
- Hematocrit
- Arterial blood gas measurement (rule out pulmonary embolism)
- Review of medications (Table 16–2 lists medications that can cause syncope)
- Toxicology screen and serum ethanol level

Step 2: Know what you are looking for. Syncope results from temporary reduction of cerebral blood flow, and in the majority of cases, the cause is a drop in systemic BP. True neurologic causes of syncope follow the same principle and result from only two basic mechanisms:

1. **Transient focal reduction of cerebral blood flow related to stenosis or embolism of a cerebral artery (i.e., TIA).** With rare exceptions, the only brain region in which transient focal ischemia can lead to loss of consciousness is the brain stem. Hence, *vertebrobasilar TIA* is the main consideration.
2. **Reduction of cerebral blood flow caused by a transient elevation of ICP.** *Subarachnoid hemorrhage* and an ICP wave associated with a *preexisting mass lesion* are the main considerations.

Seizures are not a cause of syncope. However, generalized seizures lead to sudden, temporary loss of consciousness and thus can be confused with syncope. As the consulting neurologist, you may be asked to corroborate or rule out the diagnosis.

SELECTED DISORDERS THAT CAN CAUSE OR MIMIC SYNCOPE

Non-neurologic Causes

Vasovagal (Vasodepressor, Neurocardiogenic) Syncope

Also known as "the common faint," vasodepressor syncope is apt to occur in the setting of a strong emotional or painful stimulus. A prodrome of presyncope (dizziness, pallor) is the rule. Bradycardia may be identified shortly after the episode, and recovery is usually rapid. If the clinical picture is unclear, *head-up tilt table testing* can be used to provoke vasovagal syncope and establish the diagnosis, with a sensitivity and specificity of approximately 80%. Sudden head-up tilting in patients with vasovagal syncope produces an increase in myocardial contractility, which in turn leads to excessive stimulation of left ventricular mechanoreceptors (C fibers) and an exaggerated reflex vagal response. Isolated episodes require no specific intervention, and the prognosis is excellent. Up to 80% of patients with recurrent vasovagal syncope and a positive tilt test respond to treatment with a **beta blocker** such as **(atenolol 25 to 100 mg qd)** that blunts the cardiac inotropic response to a fall in BP and thus prevents the overly sensitive reflex vagal response. Approximately half of patients who do not respond to a beta blocker or other agents will respond to **paroxetine 20 mg daily,** a selective serotonin uptake inhibitor.

Carotid Sinus Syncope

This unusual disorder is seen almost exclusively in older individuals and results from hypersensitivity of baroreceptors in the carotid sinus. External pressure of the neck (e.g., turning the head while wearing a tight collar) results in an exaggerated vagal response and fall in BP. *Carotid massage* with ECG monitoring can be used to establish the diagnosis, but this should be performed with caution.

Neurologic Causes

Transient Ischemic Attack

As stated previously, **vertebrobasilar stenosis or occlusion** is a rare cause of syncope. The diagnosis is suggested by symptoms or signs of focal brain stem ischemia (diplopia, vertigo, ataxia, nystagmus, dysarthria, facial numbness, unilateral or bilateral weakness, or sensory loss) either before or after the event. Deficits referable to the posterior cerebral artery, particularly hemianopia, may also occur. Syncope following prolonged head extension ("beauty parlor syncope") in patients with atherosclerotic vertebrobasilar disease has been described. *Transcranial and duplex Doppler ultrasonography, CT or magnetic resonance angiography*, or *conventional angiography* is required to establish the diagnosis. Management is discussed in Chapter 23.

Subclavian steal syndrome is an unusual cause of vertebrobasilar insufficiency. It results from occlusion of one of the subclavian arteries proximal to the origin of the vertebral artery. The distal subclavian artery is hence supplied by retrograde flow from the ipsilateral vertebral artery, which "steals" flow from the basilar and contralateral vertebral arteries, resulting in intermittent hemodynamic flow failure in the posterior circulation.

Unilateral **carotid stenosis or occlusion** does not cause syncope. However, in very rare instances, syncope may result from severe bilateral disease, particularly with superimposed reduction of blood pressure.

Seizures

Generalized tonic-clonic seizures always result in loss of consciousness and can easily be mistaken for syncope if the event is unwitnessed. **Atonic (akinetic) seizures** manifest as sudden loss of consciousness and muscle tone and thus are clinically indistinguishable from true syncope. They represent an unusual form of generalized-onset seizure and occur most often in children with severe epilepsy, in combination with other seizure types. Atonic seizures are exceedingly rare in adults. If seizures are suspected, identification of interictal epileptiform activity on *EEG* can establish the diagnosis. Refer to Chapter 25 for information regarding the management of epilepsy.

Subarachnoid Hemorrhage

This frequently presents with sudden loss of consciousness due to a brief surge in ICP. However, in most cases, severe headache and nuchal rigidity are the predominant symptoms once the patient awakens, and these complaints easily point to the diagnosis. *Head CT and LP* are required to establish the diagnosis. Management is discussed in Chapter 23.

Intracranial Mass Lesions

In rare instances, syncope can result from an ICP wave in a patient harboring an unsuspected intracranial mass lesion or in a patient with obstruction to cerebral venous outflow resulting from dural sinus thrombosis. The diagnosis should be evident by the presence of abnormalities on the neurologic examination and can be confirmed with *neuroimaging studies (CT or MRI)*.

Autonomic Dysfunction

Syncope or near-syncope due to autonomic impairment is *always* associated with orthostatic hypotension. **Peripheral neuropathy** from diabetes, amyloidosis, paraneoplastic disease, and other causes can involve the sympathetic nerves, which normally mediate a compensatory pressor response when BP declines upon standing. **Shy-Drager syndrome** is a multiple-system atrophy (MSA) characterized by parkinsonism (tremor, rigidity, bradykinesia, postural instability) and central autonomic failure that manifests primarily as orthostatic hypotension. Idiopathic isolated central and peripheral autonomic failure have also been described but are rare. Autonomic failure leading to orthostatic hypotension can be treated with **support stockings** and **fluordrocortisone (Florinef) 0.1 mg one to three times a day,** a pure mineralocorticoid that induces sodium retention and intravascular volume expansion. The alpha-agonist **midodrine 5 to 10 mg three times a day** can be used as an alternative to fludrocortisone.

Conversion Disorder

"Hysterical faints" generally occur as a dramatic loss of consciousness in the presence of other people, without changes in BP or pulse. Patients may betray their state by having complete or partial memory of the spell. The diagnosis should be suspected when preexisting psychiatric disease (anxiety or personality disorder) is present and the workup is negative. *Caution:* Many psychiatric medications can cause true syncope.

Hyperventilation

Hypocapnia resulting from hyperventilation leads to syncope or presyncope by decreasing cerebral blood flow because of cerebral vasoconstriction. Acute lowering of PCO_2 to 25 mm Hg is sufficient to produce symptoms. Tetany or carpopedal spasm can result from the associated alkalosis and may or may not precede the event. The diagnosis is established by a *3-minute trial of hyperventilation,* which reproduces the symptoms of presyncope or syncope. Hyperventilation usually results from **anxiety or panic disorder;** further management should be directed toward treatment of these conditions. If the problem is recurrent, acute episodes can be managed by having the patient breathe into a paper bag (CO_2 rebreathing).

Pain Syndromes

Pain is the chief complaint in many patients. Both nociceptor and spinothalamic sensitization may contribute to the development of chronic pain. Although pain may arise from a variety of non-neurologic causes, this chapter will cover the diagnosis and management of six pain syndromes that are uniquely neurologic. Headache is covered in Chapter 14. Treatment of pain, independent of the underlying cause, is usually possible with appropriate therapeutic agents, but rational management decisions can be made only after identification of the site of the pain-producing lesion and recognition of the pathophysiology of the particular pain syndrome. Figure 17–1 outlines the possible sites and mechanisms of pain. This chapter will address the following pain syndromes:

- Complex regional pain syndrome (reflex sympathetic dystrophy, causalgia, sympathetically maintained pain [SMP])
- Facial pain (tic douloureux)
- Postherpetic neuralgia
- Painful peripheral neuropathy
- Cervical or lumbar root compression
- Brachial neuritis

PHONE CALL

Questions

Questions to be asked at the time of initial contact depend on the pain syndrome. Localization will determine the subsequent path of questioning, but certain questions are pertinent to all pain syndromes. The first three questions can be asked over the phone to prepare for the history taking and examination.

1. **Where is the pain?**

   Is the pain localized, or does it radiate from one region to another, suggesting an anatomic territory?

2. **When did it begin?**

   Acute pain may respond well to specific analgesics, whereas chronic pain may require a combination of therapies, including strong psychologic support.

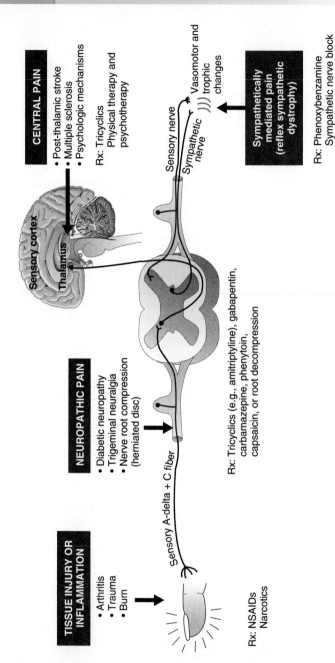

Figure 17-1 Sites of origin of pain within the nociceptive pathway.

CENTRAL PAIN
- Post-thalamic stroke
- Multiple sclerosis
- Psychologic mechanisms

Rx: Tricyclics
Physical therapy and psychotherapy

Sympathetically mediated pain (reflex sympathetic dystrophy)

Rx: Phenoxybenzamine
Sympathetic nerve block

Vasomotor and trophic changes

Sensory nerve

Sympathetic nerve

Sensory cortex

Thalamus

NEUROPATHIC PAIN
- Diabetic neuropathy
- Trigeminal neuralgia
- Nerve root compression (herniated disc)

Rx: Tricyclics (e.g., amitriptyline), gabapentin, carbamazepine, phenytoin, capsaicin, or root decompression

Sensory A-delta + C fiber

TISSUE INJURY OR INFLAMMATION
- Arthritis
- Trauma
- Burn

Rx: NSAIDs
Narcotics

3. **Is there a history of injury or underlying neurologic disease?**

Acute injury from lifting or from a mechanical task is common for radicular pain. Traumatic injury to a limb usually precedes complex regional pain syndrome. A variety of underlying medical conditions predisposes to painful peripheral neuropathies, including diabetes mellitus, alcoholism, AIDS, and exposures to environmental toxins. Some medications can produce painful neuropathies as well.

Orders

No orders should be given over the phone. Although analgesia may be required in order to obtain an adequate history and perform an adequate physical examination, it is best to evaluate the patient yourself first.

Inform RN

"Will arrive at the bedside as soon as possible."

ELEVATOR THOUGHTS

What is the differential diagnosis based on the location of pain?

Face: trigeminal neuralgia (tic douloureux), herpes zoster ophthalmicus (or herpes zoster oticus), temporomandibular joint disease, atypical facial pain, carotid artery dissection

Neck: rheumatoid arthritis, osteoarthritis, meningitis, subarachnoid hemorrhage, vertebral artery dissection, carotid artery dissection, glomus jugulare tumor, tension headache

Low back: herniated nucleus pulposus, epidural abscess, vertebral metastasis, osteomyelitis, osteoarthritis, disk infection, herpes zoster, spinal stenosis, myofasciitis, musculoligamentous strain, ankylosing spondylitis, retroperitoneal disease (referred pain from neoplasm, pancreatitis, ulcer, aortic aneurysm, etc.)

Arms/shoulders: cervical radiculopathy, brachial plexitis, SMP, ischemic heart disease, entrapment syndromes (suprascapular syndrome, radial nerve entrapment, interosseous syndrome, lateral epicondylitis)

Hands/feet (painful peripheral neuropathies): diabetes mellitus, alcoholic neuropathy, AIDS-associated neuropathy, toxin exposure (arsenic, thallium, chloramphenicol, metronidazole), amyloidosis, carpal tunnel syndrome, de Quervain's disease, SMP, paraneoplastic sensory neuropathy, multiple myeloma, inherited neuropathies (Fabry's disease, Tangier disease, dominantly inherited sensory neuropathy)

MAJOR THREAT TO LIFE

Neck pain is the only category in which a missed early diagnosis could lead to significant disability or death. Etiology of pain syndromes in this category includes carotid artery dissection, meningitis, and subarachnoid hemorrhage.

BEDSIDE

Quick Look Test

Does the patient appear acutely ill?
> Tachypnea, jaundice, or a decreased level of alertness suggests that the medical illness should be attended to before the pain syndrome is addressed.

How severe does the pain appear to be?
> Pain tolerance varies widely from individual to individual. Psychologic factors mediate the response to pain. You should try to get an impression of the relationship between the complaints and the true degree of disability. When you walk into the room, is the patient lying or sitting comfortably in bed or is he or she rolling about, grimacing, moaning, or holding the body in an unmoving posture?

Vital Signs

Fever suggests infection. Tachypnea may mean diabetic ketosis or hyperventilation in response to pain. Tachycardia and elevated blood pressure often accompany acute pain.

Selective History and Chart Review

1. **Define the character of the pain.**
   > The questions posed during the phone call should be asked directly (Where is the pain? When did the pain begin?). It is then important to try to determine whether the pain is due to involvement of neural or non-neural tissue.
   >
   > Injury to non-neural structures (muscle, bone, or joint) is often abrupt in onset, is continuous or recurrent in specific focal regions, and is usually relieved by rest. Pain caused by injury to neural structures, by contrast, can be delayed or gradual in onset, is often paroxysmal, and is often present at rest. Numbness or tingling between episodes of pain is common. The pain is often described as burning or lancinating. Particularly when the pain is caused by injury to the peripheral nervous system, the pain may be induced by normally innocuous stimuli such as the touch of a shirt or spray from a shower.

2. **What makes the pain better or worse?**

    Dysesthesias from light tactile stimuli suggest injury to peripheral nerves. "Shooting" (radiating) pains induced by movement of the arm or leg suggest cervical or lumbosacral radiculopathy.

3. **What is the patient's medical history?**

    Ask specifically about diabetes, renal disease, and risk for HIV infection when probing for causes of peripheral neuropathy. Any history of trauma may lead to a diagnosis of nerve or root compression or complex regional pain syndrome. Malignancy may produce neural pain either by compression from a mass or by neural infiltration. Chemotherapeutic agents such as vincristine can produce a painful neuropathy. A previous stroke, particularly in the thalamus, the lateral medulla, or the parietal lobe, may produce a late pain syndrome.

4. **What medications are the patient taking?**

    See Table 17–1 for a list of medications that have pain as a potential side effect.

Selective Physical Examination I

Specific points on examination are discussed under the individual pain syndromes. Certain general principles of examination hold for all pain syndromes, however.

General Physical Examination

Musculoskeletal	If there is pain in or around a joint, look for signs of inflammation, palpate for tenderness, and test the joint for active and passive range of motion. Be sure to percuss the spine to check for spinal involvement from infection or neoplastic disease.

TABLE 17–1 **Common Medications That Can Cause Pain or Paresthesia**

Antimicrobials	Psychoactive agents
Chloramphenicol	Amitriptyline
Metronidazole	Phenelzine
Streptomycin	Other medications
Nalidixic acid	Acetazolamide
Isoniazid	Pyridoxine
Antineoplastic agents	Ergotamine tartrate
Vincristine	Sulindac
Procarbazine	
Cisplatin	
Cytosine arabinoside	

Skin	Rash may accompany an infection or a drug reaction. Vesicles of herpes zoster may precede or follow the associated neuralgia.
Abdomen	Organomegaly may suggest chronic ethanol abuse. Abdominal or pelvic masses may produce pain that is referred to the back or the legs.

Neurologic Examination

Focus on the motor and sensory examinations in the location of the pain. A straight leg raise test should be done when there is low back or leg pain (Fig. 17–2). A straight leg raise test is positive when raising the leg reproduces the pain (by stretching the nerve root), particularly if the pain occurs with straight leg raise of the contralateral leg. Look for muscular atrophy in the distribution of the pain to suggest chronic sensorimotor neuropathy or local nerve entrapment or compression. Sensory loss will often map to the same territory as the pain. Hyporeflexia usually accompanies peripheral neuropathy.

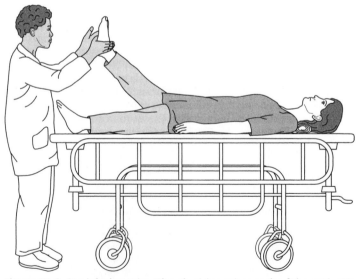

Figure 17–2 Straight leg raise. The physician raises each of the patient's legs, in turn, while the patient is supine. A positive test occurs when the pain is reproduced as a result of stretch on a nerve root. Pain of muscle stretch in the posterior thigh does not constitute a positive test.

MANAGEMENT

Management of individual pain syndromes is discussed later. There are, however, some general principles of pain management that apply in any symptomatic treatment of pain.

1. **Treat acute pain aggressively and early.**

   A common error in managing pain is to wait to see whether the pain will go away or become less intense on its own. The problem with this approach is that peripherally induced central mechanisms may intensify and prolong the pain. Partial treatment of acute pain may also be counterproductive. **For severe, acute pain, opioids are the drug of first choice** (Table 17–2). They are quick acting, and their actions may be reversed pharmacologically if necessary. Doses should be increased for maximal pain control and should be limited only by undesirable side effects. **NSAIDs, tricyclic antidepressants (TCAs), amphetamine, or hydroxyzine** may be useful adjuncts to opioids if only partial pain control is achieved (see Table 17–2 for opioid dosing).

2. **Avoid as-needed dosing for chronic or frequently recurring pain.**

   Regular dosing schedules achieve better pain control in chronic pain and minimize the anxiety from uncertainty about the next attack.

3. **Tailor the therapy to the type, location, and duration of pain.**

   Specific pharmacologic therapy remains the cornerstone of treatment, but nonpharmacologic treatment such as transcutaneous electric nerve stimulation (TENS), local or regional

TABLE 17–2 **Narcotic Equivalence Doses**

Drug	IM/IV Dose (mg)	PO Dose (mg)	Duration of Action (Hours)
Codeine	130	200	4-6
Fentanyl	0.1	—	1-2
Hydrocodone	—	5-10	4-5
Hydromorphone (Dilaudid)	1.3	7.5	4-5
Meperidine (Demerol)	75	300	3-5
Methadone	10	20	4-6
Morphine	10	60	4-5
Oxycodone (Percocet)	—	5-10	4-5
Oxymorphone	1	—	4-6
Pentazocine (Talwin)	30	—	4-6

anesthetic blocks, or physical therapy may be useful in specific instances. Psychologic support is especially important in management of chronic pain.

SELECTED PAIN SYNDROMES

Complex Regional Pain Syndrome (Reflex Sympathetic Dystrophy, Causalgia)

Clinical Presentation

This relatively rare entity usually occurs after trauma to a limb, either soft-tissue injury (type 1, formerly called reflex sympathetic dystrophy) or neural injury (type 2, formerly called causalgia). The natural history is one of persistent pain, with the development of signs of sympathetic involvement occurring days to weeks later. Sympathetic signs may include vasoconstriction and sweating, with red, glossy skin and abnormalities of the hair and nails. Hyperpathia or allodynia to light touch or cold are present on examination. Long-term consequences may be fixed joints and osteoporosis.

Diagnosis

The symptoms and signs resolve following sympathetic blockade. Blockade may be achieved by sympathetic ganglion blocks with local anesthetic, regional alpha-adrenergic blockade with guanethidine, or systemic alpha-adrenergic blockade with IV phentolamine.

Treatment

1. Pharmacologic: begin with **phenoxybenzamine** (systemic alpha-adrenergic blocker) **10 mg two times a day, tapering up to 120 mg per day** maximum or until unacceptable side effects (impotence, postural hypotension) occur. Alternatives are **clonidine 0.1 mg up to three times a day** or **prazosin 2 mg two times a day.**
2. Repeated regional sympathetic blockade with guanethidine.
3. Surgical sympathectomy.
4. Treatment with **gabapentin 900 mg to 3600 mg divided into three doses** is often effective for neuropathic pain in general. Gabapentin or another antiepileptic drug such as phenytoin or carbamazepine may be helpful as an adjunct in any of the first three treatments.

Trigeminal Neuralgia (Tic Douloureux)

This disorder of the sensory division of the trigeminal nerve usually occurs in the middle and late stages of life. The cause is unknown. Degenerative or fibrotic changes in the gasserian ganglion have been reported. In some cases, the trigeminal nerve has been found to be compressed by a tumor or a blood vessel.

Clinical Presentation

Paroxysmal unilateral lightning-like jabs of pain occur in one or more divisions of the trigeminal nerve, most commonly in the second or third division. Paroxysms usually last 1 to 2 minutes but may last up to 15 minutes. The frequency of pain ranges from several times daily to once or twice a month. Typically, patients describe a trigger that induces the paroxysm, for example, chewing, facial movements, or light touch. Patients may avoid nourishment or conversation in a desperate attempt to avoid triggering an attack. There is generally no objective sensory loss or weakness in the distribution of the pain, although patients may refuse to be examined for fear of inducing a paroxysm.

Diagnosis

Because of an absence of signs, the diagnosis of trigeminal neuralgia is made on the basis of history and observation. The differential diagnosis includes dental and sinus pain, as well as herpes zoster. Herpes (and postherpetic neuralgia) most commonly involves the first division, however. The appearance of vesicles verifies the diagnosis of herpes infection.

Treatment

Carbamazepine 200 mg two to five times a day is the first-line treatment, and it induces remissions in a high percentage of patients. **Phenytoin** or **lamotrigine** may be a medical alternative. Radiosurgery of the trigeminal ganglion may be successful in refractory cases.

Herpetic Neuralgia (Shingles), Postherpetic Neuralgia

Clinical Presentation

Herpes zoster infection causes a painful neuropathy in a dermatomal distribution, thought to result from the reactivation of a latent infection of the virus in sensory ganglion cells (i.e., from childhood chickenpox). It occurs during the lifetime of 10% to 20% of the general population, but this incidence is mostly in the elderly and in those who are immunocompromised. A thoracic dermatome is the most common site of occurrence, followed by the cervical and then the lumbosacral dermatome. Herpes zoster ophthalmicus results from infection in the first division of the trigeminal ganglion, producing a painful vesicular eruption over the upper face and the eyes. The rash of herpes zoster appears 1 to 4 days after a prodrome of fever, malaise, and dysesthesias. The vesicular eruption becomes pustular in 3 to 4 days and then crusts over by 7 to 10 days. In the normal host, the lesions resolve without sequelae in 2 to 3 weeks. In immunocompromised hosts, however, the infection may linger.

Postherpetic neuralgia is the persistence of pain after the resolution of the rash. This occurs in 10% to 20% of patients with herpes zoster, with the bulk of occurrences in the elderly and the immuno-compromised. Fifty percent of patients with postherpetic neuralgia will have a resolution of the pain in 2 months, and 70% of patients are better in 1 year. In some patients, however, the neuralgia may persist for many years.

Diagnosis

You can make the clinical diagnosis on the basis of the typical dermatomal rash. Pain and mild sensory loss should follow the same dermatomal distribution. For confirmatory diagnosis, consultation from the infectious disease or dermatology service may be helpful. Vesicles may contain polymorphonuclear leukocytes. A scrape biopsy may show giant cells and intranuclear inclusions. Varicella-zoster virus antibody titers may increase fourfold.

Treatment

1. **Acute herpes zoster infection**
   Acyclovir 5 mg/kg IV (infuse over 1 hour) three times a day for 7 days will shorten the period of acute dermatomal pain and accelerate healing of the rash but will not reduce the incidence or severity of postherpetic neuralgia. A newer antiviral agent, **famciclovir, given orally for 7 days** may reduce the duration and severity of the neuralgia. **Prednisone 60 mg PO per day for 7 days** may reduce acute pain and potentially reduce the incidence of postherpetic neuralgia. Beware of using prednisone in immunocompromised hosts.
2. **Postherpetic neuralgia**
   This condition is notoriously difficult to treat, and a variety of anticonvulsants and antidepressants have been tried. Amitriptyline 50 to 150 mg PO per day in divided doses, gabapentin 300 to 900 mg PO three times a day, and oxycodone/acetaminophen (Percocet) 1 to 2 tablets every 6 hours may reduce the burning pain. Lidoderm (5% lidocaine) patch has been shown to be an effective topical treatment. Intrathecal treatment with methylprednisolone (60 mg) plus 3% lidocaine (3 ml) has been shown to be effective in patients with refractory pain.

Painful Peripheral Neuropathy

Clinical Presentation

Systemic disease affecting the peripheral nervous system produces symptoms in the longest nerves first. Dysesthesias and sensory loss in a symmetric, stocking-glove distribution are typical for early peripheral neuropathy. The patient may describe "burning" on the soles of the feet or hypersensitivity to touch in the feet more than in the hands. There may be gait disturbance from the pain of walking or from early sensory loss.

During the examination, look for wasting of the muscles, sensory loss (vibratory sense may be the first to be lost), and hyporeflexia in the distal extremities.

Diagnosis

The clinical diagnosis may often be made from the history and physical examination. Be sure to ask about diabetes mellitus, alcohol use, renal disease, and HIV risks. Occupational history may reveal exposure to toxins.

If the patient has an obvious cause (e.g., postvincristine chemotherapy), no further workup may be needed. *EMG and nerve conduction studies* can confirm a diagnosis of peripheral neuropathy and distinguish between demyelinating and axonal pathology (most painful neuropathies are axonal). Initial laboratory tests to order should include fasting glucose level with full chemistry panel including liver and thyroid function tests, rheumatologic screen (ESR, ANA, and RF) SPEP (screen for multiple myeloma), CBC, and serum vitamin B_{12} level.

Treatment

1. Treat any underlying metabolic disorder or malignancy or remove any offending neurotoxins.
2. Symptomatic treatment of painful peripheral neuropathy consists of anticonvulsants, tricyclic antidepressants, or topical agents. Begin with **gabapentin 100 mg three times a day** (lower dosage for elderly patients) and taper up to 1800 to 3600 mg per day divided in three doses. **Pregabalin 150 to 300 mg bid** may have greater analgesic properties than its predecessor, gabapentin, particularly with painful diabetic neuropathy. Tricyclic antidepressants, such as amitriptyline 25 to 100 mg daily, are an alternative.
3. For topical treatment, use **capsaicin (0.075% to 0.25%) three to four times per day or Lidoderm (5% lidocaine)-impregnated occlusive dressing.**
4. Anti-inflammatory agents such as **ibuprofen 400 to 800 mg PO every 6 hours** may be a useful adjunct to more specific therapies, particularly when the cause of the neuropathy may be inflammatory. A 10- to 14-day tapering course of oral steroids such as **dexamethasone 6 mg PO four times a day** can be a useful analgesic while chemotherapy is being initiated.
5. Nonpharmacologic therapies such as TENS can supplement the treatment regimen.

Cervical or Lumbosacral Root Compression

Clinical Presentation

Acute low back or neck pain from root compression is often precipitated by a specific physical event such as lifting a heavy weight or twisting in an unusual way during housework or gardening. The differential diagnosis includes neck or back strain without neural injury. Radicular pain usually presents as shooting pain into an arm or leg. There is almost always perispinal pain because of reactive muscle spasm. With lumbosacral disk herniation, the pain is often increased by coughing or sneezing. Lumbar disks tend to herniate posterolaterally, and cervical disks tend to herniate centrally. Disk herniation is therefore more likely to produce radicular syndromes in the low back as opposed to signs of myelopathy in the neck. Root compression in the neck, therefore, is more often seen with cervical degenerative disease. Osteoarthritis can produce cervical spondylitic ridges and osteophytes, facet joint arthritis, and neural foraminal narrowing.

Diagnosis

The typical symptom for lumbar radiculopathy is **sciatica**, or radiation of pain into the back and side of the leg. The most commonly affected roots are L5 (produced by herniation of the L4-L5 disk) and S1 (produced by herniation of the L5-S1 disk). Upper lumbar root compressions are less common. In the cervical region, C5 and C6 are the roots most affected by cervical spondylosis; C7 is the root most affected by disk lesions. Higher cervical involvement or thoracic radiculopathies warrant further investigation for neoplastic disease or neurofibromatosis. Table 17–3 lists the pain, sensory, and reflex changes for common cervical and lumbosacral radicular syndromes. Also see the **dermatome and myotome charts** in Appendices A-1, A-2, and A-5. Clinical diagnosis can usually be made from the history and examination. Be sure to check motor, sensory, and reflex function in the distribution of the pain. For lumbosacral pain, putting stretch on the root with a straight leg raise test (the exact pain syndrome should be reproduced by ipsilateral or contralateral straight leg raise) supports the diagnosis of radiculopathy (see Fig. 17–2). *Cervical or lumbosacral spinal MRI* is the diagnostic test of choice to visualize the spinal cord, the vertebrae, the disks, and the nerve roots. If there is any suspicion of a neoplastic or infectious lesion, a gadolinium MRI should be obtained.

Treatment

1. **Conservative management** with rest and analgesia usually suffices to achieve good recovery. Even if there is evidence for disk herniation, long-term recovery will be better if the condition resolves without operation. For cervical radiculopathy, a soft collar in combination with **ibuprofen 600 mg PO every 4 to 6 hours** may be enough to promote recovery. For cervical or lumbosacral root disease, the addition of narcotics such as **acetaminophen with codeine 1 to 2 tabs PO every 4 to 6 hours** may be necessary, particularly in the first

TABLE 17–3 Clinical Features of Cervical and Lumbosacral Root Compression Syndromes

Root	Area of Pain	Sensory Loss	Motor Loss	Reflex
C5	Lateral upper arm and medial scapula	Lateral upper arm	Shoulder abduction, internal and external rotation, and elbow flexion	Biceps jerk
C6	Lateral forearm, thumb, and index finger	Lateral forearm and thumb	Elbow supination	Supinator jerk
C7	Over the triceps, midforearm, and middle finger	Middle fingers	Elbow extension and wrist extension	Triceps jerk
C8	Medial forearm and little finger	Medial forearm and little finger	Finger flexion and finger extension	Finger jerk
L4	Knee to medial malleolus	Medial knee and leg	Foot inversion and knee extension	Knee jerk
L5	Back of thigh, lateral calf, and dorsum of foot	Dorsum of foot	Foot and toe dorsiflexion	None
S1	Back of thigh, back of calf, and lateral foot	Behind lateral malleolus, sole of foot	Foot plantar flexion and foot eversion	Ankle jerk

few days. The addition of **diazepam 2 to 5 mg every 6 hours** may also be helpful in the short term to relieve reactive muscle spasm.

2. **Surgical intervention** should be reserved for three indications: (1) bowel or bladder involvement with lumbosacral radiculopathy, (2) severe neurologic deficit, such as a complete footdrop or more than mild weakness in the upper extremity, and (3) failure to control pain or reverse a neurologic deficit with medical management for at least 3 weeks. Referral should be made to a neurosurgeon experienced with spine disease.

3. Local injections of **corticosteroids** at the nerve roots may obviate the need for surgery.

Brachial Neuritis (Neuralgic Amyotrophy, Brachial Neuralgia, Parsonage-Turner Syndrome)

Clinical Presentation

This rare syndrome typically begins with pain localized to the C5 and C6 dermatomes. Pain in the shoulder may have an aching quality that radiates into the arm. Some patients have mild sensory loss in the distribution of the axillary nerve. Within a few days, the shoulder girdle musculature becomes weak and atrophic, affecting the C5 and C6 myotomes. The disease is idiopathic and sporadic, affecting men more than twice as frequently as women. Most cases occur after the third decade. The syndrome may be associated with trauma, infection, or vaccination and is usually unilateral, rarely bilateral. Guarding of the shoulder may lead to a frozen shoulder.

Diagnosis

The clinical pattern of relatively rapid onset of pain followed by weakness is typical for brachial neuritis. The differential diagnosis at the early stage in which pain is the only complaint includes inflammatory and orthopedic involvement, as well as cervical radiculopathy and root compression from a rudimentary cervical rib. **EMG/nerve conduction studies usually show evidence of denervation in the affected myotomes and decreased amplitude of sensory nerve action potentials.** Subtle signs may also be present on the unaffected side in up to 25% of patients.

Treatment

Because the cause of brachial neuritis is unknown, there is no specific therapy. *Immobilization of the shoulder girdle* can help minimize the pain caused by movement, but gentle physical therapy with **passive range-of-motion exercises** should be used to avoid a frozen shoulder. **Ibuprofen 600 mg every 4 to 6 hours** may be used as the first therapy for analgesia. If there is no relief in 24 hours, **acet-aminophen with codeine 1 to 2 tabs PO every 4 to 6 hours,** or a 2-week, tapering course of steroids, beginning with **prednisone 60 mg PO per day,** may be used. The prognosis is good, with 90% of patients making a good recovery. The prognosis is poor if the EMG shows no voluntary motor units.

Brain Death

Brain death describes a condition of complete and irreversible cessation of all cortical and brain stem activity. Although death has traditionally been defined by the irreversible cessation of cardiorespiratory function, technologic advances have led to formal recognition of death on the basis of complete and permanent brain destruction in individuals on life support. In turn, legislative and hospital policies recognizing cerebral death as the equivalent of cardiac death have enabled physicians to save thousands of lives through organ transplantation.

The most common causes of brain death are trauma, intracranial hemorrhage, and hypoxic-ischemic injury from cardiac arrest. Whatever the inciting cause, in the end, brain death ultimately results from widespread cerebral necrosis and edema, herniation, increased ICP, and the complete absence of cerebral blood flow.

CLINICAL SIGNIFICANCE OF BRAIN DEATH

It is important to identify and diagnose brain death **quickly** for the following reasons:

1. To prevent prolonged anguish and suffering on the part of the patient's loved ones
2. To avoid the needless waste of valuable medical resources in an unequivocal no-win situation
3. To create an opportunity for organ donation. Because circulatory collapse and homeostatic disarray begin as soon as brain death occurs, delays in declaration of brain death can lead to the loss of organ viability.

Although the clinical criteria for brain death outlined in the following section are widely agreed upon, policies vary by state and institution regarding (1) the need for examination by a concurring physician, (2) the timing of examinations or a required observation period, and (3) the requirements for confirmatory testing. If you are unsure of the policy at your institution, find out. The declaration of death is a serious issue and must be made with care and precision.

CRITERIA FOR THE CLINICAL DIAGNOSIS OF BRAIN DEATH

To make the clinical diagnosis of brain death, the following conditions must be met:

1. **CEREBRAL FUNCTION MUST BE ABSENT.**

   This means that the patient must be in deep coma, with no behavioral or reflex responses to painful stimuli mediated above the level of the foramen magnum. Triple flexion responses, deep tendon reflexes, or other primitive movements (back arching, extensor plantar responses) resulting from spinal reflex activity are compatible with brain death. In most cases, the patient with brain death is in a state of flaccid and areflexic paralysis, with isolated lower-extremity triple flexion responses to deep pain. Decerebrate or decorticate posturing is incompatible with brain death, because these reflexes are mediated at the brain stem level.

2. **BRAIN STEM FUNCTIONS MUST BE ABSENT.**

   a. **Pupils**

      The pupils must be unreactive to bright light. Size is not critical, as pupils may be small, midposition, or large. Exposure to mydriatic agents must be excluded.

   b. **Ocular movements**

      Ocular responses must be absent to passive head turning (the oculocephalic or "doll's eye" reflex) and caloric irrigation of the ear canals with 50 ml of ice water (the oculovestibular reflex). Care must be taken that the stimulus reaches the tympanic membrane. Testing using passive head turning alone is not adequate.

   c. **Facial sensation and motor response**

      Corneal reflexes should be tested with a cotton-tipped applicator. Reflex or spontaneous facial or eyelid movements must be completely absent.

   d. **Pharyngeal and tracheal reflexes**

      Cough and gag responses must be absent in response to manipulation of the endotracheal tube or bronchial suctioning.

3. **THE PATIENT MUST BE APNEIC.**

   Spontaneous respirations must be absent in response to a hypercarbic stimulus, as documented by formal apnea testing (Box 18–1).

4. **A PROXIMATE AND UNTREATABLE CAUSE OF BRAIN DEATH MUST BE ESTABLISHED.**

   a. **The cause of coma should be clearly evident and sufficient to account for the loss of brain function.**

      Examples include documented structural disease (e.g., massive intracranial hemorrhage) or severe brain anoxia resulting from cardiopulmonary arrest.

BOX 18–1 **Protocol for Apnea Testing**

1. Adjust minute ventilation to attain PCO_2 levels of 35 to 45 mm Hg and document with a **baseline arterial blood gas measurement.**
2. **Preoxygenate** with 100% oxygen for 5 minutes.
3. Place the patient on a **T-piece with 100% oxygen flow-by** at 6 to 10 L/min for **4 to 6 minutes.** Because PCO_2 increases 3 to 4 mm Hg per minute of apnea, a *4- to 6-minute period of observation* should allow the PCO_2 to rise to levels of hypercarbia (greater than 55 mm Hg) sufficient to provide an adequate respiratory stimulus.
4. **Observe for respiratory movements.** Abort the test and place the patient back on mechanical ventilation if cardiac arrhythmia, hypotension, or significant oxygen desaturation occurs.
5. At the end of the observation period, **perform a second ABG measurement** to document the level of hypercarbia attained and place the patient back on **mechanical ventilation.**
6. **Write a note** in the chart documenting that no respiratory movements were observed. Record the duration of the observation period and the postobservation arterial blood gas level.

b. **Potentially reversible conditions must be excluded.**

These conditions may include *hypothermia* (core temperature less than 34° C), *intoxication, drug hypotension* (systolic BP less than 90 mm Hg), and *severe acid-base or electrolyte abnormalities.* If these conditions are present, the patient may require rewarming, treatment with IV pressors, or correction of acid-base and electrolyte disorders in order to proceed with the declaration of brain death. A toxicology screen should be performed in all patients to exclude intoxication or poisoning. A common clinical scenario is brain death in the setting of barbiturate coma with pentobarbital or a similar agent for ICP control or management of status epilepticus. In this scenario, the diagnosis of brain death can still be established by demonstrating complete intracranial circulatory arrest with cerebral angiography, a nuclear cerebral perfusion scan, or transcranial Doppler, despite the presence of pentobarbital anesthesia.

c. **Loss of all brain function should persist for an appropriate period of observation.**

If the cause of coma is established and is adequate to account for brain death, an extended period of observation is not required. A period of observation of 6 to 24 hours may be appropriate if the cause of brain death is not absolutely clear (for example, suspected but unwitnessed cardiac arrest). Some institutions require a period of observation of 6 to 24 hours in all patients.

CONFIRMATORY TESTING

Brain death is a clinical diagnosis. Confirmatory tests such as EEG are not essential to the declaration of brain death but may be required according to state laws or institutional policy. In circumstances in which the clinical diagnosis of brain death cannot be made with certainty, a confirmatory test may be needed (Fig. 18–1). Examples may include severe facial or limb trauma, preexisting pupillary abnormalities, severe pulmonary disease resulting in chronic retention of carbon dioxide, or recent treatment with a barbiturate.

Tests Commonly Used for the Confirmation of Brain Death

1. **EEG**

   Confirmation of neocortical death can be documented by at least 30 minutes of electrocerebral silence, using a 16-channel instrument with increased gain settings, according to guidelines developed by the American Electroencephalographic Society. If any brain wave is present, the diagnosis of brain death cannot be made. EEG confirmation of brain death is also not valid in patients exposed to sedatives or toxins, since they can directly suppress the brain electrical activity.

2. **Angiography**

   Complete absence of intracranial blood flow in a four-vessel angiogram confirms the diagnosis of brain death.

3. **Radioisotope cerebral imaging**

   The complete absence of cerebral perfusion can also be established using radionuclide angiography or single photon emission computed tomography (SPECT).

4. **Transcranial Doppler ultrasonography**

   A velocity profile showing systolic spikes with absent or reversed diastolic flow is consistent with the cessation of cerebral blood flow and brain death.

PSYCHOSOCIAL ISSUES

The emotional and psychosocial impact of death is always stressful for those who survive the patient; this can be even more difficult in the setting of brain death. Communication of the concept and meaning of brain death to the patient's family is paramount. This communication, however painful, should be initiated as early as possible in order to give those involved time to adjust to the situation. Although family permission is generally *not* required to discontinue life support once a patient is declared legally brain dead, their consent and understanding is extremely important. Misunderstanding, bereavement, emotional upset, and religious or moral beliefs

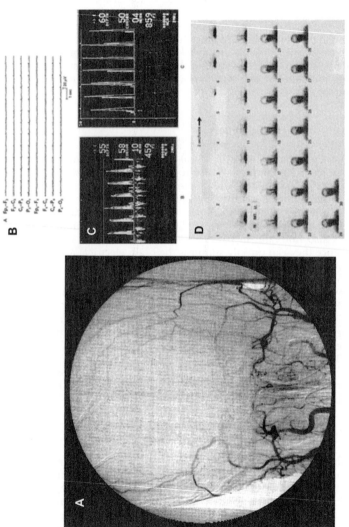

Figure 18–1 Diagnostic tests for the confirmation of brain death. A, Anteroposterior view of a cerebral angiogram demonstrating complete intracranial circulatory arrest at the level of the petrous internal carotid arteries. Note the persistence of external carotid artery flow. B, Flat electrocerebrosilence EEG demonstrating artifactual electrocardiographic activity generated by the heart. C, Transcranial Doppler sonography of the middle cerebral arteries demonstrating isolated systolic spikes with reversed (left panel) or absent (right panel) diastic flow. D, Radionuclide cerebral perfusion scan demonstrating the complete absence of blood flow to the brain.

may lead family members to object to "pulling the plug" in some cases. In these instances, third-party mediation by a medical ethics consultant or member of the clergy may be desirable.

ICU MANAGEMENT OF THE POTENTIAL ORGAN DONOR

Brain death eventually leads to severe homeostatic derangements and cardiac arrest despite mechanical ventilation and aggressive life-support measures. This inexorable progression toward multisystem organ failure creates a challenge in managing the potential organ donor, in whom the goal is to maintain and optimize organ viability for transplantation.

Most patients become hypotensive due to sudden loss of resting sympathetic tone and require IV pressors at the time brain death occurs, and soon thereafter they develop diabetes insipidus (because antidiuretic hormone secretion ceases). Adrenergic vasopressors such as dopamine or arginine vasopressin, both of which cause peripheral vasoconstriction in this setting, are considered the first-line interventions for hypotension. In some cases, continued hypotension will respond to thyroid and glucocorticoid hormone replacement, indicating a relative deficiency of these hormones.

The situation usually deteriorates when brain dead patients are maintained on a ventilator for a prolonged period of time. Hypothermia, refractory hypoxia, disseminated intravascular coagulation, metabolic acidosis, renal failure, and adult respiratory distress syndrome may all occur. The key to management is to be ready for these complications. Even with meticulous attention to cardiovascular, acid-base, and electrolyte homeostasis, organ viability in most adult patients with brain death can be maintained for only 72 to 96 hours.

Protocol for Management of the Potential Organ Donor in the Intensive Care Unit

1. Insert a central venous catheter or two large-bore peripheral IV lines.
2. Insert an arterial line for continuous BP monitoring.
   a. Maintain systolic BP at or higher than 100 mm Hg with stepwise intervention:
      (1) **500 ml 0.9% saline fluid bolus (two times at 10-minute intervals)**
      (2) **Dopamine 800 mg/500 ml NS (start at 13 ml/hr, 5 μg/kg/min), titrated to maintain systolic BP at or higher than 100 mm Hg**
      (3) If refractory hypotension (systolic BP less than 90 mm Hg) or tachyarrhythmia occurs with dopamine treatment, start **vasopressin (Pitressin) 4 U/hr**

(4) If hypotension is refractory to dopamine and/or IV Pitressin, perform thyroxine (T_4) replacement protocol:

a. Administer as IV boluses:
   i. **Dextrose 50% (1 amp)**
   ii. **Methylprednisolone 1 g**
   iii. **Regular insulin 10 U**
   iv. **Levothyroxine 20 μg**
b. If the BP responds to the above boluses, start **levothroxine 5 μg/hr as a continuous infusion (200 μg/500 ml NS at 12.5 ml/hr)** and titrate to maintain the SBP >100 mm Hg. Note that throxine can precipitate cardiac arrhythmias, particularly in younger, hypokalemic patients.

3. Start baseline IV flow: **0.9% saline at 150 to 200 ml/hr.**
   a. Check serum sodium levels every 6 hours:
      (1) If sodium level is 150 to 159 mmol/L, change baseline IV to 0.45% saline.
      (2) If sodium level is >160 mmol/L, change baseline IV to 0.25% saline.

4. Transfuse if hematocrit is lower than 24%.

5. Adjust fraction of inspired oxygen and positive end-expiratory pressure to maintain PaO_2 >100 mm Hg and oxygen saturation higher than 92%.

6. Insert a Foley catheter. Measure fluid input and urine output and monitor urine specific gravity every 2 hours.
   a. If the urine output over 2 hours is greater than 500 ml with specific gravity of 1.005 or lower, begin treatment for DI:
      (1) Administer **aqueous Pitressin 6 to 10 U IVP.**
      (2) Start **IV Pitressin 2 to 4 U/hr titrated to maintain SBP >100 mm Hg and UO <200 ml/hr.**
      (3) Replace hourly urine output milliliter for milliliter with D5W.

7. Check the finger stick glucose level every 4 hours.
   a. If finger stick glucose level is higher than 140 mg/dl, begin **insulin drip (100 U regular insulin in 1000 ml 0.9% saline) starting at 20 ml/hr (2 U/hour), titrated to maintain blood glucose between 80 and 120 mg/dl.**

Selected
Neurologic
Disorders

Nerve and Muscle Diseases

Patients with neuromuscular disease generally present with weakness, sensory loss, or both of these conditions. Your approach should initially focus on localizing the problem to a specific component of the peripheral nervous system that is involved (e.g., neuropathy or myopathy) and then be directed toward identifying a specific disease process. The major anatomic components of the peripheral nervous system are listed in Table 19–1.

APPROACH TO THE PATIENT WITH SUSPECTED NEUROMUSCULAR DISEASE

History

1. **Clarify the pattern of weakness.** Proximal weakness suggests myopathy; distal weakness suggests neuropathy.
2. **Characterize any sensory symptoms.** Have the patient identify the exact regions involved and symptom character (sensory loss or unpleasant sensation).
3. **Ask about cramps and muscle twitches (fasciculations).** These symptoms point to disease of the motor neuron (amyotrophic lateral sclerosis, ALS) or muscle (myopathy).
4. **Ask about pain.** Pain may be related to a musculoskeletal structure (e.g., herniated disk), or it may be neuropathic or muscular.
5. **Is there any autonomic involvement?** Ask about orthostatic dizziness, anhidrosis, visual blurring, urinary hesitancy or incontinence, constipation, and impotence. These symptoms can result from autonomic neuropathy.

Examination

1. **Determine whether the patient has true weakness.** Decreased strength needs to be differentiated from limitation arising from pain, and from submaximal effort. Effort-limited weakness is inconsistent and tends to "give way" suddenly.

TABLE 19–1 Basic Anatomic Subtypes of Neuromuscular Disease

Anatomic Site	Typical Pattern of Motor and Sensory Deficit	Examples
Motor neuron disease	Weakness, wasting, fasciculations; no sensory deficits; hyper-reflexia with ALS	Amyotrophic lateral sclerosis, spinal muscular atrophy, polio
Monoradiculopathy	Distribution of a single nerve root (dermatomal pattern)	L5 or S1 root compression herniated disk form
Polyradiculopathy	Distribution of multiple nerve roots	Cauda equine syndrome; carcinomatous meningitis
Plexopathy	Distribution of a nerve plexus	Acute brachial neuritis
Mononeuropathy	Distribution of a single peripheral nerve	Carpal tunnel syndrome
Mononeuropathy multiplex	Multifocal process affecting several discrete peripheral nerves	Vasculitis, leprosy
Polyneuropathy	Diffuse, symmetric, distal stocking-glove pattern; distal hyporeflexia	Diabetic polyneuropathy
Neuromuscular junction disease	Fluctuating weakness with fatigability; no sensory deficits; reflexes preserved	Myasthenia gravis
Myopathy	Diffuse proximal muscle weakness; no sensory deficits; preserved reflexes until late	Polymyositis; muscular dystrophy

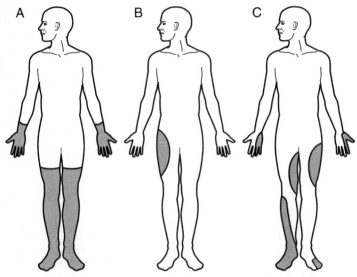

Figure 19–1 Patterns of sensory loss in patients with neuropathy. *A*, Polyneuropathy: diffuse stocking-glove pattern. *B*, Mononeuropathy: focal involvement corresponding to a single peripheral nerve. *C*, Mononeuritis multiplex: pattern of multiple, asymmetric regions of sensory loss, corresponding to multiple peripheral nerves.

2. **Map out any sensory deficits.** Think in terms of identifying *diffuse, distal sensory loss* (stocking-glove pattern), as seen in polyneuropathy; *focal sensory loss* restricted to a single root dermatome or peripheral nerve; or *multifocal sensory loss*, which suggests mononeuropathy multiplex or a plexus lesion (Fig. 19–1).
3. **Test the reflexes.** Loss of deep tendon reflexes suggests peripheral nerve involvement.
4. **Undress the patient to check for wasting and fasciculations** (irregular individual muscle twitches). These findings indicate lower motor neuron disease.

MOTOR NEURON DISEASE

The clinical hallmarks of anterior horn cell disease are the lower motor neuron signs of **weakness, wasting (atrophy), and fasciculations.** These signs may be seen alone or in combination with upper motor neuron signs (hyper-reflexia, upgoing toes) in the case of ALS. Sensory disturbances are absent. There are several distinct forms of motor neuron disease:

1. **Amyotrophic lateral sclerosis**

   Also known as Lou Gehrig's disease, ALS is the most common form of motor neuron disease. It is easily recognized on the basis of progressive weakness, wasting, fasciculations, and upper motor neuron signs. It is familiar in 5% to 10% of cases. The presence of bulbar involvement (dysarthria, dysphagia) carries a worse prognosis. Median survival after diagnosis is 3 years. Approximately 5% of patients have a circulating paraprotein, and in these cases an underlying lymphoma or plasma cell dyscrasia may be detected. ALS is a clinical diagnosis, which is supported by the finding of diffuse, chronic partial denervation in at least three limbs on EMG.

2. **Spinal muscular atrophy**

   This condition resembles ALS but is limited to pure lower motor neuron degeneration (e.g., no upper motor neuron signs are seen). Spinal muscular atrophy typically has infantile or childhood onset, but adult forms also occur. Adult onset progression is slower than ALS and is more often hereditary. Genetic confirmation of some forms is available.

3. **Multifocal motor neuropathy**

   This is an immune-mediated motor neuropathy, differentiated by the presence of **conduction block** on nerve conduction studies. The course is protracted over many years, and the weakness is asymmetric. Some patients have anti-GM1 antibodies. The disorder is important to recognize because it is treatable with IVIG.

4. **Other motor neuron diseases**

   These diseases include poliomyelitis, hereditary neurodegenerative diseases, and metabolic systemic storage disorders.

Diagnosis

Diagnostic testing for suspected motor neuron disease should include the following: EMG/NCS, serum and urine electrophoresis, serum immunoelectrophoresis, quantitative immunoglobulins, and anti-GM1 antibody levels. Cervical spine MRI and lumbar puncture should be considered. In patients with a paraprotein, bone marrow biopsy may be indicated.

Treatment

ALS is incurable, but **riluzole 50 mg PO twice per day,** a glutamate antagonist, may slow the progression of the disease. Clinical trials of additional agents are ongoing. Patients with multifocal motor neuropathy may improve with treatment with **IVIG 0.4 g/kg given every 6 to 12 weeks.**

MONORADICULOPATHY AND POLYRADICULOPATHY

Monoradiculopathies typically result from disk herniation and nerve root compression. They present with a radicular distribution of pain and are discussed in Chapter 17. *Polyradiculopathy* involving multiple lumbosacral nerve roots (cauda equina syndrome) presents with low back pain, urinary disturbances, and gait failure.

PLEXOPATHY

Diseases that cause diffuse injury to either the brachial or the lumbosacral plexus lead to **regional motor, sensory, and reflex disturbances in one limb.** The key to identifying the syndrome is to find a pattern of deficits that cannot be explained by involvement of one nerve root or a single peripheral nerve. EMG and NCS are helpful in confirming and defining the syndrome; complex repetitive discharges on EMG are characteristic. See Appendices A-3 and A-4 for the anatomy of the brachial and lumbosacral plexus.

Brachial Plexopathy

Upper brachial plexus injury (arising from C5 to C7) results in weakness and atrophy of the shoulder and upper arm muscles (Erb's palsy). Lower brachial plexus injury (arising from C8 and T1) leads to weakness, atrophy, and sensory deficits in the forearm and hand (Klumpke's palsy). The main causes of brachial plexopathy include the following:

1. **Trauma**
2. **Idiopathic brachial neuritis (Parsonage-Turner syndrome)**
   This under-recognized syndrome presents with the sudden onset of pain in the shoulder and arm; as the pain resolves over 2 to 4 weeks, weakness and muscle wasting become evident.
3. **Tumor infiltration**
   Metastatic disease and neurofibroma are most common.
4. **Radiation plexopathy**
   High-dose irradiation for lymphoma or breast cancer can lead to painless progressive brachial plexopathy 1 to 5 years later. *Myokymia* (irregular wormlike muscle movement) may be a distinguishing feature.
5. **Cervical rib or bands (thoracic outlet syndrome)**
   This rare condition is caused by compression of the lower trunk of the brachial plexus as it passes over an abnormal first cervical rib or fibrous band. Patients complain of pain and paresthesias in the C8-T1 distribution of the hand and medial forearm when carrying heavy objects or when raising the arm above shoulder level. Surgical decompression may be helpful in rare cases.

Lumbosacral Plexopathy

Unilateral lumbosacral plexopathy is rare. The main diagnostic considerations include idiopathic neuritis, diabetic infarction, and compression from a retroperitoneal abscess, hemorrhage, or neoplasm.

Diagnosis

In many cases, the cause of brachial or lumbosacral plexopathy is readily apparent (e.g., trauma or radiation). If not, chest and cervical spine radiographs, LP, and MRI or CT of the plexus should be considered.

Treatment

Physical therapy can help speed recovery, minimize muscle wasting, and prevent contractures.

MONONEUROPATHIES

Mononeuropathies result from injury, compression, or entrapment of a single nerve, usually at a specific site. There are multiple different syndromes.

Carpal Tunnel Syndrome

Carpal tunnel syndrome is by far the most common cause of mononeuropathy; it results from compression of the median nerve at the wrist and usually presents with wrist pain and tingling of the first three digits. The pain may radiate proximally to the elbow and is almost always worse at night. Examination may reveal *Tinel's sign* (radiation of pain into the first three digits when the wrist is tapped with a hammer). Thenar muscle wasting and persistent sensory deficits in the distal median nerve distribution are advanced findings (Fig. 19-2). Risk factors include repetitive "overuse" injury, thyroid disease, pregnancy, acromegaly, diabetes, and amyloidosis.

Diagnosis

EMG and NCS show focal sensory and/or motor slowing across the wrist in the median nerve. Check thyroid function tests (TFTs) and fasting glucose level to screen for hypothyroidism and diabetes.

Treatment

Mild disease can be treated with a neutral position wrist splint; more severe disease may require surgical decompression. Repetitive stress to the wrist can be minimized with special occupational devices.

Facial Palsy (Bell's Palsy)

Facial palsy (Bell's palsy) is the most common cranial mononeuropathy. Patients present with acute unilateral facial paralysis, with equal involvement of the forehead and lower half of the face. The

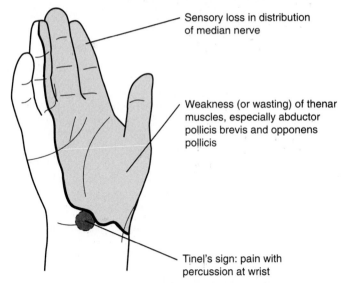

Sensory loss in distribution of median nerve

Weakness (or wasting) of thenar muscles, especially abductor pollicis brevis and opponens pollicis

Tinel's sign: pain with percussion at wrist

Figure 19–2 Sensory and motor involvement in carpal tunnel syndrome.

disorder is thought to result from inflammation of cranial nerve 7 within the facial canal. In some patients, an antecedent viral infection is identified, and approximately 25% of cases are associated with pain in the ipsilateral ear. If the injury to the facial nerve is proximal to the chorda tympani in the facial canal, loss of taste occurs on the anterior two thirds of the tongue ipsilaterally. Complete or near-complete recovery occurs in 85% of cases.

Diagnosis

The majority of cases are idiopathic (Bell's palsy). Examination should focus on searching for signs of other treatable diseases that can present with facial paralysis:

- Decreased hearing or a decreased afferent corneal reflex is suggestive of a cerebellopontine angle tumor (e.g., acoustic neuroma), which should be excluded by MRI with gadolinium.
- Vesicles in the external auditory canal are indicative of the Ramsay Hunt syndrome, which results from herpes zoster infection of the ipsilateral geniculate ganglion.
- An antecedent annular rash or tick bite is suggestive of Lyme disease. Serum Lyme antibody titers and LP with testing for CSF Lyme antibodies are required to establish the diagnosis.
- Interstitial lung disease with hilar adenopathy, uveitis, or parotitis may be a clue to neurosarcoidosis. CSF examination may

reveal a lymphocytic pleocytosis; biopsy of involved tissue is required to establish the diagnosis.

Treatment

Recovery from idiopathic Bell's palsy can be accelerated by treatment with **prednisone 80 mg PO daily for 5 days,** followed by a 7-day taper. Ramsay Hunt syndrome is treated with **acyclovir 800 mg PO five times daily for 7 days** in addition to prednisone. The likelihood of complete recovery is increased when treatment is started within 7 days of onset. Treatment for Lyme disease (see Chapter 21) and neurosarcoidosis (see Chapter 21) is discussed elsewhere. Patients with incomplete eye closure should use an ophthalmic ointment (e.g., Lacri-Lube) and a protective eye shield at night to prevent corneal abrasions.

Other Common Nerve Entrapment Syndromes

The nerves implicated in additional selected entrapment syndromes are the following:
- Ulnar nerve at the medial epicondyle of the humerus (cubital tunnel syndrome)
- Median nerve at the pronator teres (pronator syndrome)
- Radial nerve at the spiral groove of the humerus (Saturday night palsy)
- Obturator nerve at the obturator foramen (childbirth)
- Peroneal nerve at the fibular head (leg crossers and surgical malpositioning)
- Lateral femoral cutaneous nerve (meralgia paresthetica)
- Posterior tibial nerve at the tarsal tunnel (tarsal tunnel syndrome).

MONONEUROPATHY MULTIPLEX

Diseases that affect multiple peripheral nerves at different sites result in the syndrome of *mononeuropathy multiplex.* The presence of **asymmetric and multifocal motor, sensory, and reflex deficits** is the key to identifying the syndrome. The patient's history may reveal a stepwise progression of deficits. The differential diagnosis of mononeuropathy multiplex includes the following:
- *Vasculitis*

    Polyarteritis nodosa is the most common vasculitis associated with this condition. Systemic lupus erythematosus, rheumatoid arthritis, and cryoglobulinemia may occasionally produce the condition.
- *Diabetes mellitus*
- *Leprosy*
- *Sarcoidosis*
- *HIV infection*

- *Lymphoma*
- *Lyme disease*
- *Hereditary liability to pressure palsies*
- *Multifocal motor neuropathy (pure motor)*
- *Chronic inflammatory demyelinating polyneuropathy (CIDP)*

Diagnosis

Initial blood tests should include fasting glucose level with chem-20 screen, CBC, ESR, ANA, RF, antineurotrophil cytoplasmic antibody (ANCA), HIV testing, hepatitis serologies, cryoglobulins, and serum angiotensin-converting enzyme (ACE) activity. LP should be considered to rule out inflammatory conditions (e.g., chronic inflammatory demyelinating polyneuropathy, neurosarcoidosis) and carcinomatous meningitis. A comprehensive EMG and NCS examination is often needed to prove multifocal involvement. Muscle or nerve biopsy is usually necessary to rule out vasculitis, sarcoidosis, leprosy, and lymphoma.

Treatment

Therapy is directed toward treating the underlying disease.

POLYNEUROPATHY

The prototypical polyneuropathy patient presents with gradual **distal, symmetric sensorimotor deficits and hyporeflexia.** Typically, the longest nerves in the body are affected first, resulting in a stocking-glove distribution of symptoms and signs (see Fig. 19–1). Dysesthetic sensory changes are often the first symptom, with weakness developing later.

The number of entities that can cause peripheral neuropathy is vast (Table 19–2), and pinpointing a precise cause can be difficult. An organized and stepwise approach is essential. **Consideration of the following points can help narrow the possibilities and allow screening for the most common and important (i.e., treatable) causes.**

Clinical Approach to the Patient with Polyneuropathy

Diagnosis

1. **History**
   - **Is the neuropathy acute or chronic?** Acute polyneuropathy (Guillain-Barré syndrome) is discussed in Chapter 15.
   - **Ask a carefully directed set of questions to identify an obvious cause.** Ask about diabetes, renal disease, HIV infection, current medications, alcohol use, potential exposure to toxins, and family history. *The majority of polyneuropathies*

TABLE 19-2 **Causes of Peripheral Polyneuropathy**

Metabolic and Endocrine Diseases

Diabetes mellitus*
Renal failure*
Hepatic failure
Porphyria
Hypothyroidism
Critical illness polyneuropathy*

Vitamin Deficiency States

Beriberi (thiamine deficiency)
Vitamin B_6 (pyridoxine) deficiency
Vitamin B_{12} deficiency
Vitamin B complex deficiency
Pellagra (niacin deficiency)
Vitamin E deficiency

Toxins and Poisons

Alcohol
Heavy metals: arsenic, lead, mercury, thallium
Organic and industrial solvents: carbon disulfide, n-hexane, acrylamide,
    methyl-N-butyl ketone
Pyridoxine (vitamin B_6) overdose
Nitrous oxide (also causes myelopathy)

Medications

Antibiotics: dapsone, nitrofurantoin, isoniazid, ethambutol,
    metronidazole, stavudine (d4T), 3TC, didanosine (ddI), dideoxycytidine
    (ddC)
Antiarrhythmics: amiodarone, procainamide, propafenone
Chemotherapeutic agents*: vincristine, vinblastine, cisplatin, paclitaxel
    (Taxol), adriamycin, suramin, tacrolimus
Cimetidine
Chloroquine (also causes myopathy)
Colchicine (also causes myopathy)
d-Penicillamine
Disulfiram
Gold salts
Hydralazine
Podophyllin
Pyridoxine
Phenytoin
Thalidomide

Immunologic or Paraprotein-Mediated Diseases

Acute inflammatory polyneuropathy (Guillain-Barré syndrome)*
Chronic inflammatory polyneuropathy (chronic inflammatory
    demyelinating polyneuropathy)*
Paraneoplastic disease (sensorimotor or pure sensory)*
Multiple myeloma

TABLE 19–2 Causes of Peripheral
Polyneuropathy—cont'd

Anti-myelin-associated glycoprotein antibody-mediated disease
Amyloidosis
Lymphoma with paraprotein
Monoclonal gammopathy
Cryoglobulinemia
Collagen vascular disease (systemic lupus erythematosus, rheumatoid
  arthritis, etc.)
Sarcoidosis
Waldentröm's macroglobulinemia

Genetic/Hereditary Diseases

Charcot-Marie-Tooth disease*
Refsum's disease
Storage diseases (metachromatic leukodystrophy,
  adrenomyeloneuropathy, etc.)
Inherited metabolic enzyme defects

Infectious Diseases

Human immunodeficiency virus infection*
Cytomegalovirus infection*
Leprosy
Lyme disease
Human T-cell leukemia virus type I (HTLV-1) infection (also causes
  myelopathy)

*Common.

are complications of previously evident medical disorders, medications, or alcohol.
- **Do the symptoms fluctuate?** Fluctuations suggest a relapsing demyelinating neuropathy (CIDP) or repeated exposures to toxins.
2. **Examination**
   - **Determine the predominant systems involved.** Most neu-
     ropathies are sensorimotor, with the sensory component
     predominant. Identifying a predominantly motor, pure
     sensory, or particularly painful neuropathy helps to limit
     the differential diagnosis considerably (Table 19–3).
   - **Determine whether the findings are asymmetric.** Patchy
     and asymmetric motor, sensory, and reflex deficits suggest
     mononeuropathy multiplex or *polyradiculopathy* (see earlier
     discussion).
   - **Check for palpably enlarged nerves.** Although it is unusual,
     a finding of enlarged nerves can help pinpoint the diagnosis
     (see Table 19–3).
3. **Electrodiagnostic studies: EMG and NCS**

TABLE 19–3 **Features Helpful in Narrowing the Cause of Peripheral Neuropathy: Syndromes Other Than Distal Axonal Neuropathies**

Pure (or predominantly) motor neuropathy	Lymphoma, multifocal motor neuropathy (with or without anti-GM 1 antibodies)
	Toxic: dapsone, lead, organophosphates
	Porphyria
	Guillain-Barré syndrome
	Tick paralysis
	Diphtheria
Pure (or predominantly) sensory neuropathy*	Acute idiopathic sensory neuropathy
	Primary biliary cirrhosis
	Sjögren's syndrome
	Diabetes mellitus
	Human immunodeficiency virus infection
	Leprosy
	Hereditary sensory and autonomic neuropathies
	Uremia
	Paraneoplastic sensory ganglioneuritis (anti-Hu, ANNA-1 antibodies)
	Toxic: thallium, pyridoxine (vitamin B_6) intoxication
Palpably enlarged nerves	*Genetic:* Charcot-Marie-Tooth disease, Dejerine-Sottas disease, Refsum's disease, neurofibromatosis, hereditary liability to pressure palsies
	Leprosy
	Chronic inflammatory demyelinating polyneuropathy
Demyelinating neuropathies	*Immunologic:* Guillain-Barré syndrome, chronic inflammatory demyelinating polyneuropathy, paraproteinemia, anti-MAG (myelin-associated glycoprotein) antibodies
	Toxic: diphtheria, buckthorn toxin, amiodarone, perhexiline
	Genetic: Charcot-Marie-Tooth type I disease, storage diseases, hereditary liability to pressure palsies
	Paraneoplastic: osteosclerotic multiple myeloma

*Usually small-fiber sensory loss (pain, temperature) with prominent autonomic dysfunction.

- **Determine whether the neuropathy is axonal or demyelinating.** Electrodiagnosis is critical for making this distinction, which can help to narrow your differential diagnosis. *Distal axonal sensorimotor neuropathies* are the most common. *Demyelinating neuropathies* have a much smaller differential diagnosis (see Table 19–3).

TABLE 19–4 **Causes of Peripheral Neuropathy That Can Be Diagnosed by Nerve Biopsy**

- Vasculitis
- Leprosy
- Lymphoma
- Cytomegalovirus (causes polyradiculopathy or mononeuropathy multiplex)
- Storage diseases (metachromatic leukodystrophy [MLD], adrenomyeloneuropathy [AMN], Krabbe's disease)
- Amyloidosis
- Immune-mediated diseases (IgM and complement deposition)

Management

Laboratory Testing for Evaluation of Polyneuropathy

1. If an obvious cause for the neuropathy exists (e.g., postvincristine chemotherapy), no further workup may be needed. Otherwise proceed with the next steps.
2. The following initial laboratory tests should be performed: fasting glucose with full chemistry panel including liver function tests (LFTs), CBC, TFTs, initial rheumatologic screen (ESR, ANA, RF), serum protein electrophoresis, vitamin B_{12} level.
3. Other tests to consider include LP, testing of urine for paraproteins, serum immunofixation electrophoresis, quantitative immunoglobulins, testing urine for heavy metals, tests for HIV, CMV, human T-cell leukemia virus type I (HTLV-1), Lyme antibody, other vitamin levels (vitamins B and E), ANCA, ACE level, homocysteine/methionine levels (vitamin B_{12} deficiency), genetic testing (Charcot-Marie-Tooth disease), special antibody assays (anti-Hu, anti-GM1, anti-MAG, anti-sulfatide), and bone marrow biopsy.
4. Nerve and muscle biopsy is helpful for confirming several diagnoses (Table 19–4), but it is most useful in evaluating *mononeuropathy multiplex.*

Selected Causes of Neuropathy

- **Diabetes mellitus**

  Diabetes is the most common cause of neuropathy in the United States. Several different forms of neuropathy may occur, and an individual may have more than one type:

  1. **Distal axonal sensorimotor neuropathy** is most common. Sensory symptoms (small-fiber) usually predominate, including painful dysesthesias.
  2. **Autonomic neuropathy** is commonly seen in combination with axonal small-fiber sensory neuropathy. Symptoms may

include anhidrosis, orthostatic hypotension, impotence, gastroparesis, and bowel and bladder disturbances.

3. **Mononeuropathy** may occur from either nerve infarction or entrapment (e.g., carpal tunnel syndrome).

4. **Mononeuropathy multiplex**

5. **Diabetic amyotrophy (asymmetric proximal motor neuropathy)** presents with dull, aching proximal pain, followed by asymmetric proximal leg weakness and wasting not limited to a root, plexus, or nerve territory.

- **Ethanol**

  Ethanol is a very common cause of axonal sensorimotor neuropathy with prominent distal paresthesias and numbness. Vitamin B complex supplements and alcohol cessation can lead to improvement.

- **Uremia**

  Renal failure often leads to a distal, axonal, sensorimotor neuropathy with prominent cramps and unpleasant dysesthesias. Improvement may occur with dialysis or kidney transplantation.

- **Chronic inflammatory demyelinating polyneuropathy**

  CIDP presents as a chronic relapsing sensorimotor polyneuropathy or, rarely, as mononeuropathy multiplex. The diagnosis is confirmed by *elevated CSF protein* and *a demyelinating pattern on EMG/NCS*. In some cases, a plasma cell dyscrasia or paraprotein may be identified. **Prednisone, starting at 60 mg/ day,** is the treatment of first choice. Long-term daily maintenance doses of 5 to 20 mg may be required in responders. **Plasmapheresis, IVIG (0.4 g/kg per treatment),** and **azathioprine 150 mg per day** are other treatment options.

- **Paraprotein-associated neuropathy**

  These neuropathies can result in a demyelinating or axonal sensorimotor neuropathy. CSF protein is elevated in 80% of demyelinating cases. The protein can be identified by either serum or urine protein electrophoresis or immunofixation electrophoresis. Bone marrow biopsy may be helpful in the two thirds of cases with plasma cell dyscrasia; in the remaining patients, multiple myeloma (in 12%), amyloidosis (in 9%), lymphoma (in 5%), leukemia (in 3%), or Waldenström's macroglobulinemia (in 2%) may be identified. **Prednisone 40 to 100 mg per day** or **azathioprine 150 mg per day** may benefit some patients; **plasmapheresis** and **IVIG** are other treatment options.

- **Critical illness polyneuropathy**

  This polyneuropathy is associated with sepsis and multisystem organ failure. It often presents as failure to wean from mechanical ventilation. EMG/NCS is consistent with severe sensorimotor axonal neuropathy. There is no specific treatment, but if the patient survives, recovery is the rule.

- **Paraneoplastic neuropathy**

  Paraplastic neuropathy most often manifests as an axonal sensorimotor neuropathy, but it can also take the form of a large-fiber pure sensory neuropathy, a demyelinating sensorimotor neuropathy, or a pure motor neuronopathy (usually seen with lymphoma). These and other paraneoplastic syndromes (see Chapter 22) are mediated by autoimmune responses against peripheral nerve.

- **Genetic (hereditary) neuropathies**

  These neuropathies are unusual except for **Charcot-Marie-Tooth disease,** which comes in two forms: type I (demyelinating) and the less common type II (axonal). The disease is autosomal dominant, with variable expression from one generation to the next. Patients present with insidious distal lower extremity weakness and wasting ("stork leg deformity"), high arches, pes cavus, and minimal sensory symptoms.

General Care of the Patient with Neuropathy

1. *Remove any potential neurotoxic medications,* even if these are not the primary cause (see Table 19–2 for a list).
2. *Treat neuropathic pain* with **gabapentin (300 to 3600 mg daily),** tricyclic antidepressants **(amitriptyline 25 to 100 mg daily** or **nortriptyline 10 to 25 mg daily), pregabalin (50 to 100 mg tid),** or the selective serotonin reuptake inhibitors **tramadol (50 mg qd to 100 mg qid)** or **duloxetine (20 to 60 mg qd).**
3. *Initiate occupational and physical therapy* in patients with moderate to severe disability for gait training, prevention of contractures, orthoses, and assistive devices.
4. *Skin care* is important in patients with severe sensory neuropathy to prevent trophic ulcers, infections, and neuropathic (Charcot) joints.
5. *Autonomic neuropathy* may require treatment for orthostatic hypotension **(fludrocortisone 0.1 to 0.3 mg a day** or **midodrine 5 to 10 mg two to three times a day)** or gastroparesis (treat with **metoclopramide 5 to 10 mg three times a day).**

NEUROMUSCULAR JUNCTION DISEASE

Myasthenia gravis and **botulism,** both of which can lead to respiratory failure, are discussed in Chapter 15.

Lambert-Eaton myasthenic syndrome (LEMS) is an autoimmune disease caused by antibodies directed against voltage-gated calcium channels of the presynaptic nerve terminals, causing impaired neuromuscular transmission. Most cases are paraneoplastic; LEMS occurs in up to 60% of patients with small cell lung carcinoma. The disease is initially identified with proximal limb weakness.

Lower extremity areflexia, myalgias, dry mouth, and impotence may also occur, but diplopia, dysphagia, and dyspnea do not occur. The disease is diagnosed by the presence of an incremental response on repetitive nerve stimulation (>10 Hz). LEMS is treated with drugs that facilitate the release of acetylcholine: **guanidine 20 to 30 mg/kg daily or 3,4-diaminopyridine 20 mg tid.** Pyridostigmine, plasmapheresis, and IVIG may also be tried.

MYOPATHY

Diseases of muscle typically lead to **proximal, symmetric weakness** without sensory deficits or bowel or bladder symptoms. The patient may complain of difficulty reaching above the head, getting out of a chair, or climbing stairs.

Questions to Ask the Patient with Suspected Myopathic Disease

1. Does the patient have muscle aches or tenderness, suggestive of muscle inflammation or necrosis?
2. Has the patient noticed darkened, cola-colored urine (*myoglobinuria*)?
3. Does the weakness fluctuate or worsen with exercise, suggestive of myasthenia gravis or periodic paralysis?
4. Are there any sensory or bowel or bladder symptoms? (Such symptoms would make a myopathic disease unlikely.)
5. Have there been any new cardiac symptoms? (Many entities affect both skeletal and cardiac muscle.)

Examination

1. Map out the pattern of weakness (proximal versus distal). Most myopathies cause proximal weakness; exceptions include myotonic dystrophy, inclusion body myositis, and rare genetic causes.
2. Check for *myotonia* (prolonged muscle contraction after voluntary contraction or percussion), which can be tested by handgrip, forced eye closure, or muscle percussion.
3. Palpate for muscle tenderness.
4. Undress the patient to evaluate for a pattern of muscle wasting.

Management

Diagnostic Testing

1. **Initial laboratory tests**—creatine kinase (CK) level, chem-20 screen, TFTs, sedimentation rate, ECG
2. **EMG/NCS:** Needle electromyography in patients with myopathy shows abnormal, short-duration, low-amplitude, polyphasic motor unit potentials and overly rapid recruitment of

motor units with an excessively low amplitude interference pattern (see Chapter 3).
3. **Muscle biopsy** is often needed to establish a diagnosis.
4. **Other tests to consider** include ACE level, serum cortisol level, serum and CSF lactate (mitochondrial myopathy), genetic testing (for muscular and myotonic dystrophy), and toxicology screen.

Causes of Myopathy

Causes of myopathy can be categorized into five main groups: **inflammatory, endocrine, toxic, hereditary, and infectious.**
1. Inflammatory myopathies
   a. *Polymyositis*
      This inflammatory autoimmune muscle disease is characterized by chronic and relapsing proximal limb weakness. Although the eyes and face are almost never affected, pharyngeal and neck weakness is common (in approximately 50% of patients). Cardiomyopathy, interstitial lung disease, and other systemic autoimmune diseases (e.g., systemic lupus erythematosus, Crohn's disease) are also found in a significant proportion of patients.
      (1) *Diagnosis:* CK levels are elevated in almost all cases, and EMG shows myopathic findings with denervation secondary to segmental muscle necrosis. Muscle biopsy reveals endomesial lymphocytic infiltrates, necrotic and atrophic muscle fibers, and connective tissue deposition.
      (2) *Treatment:* Prednisone 60 to 100 mg daily leads to improvement in most patients within 2 to 3 months and is most effective early in the disease course. Azathioprine 1 to 3 mg/kg per day or methotrexate 25 to 50 mg per week can be used for disease suppression in steroid nonresponders.
   b. *Dermatomyositis*
      Dermatomyositis is similar to polymyositis but is accompanied by a characteristic rash that precedes or accompanies muscle weakness. Skin manifestations include a heliotrope (bluish) rash on the upper eyelids, erythematous rash on the face and trunk, violaceous scaly eruptions on the knuckles (Gottron's papules), and subcutaneous calcifications.
      (1) *Diagnosis:* Muscle biopsy findings differ from polymyositis in showing perivascular inflammation and *perifascicular atrophy.* A malignancy screen is prudent with a later age of onset.
      (2) *Treatment:* Treatment is the same as for polymyositis.
   c. *Inclusion body myositis*
      This entity differs from polymyositis in that it tends to produce distal and asymmetric weakness, it occurs

primarily at an older age, and it responds poorly to steroids. Muscle biopsy reveals rimmed vacuoles, and eosinophilic cytoplasmic inclusions with amyloid. IVIG (0.4 mg/kg per treatment) may improve strength in isolated cases. Finger flexor and quadriceps weakness is a hallmark.

    d. *Sarcoidosis*

        Patients with sarcoidosis can develop focal or generalized myopathy. Biopsy shows noncaseating granulomas. Steroids usually produce clinical improvement.

2. **Endocrine myopathies**

    Patients with endocrine myopathy usually show systemic signs of endocrine disease before the onset of weakness, but in some instances, myopathy is the presenting feature. CK levels are usually normal or only mildly elevated. In all cases, weakness is reversed by treating the underlying endocrinopathy, which includes thyroid disease, Cushing's disease (hyperadrenalism), or parathyroid disease.

3. **Toxic myopathies**

    a. *Medications*

        Drugs and medications produce subacute, generalized proximal muscle weakness through a variety of mechanisms. Table 19–5 lists some medications and toxins commonly associated with myopathy.

    b. *Critical illness myopathy*

        This myopathy presents as a failure to wean from mechanical ventilation in ICU patients treated with steroids and nondepolarizing paralyzing agents (e.g.,

TABLE 19–5 **Drugs That Can Cause Myopathy**

Rhabdomyolysis	**Myopathy (Weakness and Myalgia)**
Amphotericin B	Colchicine
ε-Aminocaproic acid	Zidovudine
Fenfluramine	Steroids
Heroin	Clofibrate
Phencyclidine	Chloroquine
Alcohol	Emetine
Barbiturates	Labetalol
Cocaine	Statin class anticholesterol
	Vincristine
Hypokalemic Myopathy	
Diuretics	
Azathioprine	
Myositis (Inflammatory)	
Penicillamine	
Procainamide	
Cimetidine	

vecuronium); however, neither precipitant is necessary for disease development. Muscle biopsy shows selective loss of thick myosin filaments. This condition is much more common than typically diagnosed. There is no treatment, but recovery over weeks to months is the rule.

c. *Neuroleptic malignant syndrome*

Dopamine blockers (e.g., haloperidol, chlorpromazine [Thorazine]) can produce this rare, idiosyncratic response characterized by generalized muscle rigidity with rhabdomyolysis, fever, altered mental status, tremor, and autonomic instability (especially hypertension). CK levels are always elevated; white blood cell counts are usually increased. Treatment includes discontinuation of the offending agent, surface cooling, dantrolene 1 to 10 mg/kg per day IV every 4 to 6 hours as needed to attain muscle relaxation, and bromocriptine 2.5 to 5 mg three times a day.

d. *Malignant hyperthermia*

This autosomal dominant condition predisposes to severe muscle rigidity, rhabdomyolysis, fever, and metabolic acidosis following exposure to inhalation anesthetics or succinylcholine. Treatment is with dantrolene 2.5 to 10 mg/kg IV in repeated doses.

4. **Hereditary myopathies**

a. *Muscular dystrophy*

Muscular dystrophy is a progressively degenerative genetic myopathy. Weakness is usually present in early life, gets worse over time, and often leads to early death.

(1) Duchenne's muscular dystrophy (X-linked). The onset is by age 5 with inability to walk occurring by age 10 and with eventual respiratory failure. Features include calf pseudohypertrophy, cardiomyopathy, and occasional mental impairment. *Becker's muscular dystrophy* is a later-onset form of the disease with less severe manifestations. **Prednisone 20 to 40 mg per day** can increase strength and function, but it does not alter the overall course. Diagnosis is confirmed by abnormal dystrophin staining on biopsy.

(2) Myotonic dystrophy (autosomal dominant). This most common form of muscular dystrophy leads to progressive *distal* myopathy. The disease occurs earlier and is more severe with successive generations (genetic anticipation). Besides myotonia, features include a distinctive facies with ptosis and frontal balding, cataracts, cardiac conduction defects, gonadal atrophy, and mental impairment. **Phenytoin 300 mg per day PO and procainamide 20 to 50 mg/kg per day three times a day** occasionally are used to treat the myotonia, if clinically necessary. ECGs performed at least yearly are

prudent to assess for evolving heart block. Definitive genetic triple repeat analysis is available for diagnosis confirmation.

(3) Other hereditary myopathies. These entities include facioscapulohumeral (autosomal dominant), limb girdle (autosomal recessive), oculopharyngeal (autosomal recessive), and Emery-Dreifuss (X-linked) myopathies. Many of these myopathies now have precise genetic diagnoses.

b. *Metabolic myopathies*

Seen mostly in the pediatric population, these diseases result from deficiencies of specific enzymes involved in utilization of glucose or lipid (the two main sources of skeletal muscle energy). Besides muscle weakness, patients with metabolic myopathies often experience *rhabdomyolysis* and *myoglobinuria*. Muscle biopsy is necessary to establish the diagnosis. The most common metabolic myopathy is McArdle's disease, an autosomal recessive disorder resulting from myophosphorylase deficiency. It presents in childhood with painful muscle cramps and myoglobinuria after intense exercise. A lack of increase in lactate levels with ischemic forearm testing is characteristic. Laboratory confirmation of urinary or serum myoglobin in an acute phase is key.

c. *Periodic paralysis*

These rare disorders are caused by genetic abnormalities of membrane ion channels. The majority are inherited in autosomal dominant fashion. Patients are usually normal between attacks of severe weakness. Hypokalemic and hyperkalemic forms have been described.

d. *Congenital myopathies*

This group of rare disorders presents mostly at birth with floppy infant syndrome, and the disorders are usually nonprogressive. Examples include nemaline (rod) body myopathy, myotubular (centronuclear) myopathy, and central core disease. Adult onset cases may be seen.

e. *Mitochondrial myopathy*

These diseases result from defects in the mitochondrial genome and hence are maternally inherited. Muscle biopsy shows "ragged red fibers." Suspicious signs for mitochondrial diseases include ptosis, ophthalmoparesis, and high serum lactate levels. Variants include myoclonic epilepsy with ragged red fibers, also known as *MELAS* (mitochondrial encephalomyopathy, encephalopathy, lactic acidosis, and strokelike episodes), and *Kearns-Sayre syndrome* (pigmentary retinopathy, cardiac conduction defects, high CSF protein). Genetic analysis is available for many types of mitochondrial myopathies.

5. Infectious myopathies

Muscle infiltration with the organisms that cause *trichinosis*, *toxoplasmosis*, and *cysticercosis* can lead to a widespread or a localized inflammatory myopathy. Acute rhabdomyolsis and myoglobinuria can occur as a result of infection with influenza virus, rubella virus, coxsackievirus, echoviruses, and mycoplasma. HIV myopathy is not uncommon and must be distinguished from zidovudine toxicity.

Demyelinating and Inflammatory Disorders of the Central Nervous System

Demyelinating and inflammatory diseases of the CNS are varied and often enigmatic. *MS*, the prototype inflammatory demyelinating disease, is a chronic autoimmune disorder characterized by loss of myelin and relative preservation of axons. *Acute disseminated encephalomyelitis (ADEM)* is a monophasic illness that is pathologically similar to MS but is typically triggered by an antecedent viral infection. *Central pontine myelinolysis (CPM)* refers to osmotic demyelination in the setting of rapid correction of hyponatremia. *Sarcoidosis* and *Behçet's disease* are idiopathic systemic inflammatory diseases that may involve the CNS. Dysmyelinating diseases, such as Alexander's and Canavan's diseases, are genetic disorders in which there is an intrinsic abnormality of myelin; they present in childhood and will not be discussed in this chapter.

MULTIPLE SCLEROSIS

The hallmark of MS is episodic or progressive multifocal deficits affecting the CNS in otherwise young healthy adults. The most common initial clinical manifestations of MS are sensory disturbances, visual loss, and weakness. Diagnosis relies on recognition of the clinical patterns of disease and is supported by MRI studies of the brain and spinal cord, analysis of cerebrospinal fluid, and electrophysiological studies. Systemic illnesses that can mimic the symptoms of MS must be excluded.

General Considerations

Next to trauma, MS is the most common cause of disability in young adults. MS affects approximately 350,000 to 500,000 Americans and more than 1 million individuals worldwide. The cause of MS is unknown, and because there is no single diagnostic test, accurate diagnosis relies on clinical recognition of the disease. The hallmarks of MS are multifocal waxing and waning, or progressive neurologic deficits, that localize to the central nervous system. *The signs and symptoms of MS are separated in space (multiple areas of the central nervous system) and evolve over time (during the life of the patient).* MS affects only the central nervous system and spares the peripheral nerves.

MS has a distinct pathology characterized by focal demyelination within the brain and spinal cord. MS is considered an autoimmune disease because inflammatory infiltrates are present within the damaged myelin. However, it is not known whether the immune response is a primary process or is triggered by infectious, toxic, or metabolic etiologies. There is no cure for MS, and current treatments are only partially effective.

Epidemiology

MS affects women two to three times as often as men. MS is rare in the pediatric population, but its risk increases steadily from adolescence up to the age of 35, then gradually decreases and is rarely diagnosed after the age of 65. MS is uncommon in equatorial climates, and its prevalence increases with northern distance from the equator.

Genetics

The risk of MS is much higher in populations of Northern European ancestry than in other ethnic groups residing at the same latitudes. Twin studies demonstrate concordance rates of approximately 30% in identical twins and 5% in fraternal twins. The rate for first-degree relatives of MS patients is also 5%. Genetic linkage studies show a consistent association of MS susceptibility with the major histocompatibility class II locus on chromosome 6p. This locus encodes the genes that present peptide antigens to T cells.

Pathology

The term multiple sclerosis refers to discrete hard or rubbery plaques within the white matter of the brain and spinal cord. These lesions are composed of areas of myelin and oligodendrocyte loss accompanied by infiltrates of macrophages and lymphocytes. The focal loss of myelin indicates a highly specific demyelinating process and distinguishes MS from leukodystrophies. In addition, preserved axons and neurons discern MS from other destructive processes. Although axons in MS plaques are relatively spared, axonal transection occurs, is irreversible, and presumably leads to neuronal death by Wallerian degeneration.

Clinical Features

Symptomatic Onset

The initial focal manifestations may be acute or insidious and can vary in severity. Acute neurologic deficits caused by MS are called *relapses* and are also known as flares, attacks, or exacerbations. The most common initial symptoms are sensory disturbances, visual loss, and weakness, although abnormal gait, loss of dexterity, diplopia, ataxia, vertigo, or sphincter disturbances can occur. Nonspecific symptoms such as malaise, fatigue, or headache often precede the initial focal disturbance.

Sensory Disturbance

The most common presenting symptom of MS is paresthesia (tingling, pins and needles), dysesthesia (burning, gritty, sandy, electrical, or wet sensations), or hypesthesia (loss of sensation or procaine-like numbness). Some patients describe a squeezing sensation as if a limb or the trunk were tightly wrapped. These symptoms can be intermittent or constant and can spread from one location to adjoining areas. Spinal cord involvement is implied by ascending numbness with a sensory level. A Lhermitte symptom, an electrical or shocklike paresthesia that radiates down the spine and into one or more limbs following neck flexion, localizes the lesion to the cervical spine. Sensory disturbances associated with MS flares usually resolve spontaneously but sometimes evolve into chronic neuropathic pain. Trigeminal neuralgia also occurs in MS.

Optic Neuritis

The next most common presenting manifestation of MS is optic neuritis: loss of vision affecting usually one eye evolving over hours or days. Bilateral simultaneous optic neuritis is much less frequent. Loss of vision can be complete or partial; patients will often report a scotoma, an area of diminished or blurred vision in the monocular field. Optic neuritis is often associated with periorbital pain elicited by eye movements. Loss of vision can be subtle and affect only color vision. Red desaturation, the inability to distinguish shades of red, can be quantified using Ishihara color plates. Demyelination of the optic nerve close to the retina causes optic disc pallor. The differential diagnosis of acute visual loss is shown in Table 20–1.

TABLE 20–1 Differential Diagnosis for Acute Visual Loss

V (vascular): nonarteritic anterior ischemic optic neuropathy, giant cell arteritis, diabetic retinopathies, Susac's syndrome (microangiopathy of the brain, retina, and inner ear, cute posterior multifocal placoid pigment epitheliopathy, Eale's disease (noninflammatory occlusive disease of the retinal vasculature), Cogan's syndrome (interstitial keratitis, vestibular dysfunction, and deafness), amaurosis fugax, central retinal vein occlusion, aneurysms and arteriovenous malformations, systemic hypercoagulable states including anticardiolipin syndrome

I (infectious): rarely cause such rapid visual loss without other symptoms and can be local (retinitis, periostitis, meningitis) or systemic (syphilis, toxoplasmosis, typhoid fever, leptospirosis)

T (trauma): rare A (autoimmune): sarcoidosis

M (metabolic /toxic): vitamin B_{12} deficiency, toxins (e.g., ethyl alcohol, ethambutol, methanol, amiodarone, clioquinol, chemotherapeutic agents, benzene, tropical ataxic neuropathy (cassava diet, tobacco use associated with a defect in cyanide detoxification), radiation-induced optic neuropathy

I (idiopathic/hereditary): Leber's hereditary optic neuropathy, Kearns-Sayre syndrome, MELAS (mitochondrial encephalopathy with lactic acidosis and strokes), NARP (neuropathy, ataxia, and retinitis pigmentosa syndrome), Friedreich's ataxia

N (neoplastic/paraneoplastic/infiltrative): infiltrating neoplasms (e.g., lymphoma, leukemia, myeloma, carcinomatous meningitis), optic nerve glioma, optic nerve glioblastoma, optic sheath meningioma, cancer-associated retinopathy (CAR), cancer-associated cone dysfunction (CACD), melanoma-associated retinopathy (MAR), diffuse uveal melanocytic proliferation (DUMP), paraneoplastic ganglion cell neuronopathy (PCGN), Langerhans' cell disorders

S (psychiatric): conversion reaction

Others: central serous chorioretinopathy, optic disc drusen, ophthalmic migraine, big blind spot syndromes (acute zonal occult outer retinopathy, acute macular neuroretinopathy, multiple evanescent white dot syndrome, acute idiopathic blind spot enlargement syndrome)

Motor Symptoms

Motor symptoms are as common as optic neuritis as initial manifestations of MS and include limb weakness, loss of dexterity, and gait disturbance. Symptoms typically evolve over hours or days; sometimes patients will awaken with a motor deficit. Weakness can affect a single limb or cause hemiparesis or paraparesis. The hemiparesis of MS usually spares the face. Sometimes weakness becomes apparent only during exertion. Weakness is usually accompanied by spasticity and hyperreflexia.

Diplopia

Disconjugate eye movements resulting in diplopia are common in MS. Intranuclear ophthalmoplegia (INO) is caused by demyelinating plaques within the medial longitudinal fasciculus (MLF). Lesions in the MLF typically occur ipsilateral to the affected third nucleus and result in impaired ipsilateral adduction with compensatory nystagmus of the abducting eye. MS can also cause vertical diplopia and isolated impairments of the sixth, third, and fourth nerves.

Ataxia and Tremor

Dyscoordinated movements of the limbs or trunk are common in MS due to plaques affecting the cerebellar afferent or efferent pathways and range in severity from subtle to disabling. Tremor and dysmetria, an error in measurement of movement, are often observed on finger-nose-finger and heel-knee-shin tests. Dysrhythmia can be demonstrated by finger or toe tapping. *Romberg sign,* truncal swaying on standing with the feet together and eyes closed, can be caused by impaired proprioception from spinal cord dorsal column lesions.

Neuropsychiatric Dysfunction

Cognitive impairments are present in 40% to 65% of MS patients and can result in loss of vocation and impairment of activities of daily living. Patients often report difficulties with short-term memory, attention, information processing, problem solving, multitasking, and language function. Cognitive deficits may not be detected by the mini mental status exam and often require neuropsychiatric testing. Emotional lability is common; up to 60% of MS patients suffer from depression.

Bladder and Bowel Dysfunction

Patients often complain of urinary urgency, frequency, hesitancy, and incontinence. Incontinence can occur in the setting of a tonically contracted (spastic) bladder that is incapable of filling completely or with a denervated distended (denervated) bladder that overflows. It is often not possible to determine the nature of bladder dysfunction by history. Measurement of the volume of postvoiding residual urine, either by catheterization, by ultrasound, or by urodynamic studies, is essential for distinguishing between a spastic and denervated bladder. Bladder dyssynergia, an impairment of sphincter and detrusor coordination, is also a cause of hesitancy and incomplete voiding. Patients with urinary retention are susceptible to urinary tract infections, and such infections may trigger MS relapses by stimulating the immune system.

Bowel dysfunction is common in MS and is presumably caused by spinal cord plaques. Chronic constipation can worsen spasticity. Incontinence occurs either as a consequence of sphincter dysfunction or from bowel spasticity and fecal urgency.

Vertigo

Vertigo caused by MS is sometimes associated with other signs or symptoms of brain stem pathology such as facial sensory loss or diplopia. Vertigo can be fleeting or last for days or even weeks. Although uncommon, unilateral hearing loss occurs in MS, sometimes in conjunction with vertigo. Vertigo caused by labyrinthine pathology identified by the Dix-Hallpike maneuver (see Chapter 13) is not due to MS.

Dysarthria

Impairments of speech are common in MS and can be caused by tongue weakness from lower brain stem dysfunction, spastic dysarthria from corticobulbar injury, or scanning dysarthria from cerebellar dysfunction.

Dysphagia

Impairment of swallowing occurs in MS, particularly later in the course of the disease. Choking on thin liquids is consistent with neurologic injury as opposed to solid food dysphagia, which is typically caused by a pharyngeal structural abnormality. Barium swallow and fiberscope endoscopic evaluation of swallowing are helpful in assessing aspiration risk.

Facial Weakness

Lower motor neuron facial weakness, similar to Bell's palsy, can occur when MS plaques affect intraparenchymal emerging fibers of the seventh cranial nerve. Ipsilateral loss of taste, hyperacusis, retroauricular pain, and synkinesis are hallmarks of peripheral facial neuropathy and do not occur with central facial weakness. Facial myokymia is a chronic flickering contraction of the orbicularis occuli or other muscles of facial expression caused by injury to the facial nerve or corticobulbar tracts within the brain stem.

Fatigue

Fatigue is the most common symptom of MS and contends with cognitive impairment as the major cause of loss of vocation. Fatigue can occur as a consequence of exertion (neuromuscular weakness), as a manifestation of depression, as a consequence of insomnia (daytime drowsiness), or as a generalized lassitude. Fatigue is often worse in the afternoon but can be present on awakening and persist throughout the day.

Paroxysmal Symptoms

Virtually all symptoms of MS, including the Lhermitte symptom, sensory disturbances, weakness, ataxia, vertigo, and diplopia, can occur as transient paroxysms lasting for seconds to minutes, sometimes in clusters. *Flexor spasms* are brief tonic spasms of a limb or the face and often occur at night and in clusters. Flexor spasms are frequently preceded by paresthesias and can be elicited by movements, hyperventilation, or other precipitating factors.

Disease Course

Relapsing Remitting Multiple Sclerosis

Because there is no specific test for MS, diagnosis of the disease relies on the clinical history. Patients experience relapses when an acute plaque develops in an area likely to cause symptoms such as the optic nerves, spinal cord, brain stem, and cerebellum. However, many plaques evolve in clinically silent areas such as the corpus callosum and the periventricular white matter. Often patients gradually recover after resolution of the acute inflammation, possibly through myelin repair and plastic reorganization. These periods of recovery of neurologic function are termed remissions, and the term relapsing remitting multiple sclerosis (RRMS) describes this pattern of episodic attacks and recoveries. Patients with RRMS initially have on average one attack per year, although the range is broad. Approximately 85% of patients will follow this disease course (Fig. 20–1). Although complete recovery of neurologic function may follow acute attacks, patients may suffer sustained neurologic deficits.

Secondary Progressive MS

Approximately 85% of subjects with RRMS will develop secondary progressive MS (SPMS), the insidiously progressive accumulation of neurologic impairments that lead to ambulatory and cognitive disability. The median time from disease onset to SPMS is 10 years. Relapses can still occur in SPMS; however, the frequency of relapses declines and eventually most patients stop experiencing attacks. Though some patients with SPMS plateau with stable deficits, disability relentlessly continues in most cases.

Primary Progressive Multiple Sclerosis

Ten to fifteen percent of MS patients have a primary progressive MS (PPMS): a disease course that is progressive from onset without relapses or remissions (Fig. 20–2). PPMS typically presents with insidious onset of asymmetric leg weakness; however, sensory, brain stem/cerebellar, or sphincter dysfunction can be initial manifestations. In contrast to RR and SPMS patients, men are affected about as often as women, and the mean age of onset is 40 years compared with 30 years for RRMS. PPMS patients develop ambulatory disability similar to that of the progressive phase of SPMS. The pathology of PPMS lesions is identical to that of RRMS and SPMS. On brain

Natural History of MS

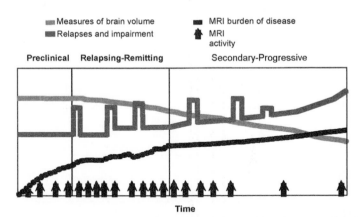

Figure 20–1 The natural history of MS. Approximately 85% of MS patients follow a similar disease course. Brain MRI scans show that MS begins prior to the onset of the first focal neurologic deficit of which the patient is aware. Relapses occur during the relapsing-remitting phase of the disease, and each relapse is followed by varying degrees of neurologic recovery. The secondary progressive phase of the disease is characterized by progressive neurologic deterioration independent of relapses. Relapses occur during the secondary progressive phase of the disease but are less frequent and eventually stop. MRI activity, measured by new, contrast-enhancing lesions, decreases during the secondary progressive phase of MS. The MRI burden of disease increases and the extent of brain atrophy increases during the course of the disease.

MRI, PPMS patients tend to have fewer plaques compared with RRMS and SPMS, and these rarely enhance on MRI. Approximately 5% of MS patients have progressive symptoms from onset and experience rare relapses. This disease course is termed progressive relapsing MS (PRMS).

Diagnosis

MS is said to evolve over space and time because it afflicts multiple areas of the central nervous system during an affected individual's life span. The recognition of this pattern accompanied by corresponding physical findings forms the basis of the diagnostic criteria used to define the disease (Table 20–2).

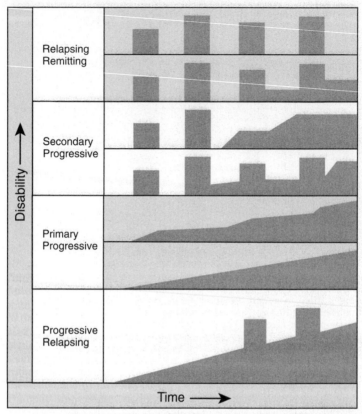

Figure 20–2 Clinical patterns of MS. Relapsing-remitting MS is characterized by complete or incomplete recovery after attacks, with a stable course between attacks. Secondary progressive MS begins with a relapsing-remitting course and later evolves into a progressive deteriorating course, with or without superimposed relapses. Primary progressive MS begins with continual or stepwise progressive deterioration. Progressive-relapsing MS, which is rare, starts as progressive deterioration, with later superimposed relapses.

Magnetic Resonance Imaging

Magnetic resonance imaging is particularly helpful in confirming the clinical diagnosis. The brain MRI is abnormal in 95% to 99% of cases of RRMS. Although sensitive, the specificity of the brain MRI is 50% to 65%, because other disease states can present with a similar pattern (Table 20–3). Typically, there are multiple areas of increased signal intensity on T2-weighted brain MRI (T2, proton density, and fluid attenuation inversion recovery sequences) that

TABLE 20–2 **Multiple Sclerosis Diagnostic Criteria**

Diagnosis of MS requires that one of five sets of criteria be fulfilled and that other etiologies be excluded.

1. Two or more clinical attacks and two or more objective lesions
2. Two or more clinical attacks and one objective lesion
   and dissemination in space by MRI*
   or positive CSF‡ and two or more MRI* lesions consistent with MS
   or await an additional attack implicating a different site
3. One clinical attack and two or more objective lesions
   and dissemination in time by MRI† or second clinical attack
4. One clinical attack and one objective lesion (clinically isolated syndrome)
   and dissemination in space by MRI*
   or positive CSF‡ and two or more MRI* lesions consistent with MS
   and dissemination in time by MRI†
   or second clinical attack
5. Progression from onset and one objective lesion
   and positive CSF‡
   and dissemination in time by MRI† or continued progression for 1 year
   and dissemination in space by MRI* evidence of nine or more brain lesions
   or two or more cord lesions and four to eight brain lesions and one cord lesion
   or positive VEP§ with four to eight MRI lesions
   or positive VEP§ with fewer than four brain lesions plus one cord lesion

*Positive MRI criteria:
  Three out of four of the following:
  1. One gadolinium-DPTA-enhancing lesion
     or nine T2 hyperintense lesions if no gadolinium-DPTA-enhancing lesion
  2. One or more infratentorial lesions
  3. One or more juxtacortical lesions
  4. Three or more periventricular lesions
  Note: One cord lesion can substitute for one brain lesion
†MRI evidence for dissemination in time:
  A gadolinium-enhancing lesion demonstrated in a scan done at least 3 months following onset of clinical attack at a site different from attack
  or follow-up scan after an additional 3 months showing a gadolinium-DPTA lesion or new T2 lesion
‡Positive CSF criteria:
  Two or more oligoclonal IgG bands in CSF (not present in serum) or elevated IgG index
§Positive VEP criteria:
  Delayed but well-preserved waveform
N.B.: An attack is an episode of neurologic disturbance of the kind typically seen in MS, lasting at least 24 hours. The time between attacks must be separated by 30 days. There must be *no better explanation* for the attacks or abnormalities identified by physical examination and by ancillary studies (MRI, CSF, and VEP).
  Adapted from McDonald WI, et al. Ann Neurol 2001;50(1):121-127.

TABLE 20–3 Differential Diagnosis for Multifocal White Matter Changes on MRI

V (vascular): microvascular ischemic leukoariosis, cerebral autosomal dominant arteriopathy with subcortical infarcts and leukoencephalopathy (CADASIL), primary angiitis of the central nervous system, migraine

I (infectious): Lyme disease, syphilis, progressive multifocal leukoencephalopathy

T (trauma): perinatal trauma or hypoxia

A (autoimmune): systemic lupus erythematosus, Sjögren syndrome, Behcet's disease, sarcoidosis

M (metabolic/toxic): central pontine myelinolysis, hypoxia (Grinker's encephalopathy), hexachlorophene poisoning, Marchiafava-Bignami disease, subacture combined degeneration (vitamin B_{12} deficiency), radiation

I (idiopathic/genetic): adrenoleukodystrophy and adrenomyeloneuropathy, metachromatic leukodystrophy, eukaryotic initiation factor leukodystrophies, Krabbe's disease, Lafora body disease, globoid leukodystrophy

N (neoplastic): CNS lymphoma, glioma, paraneoplastic encephalopmyelitis

often have a round or ovoid appearance and are characteristically located within the corpus callosum and the periventricular and sub-cortical white matter (Fig. 20–3). On sagittal views, these plaques appear as linear or flame-like streaks oriented perpendicularly to the lateral ventricles and are called Dawson fingers after the British pathologist who described similar findings at autopsy. The white matter of the brain stem and cerebellum are also often affected. Less often gray matter structures such as the thalamus and basal ganglia are affected. Although cortical plaques occur, they are not well visu-alized by MRI. On T1-weighted imaging, areas of relative hypoin-tensity can be identified that correspond to some of the areas of increased T2 signal. These so-called T1 "black holes" correspond to chronic MS plaques and are associated with axonal loss. Acute plaques show contrast uptake on gadolinium DPTA-enhanced T1-weighted imaging. The pattern of enhancement can be homogenous or ring enhancing, typically persists for 2 to 8 weeks, and then sub-sides. The presence of new lesions on a follow-up brain MRI can help confirm the diagnosis of MS in patients who have suffered from only one clinical attack (see Table 20–2). Brain MRI is also useful for evaluating a patient's response to treatment.

Although not as sensitive as brain MRI, plaques within the paren-chyma of the spinal cord can be seen on T2-weighted imaging or on T1-weighted imaging after administration of gadolinium-DPTA. Typically, these plaques are oriented longitudinally along the cord, often with a dorsal location, spanning one or two vertebral cord segments.

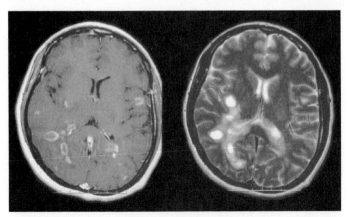

Figure 20–3 Magnetic resonance imaging findings in a 36-year-old woman with acute fulminant relapsing remitting multiple sclerosis. The T1-weighted image on the left shows multiple scattered ovoid foci of demyelination with ring enhancement. The T2-weighted image on the right shows high-intensity (white) signal changes associated with these lesions and diffuse edema affecting the deep white matter of the right parieto-occipital regions.

Cerebrospinal Fluid

In cases where the MRI is normal or shows a pattern that is consistent with other disease processes such as microvascular ischemia, cerebrospinal fluid analysis is indicated. The CSF is abnormal in 85% to 90% of MS patients. Typically, there is intrathecal synthesis of gamma globulins (increased total IgG, IgG/total protein ratio, or IgG synthesis rate) or the presence of two or more oligoclonal bands in the CSF that are not present in a simultaneously drawn serum sample. Intrathecal synthesis of gamma globulins also occurs in the setting of infections such as acute bacterial meningitis, chronic meningitis (Lyme disease, syphilis), viral encephalitis, and autoimmune disorders such as CNS vasculitis. A lymphocytic pleocytosis with cell counts >5 cells/μL is present in approximately 25% of MS patients and is usually less than 20 cells/μL. The total protein is usually normal or mildly elevated. Cell counts higher than 50 cells/μL, polymorphonuclear cells, or protein elevation >100 mg/dl should raise suspicion for alternate diagnoses such as infection, collagen vascular diseases, or neoplasm.

Evoked Potentials

Electrophysiological studies of the visual and somatosensory pathways can be useful when imaging studies or physical findings do not support the clinical impression. Delay or conduction block of the

Expanded Disability Status Scale (EDSS)

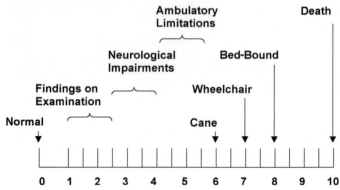

Figure 20–4 Expanded disability status scale. The EDSS scale is a non-linear rating scale with point intervals from 0 to 10. An EDSS score of 0 is normal. Scores of 1 to 2 reflect physical findings on examination. Scores of 2.5 to 3.5 correspond to impairments such as hemiparesis, paraparesis, cerebellar dystaxia, or substantial sensory loss. Scores from 4 to 5.5 usually reflect limitations in the distance a patient can walk without assistance. Scores of 6 and higher are based on the extent of ambulatory disability ability and the ability to perform activities of daily living. A score of 10 is death due to MS. (From Kurtzke: Neurology 1983;33:1444-1452 with permission.)

P100 visual evoked potential is found in 85% of MS patients. Delays or block of the N-20 potential on somatosensory evoked potentials of the median or tibial nerve are present in approximately 75% of MS patients. Evoked potential abnormalities are not specific for multiple sclerosis, which limits their diagnostic utility.

Rating Scales

The most commonly used measure of neurologic impairment in MS is the expanded disability status scale (EDSS, Fig. 20–4). The EDSS takes into account the extent of ambulatory disability and limitations in self-care and quantifies the neurologic examination as functional scale scores that quantify vision, brain stem, corticospinal, sensory, cerebellar, cognitive, and bowel and bladder functions.

Differential Diagnosis

Because MS may affect any function of the central nervous system, the differential diagnosis potentially is broad. MS is difficult to distinguish from other disorders in several settings.

Progressive Myelopathy

Although PPMS can present as an asymmetric insidiously progressive myelopathy, several other diagnoses should be considered, including neoplasm, dural AVM, subacute combined degeneration (B_{12} deficiency), sarcoidosis, Sjögren syndrome, hereditary spastic paraplegias (HSPs), adrenomyeloneuropathy (in women), syphilis, human immunodeficiency virus, and human T-cell lymphotrophic virus I and II myelitis. MRI of the spinal cord is usually able to identify neoplasms and AVMs. Blood tests help diagnose subacute combined degeneration (vitamin B_{12}, methylmalonic acid, and homocysteine), systemic sarcoidosis (angiotensin-converting enzyme), Sjögren syndrome (anti-SSA and anti-SSB autoantibodies, rheumatoid factor, antinuclear antibody), adrenomyeloneuropathy (very long-chain fatty acids), and infectious etiologies (VDRL and FTA-ABS, HIV, and HTLV I/II serologies). In cases with minimal sensory involvement, normal bladder function, and relatively symmetric presentations of leg weakness and spasticity, primary lateral sclerosis (PLS) and HSP are possibilities. Genetic testing is available for some HSP mutations. PLS is a diagnosis of exclusion.

Progressive Cognitive Impairment with Symmetric White Matter Disease

Although leukodystrophies typically present in childhood, some have adult onset variants that present with progressive cognitive impairment. White matter lesions similar to MS can be seen on brain MRI; however, MRI changes in the leukodystrophies usually have a symmetric and confluent appearance. Differential diagnoses includes adrenoleukodystrophy, metachromatic leukodystrophy, eukaryotic initiation factor mutations, Krabbe's disease, methylenetetrahydrofolate reductase deficiency, biotinidase deficiency, cerebral autosomal dominant arteriopathy with subcortical infarcts and leukoencephalopathy (CADASIL), and polyglucosan storage disease.

Cranial Neuropathies

In addition to MS, Behçet's disease and Sjögren syndrome can cause multiple cranial neuropathies. Behçet's disease should be suspected in patients with cranial neuropathies and oral ulceration (aphthous sores). Genital ulcerations, dermatographia, and an elevated erythrocyte sedimentation rate are other features of the disease. Sjögren syndrome is associated with xerostomia and xerophthalmia (dry mouth and eyes); the diagnosis is confirmed through biopsy of a minor salivary or lacrimal gland. **Glucocorticoids** and **immune suppressants** (i.e., cyclophosphamide) are used to treat Behçet's disease and Sjögren syndrome. Lyme disease and sarcoidosis may cause bilateral facial paresis. Sarcoidosis also causes optic neuropathy, which may be poorly responsive to glucocorticoids.

Disease-Modifying Therapies

Treatment for MS is divided into two categories: disease-modifying therapies and symptomatic management. Although there is no cure for MS, currently six U.S. FDA-approved drugs alter the course of the disease (Table 20–4).

Interferons

Interferons (IFN) are cytokines secreted by immune cells that inhibit viral replication. IFN beta has potent regulatory and anti-inflammatory functions on the immune system and reduces disease activity in MS. **IFN beta 1-b (Betaseron)** reduces the relapse rate and slows accumulation of new lesions on brain MR in RRMS. **IFN beta 1-a (Avonex, Rebif)** also decreases the relapse rate, slows accumulation of new lesions on brain MRI, and lessens the accumulation of neurologic impairments (see Table 20–4 for dosages and routes of administration of the IFN beta preparations). Patients treated with IFN beta are at risk for liver function abnormalities, leukopenia, thyroid disease, and depression. Liver functions (aspartate and alanine amino transferase) and white count with differential should be monitored after initiation of treatment and periodically thereafter. Most patients do not experience significant transaminemia requiring treatment discontinuation. A flulike reaction occurs in 60% of patients after IFN beta injection. With repeated treatments, the flulike reactions gradually subside over time. The flulike symptoms are reduced by coadministration with acetaminophen or a nonsteroidal anti-inflammatory drug. Erythematous skin site reactions can occur with the subcutaneously injected preparations. Long-term follow-up studies show that IFN beta is safe and well tolerated for at least 10 years.

Glatiramer Acetate

Glatiramer acetate (GA, Copaxone) is a synthesized copolymer composed of L-glutamic acid, L-lysine, L-alanine, L-tyrosine in random order and is injected 20 mg subcutaneously daily. GA resembles myelin basic protein and is thought to alter T-cell immune function, inducing "bystander suppression," so that T-cells inhibit autoreactive T-cells. GA reduces the attack rate in RRMS and reduces accumulation of contrast-enhanced lesions on brain MRI. Ten-year follow-up data demonstrate that many patients treated with GA are able to safely continue treatment. The typical flulike reaction characteristic of IFN beta does not occur with GA; however, approximately 15% of GA-treated patients will experience a self-limited, postinjection systemic reaction characterized by chest tightness, flushing, anxiety, dyspnea, and palpitations.

TABLE 20–4 FDA-Approved Disease Modifying Therapies for MS

Medication	Avonex	Betaseron	Rebif	Copaxone	Novantrone	Tysabri
Dose	6 MIU	8 MIU	12 MIU	20 mg	12 mg/m^2	300 mg
Frequency	Once weekly	Every other day	Thrice weekly	Daily	Every 3 months	Every 4 weeks
Route	IM	SC	SC	SC	IV	IV
% Relapse rate reduction, 2 years	18	34	30	29	38	68
% Reduction in disability 2 years	37	29 (NS)	30	12 (NS)	24	42

The clinical outcomes from five independent randomized, placebo-controlled trials are shown. All comparisons are versus placebo within the same study. The relapse rate reductions are for 2-year data using the intention-to-treat method of analysis. Disability is measured by a confirmed 1-point change in the EDSS at 2 years. The patient populations for each study are different; therefore direct comparisons between each medication should be interpreted with caution.
IM, intramuscular; SC, subcutaneous; IV, intravenous; NS, nonsignificant p value.

Mitoxantrone

Mitoxantrone (Novantrone) is a cytotoxic agent that intercalates into DNA and inhibits topoisomerase II activity (see Table 20–4 for dosage schedule). It is a potent immune suppressor because of its cytopathic effects on replicating cells. In a study of RRMS and SPMS patients with incomplete recovery after attacks, mitoxantrone reduced the accumulation of neurologic impairment and number of relapses compared with placebo. Mitoxantrone has cardiotoxic properties that limit its total lifetime cumulative dose to 140 mg/m^2. Patients treated with mitoxantrone should undergo echocardiographic evaluations of left ventricular function at baseline and then every 6 months during treatment. Most patients are treated for 2 years, although some patients can be treated for up to an additional year. Mitoxantrone causes leukemia in 0.25% of MS patients. Because of its toxicity, mitoxantrone is regarded as a second-line agent and is used for MS patients who continue to have relapses and disease progression despite treatment with IFN beta or GA.

Natalizumab

Natalizumab (Tysabri) is a monoclonal antibody that binds a-4 integrin on monocytes and blocks the interaction between a-4 integrin and VCAM-1, an integrin expressed on the surface of vascular endothelial cells. The interaction between VLA4 and VCAM-1 is necessary for lymphocyte adherence to vascular endothelia and subsequent transmigration of lymphocytes into body tissues. Natalizumab was shown to reduce the number of MS flares, slow accumulation of neurologic disability, and reduce the accumulation of lesions on brain MRI. Natalizumab is dosed at 300 mg and is intravenously administered every 4 weeks. Although natalizumab appeared to be more efficacious than other disease-modifying therapies, it was recently withdrawn from the market because two patients developed progressive multifocal leukoencephalopathy (PML), but has since been reintroduced with a warning that it should only be used when patients are refractory to other immunotherapy.

Glucocorticoids

Glucocorticoids are the mainstay of therapy for treatment of acute MS relapses. Intravenously administered **methylprednisolone (Solumedrol) dosed at 1 to 2 g/day** or **dexamethasone (Decadron) dosed at 2 mg/kg/day** and administered over 3 to 5 days reduces the symptoms of flares and shortens the recovery time. A rebound in disease activity can occur after discontinuation of glucocorticoid treatment, and some clinicians follow intravenous treatment with a prednisone taper, gradually reducing the dose from 100 mg daily to off over 2 to 4 weeks. Monitoring of bone densitometry is recommended for patients treated with frequent pulsed doses of glucocorticoids. Short-term risks of glucocorticoids include fluid retention, hypokalemia, flushing, acne, insomnia, psychiatric disturbance, dyspepsia, and increased appetite. Patients with preexisting psychiatric illness may experience psychotic symptoms from glucocorticoids.

Plasma Exchange

Small trials showed that plasma exchange may help resolve acute flares of severe demyelinating disease that are not responsive to glucocorticoids. Plasma exchange was shown not to be beneficial in treatment of SPMS.

Treatments for SPMS

IFN beta 1-b appears to reduce the relapse rate and disability in patients who recently transitioned from RRMS into SPMS and are still experiencing relapses. IFN beta 1-b is probably of no benefit in SPMS patients who experience disease progression without relapses. Mitoxantrone is similarly indicated in SPMS patients who experience relapses.

Treatments for PPMS

There are no FDA-approved treatments for PPMS, and trials using IFN beta, GA, and mitoxantrone have not shown benefit.

Off-Label Immunomodulatory Agents

Many other medications with immune modulating or suppressing properties are used to treat MS either alone or in combination with FDA-approved treatments and include azathioprine, methotrexate, mycophenolate mofetil, cladribine, cyclophosphamide, rituximab, alemtuzumab, and IVIG. Use of these agents is best left to experienced clinicians.

Symptomatic Therapies

Because MS affects multiple functions of the nervous system, the symptomatic treatment of MS patients can be complex, especially for patients with SPMS.

Spasticity

Spasticity is a velocity-dependent change in tone and occurs in MS as a consequence of reorganization within the spinal cord or higher centers after injury to the motor pathways. Physical therapy and daily stretching exercises are essential to prevent contracture formation. Antispasmodic treatments should start at low doses and escalate upward until symptomatic relief is obtained or until intolerable side effects occur (usually drowsiness). **Baclofen (10 mg three times daily)** and **tizanidine (2 mg three times daily)** should be the first agents prescribed. **Gabapentin started at 300 mg three times daily and rapidly escalated** is also an effective antispasmodic agent; doses of 3600 mg/day or higher are typical. **Diazepam started at 2 mg three times daily** can be titrated up to 20 mg three times daily. In patients with spasticity who experience excessive side effects or limited relief with oral medications, **intrathecal baclofen** can be administered by an indwelling pump.

Fatigue

MS patients may suffer from neuromuscular fatigue (weakness), fatigue associated with depression, daytime drowsiness secondary to insomnia, generalized lassitude, or deconditioning. MS patients are at high risk for depression, and if it is present, it should be adequately treated. Sleep disturbance is also common in MS, and patients should be educated about sleep hygiene. Some patients may require treatment with hypnotics for sleep. The lassitude associated with MS may respond to **amantadine 100 mg twice daily**. Other stimulants include **modafinil (Provigil) 100 to 200 mg twice a day**, and **methylphenidate (Ritalin) 10 to 20 mg twice a day**. All CNS stimulants can cause insomnia, which can further exacerbate fatigue, and caution must be exercised in patients who are treated with a hypnotic medication for insomnia and a stimulant for fatigue. Physical therapy and regular exercise are essential for MS patients. For patients who experience neuromuscular fatigue associated with increases in body temperature, aquatic exercise is recommended.

Pain

Acute or chronic neuropathic pain is a frequent complication of MS and usually does not respond to treatment with nonsteroidal anti-inflammatory medications. **Gabapentin** is often beneficial but usually requires doses of **1800 mg/day or higher** (see Table 20–5 for dosage ranges and side effects of commonly used medications). **Carbamazepine (Tegretol)** or **oxcarbazepine (Trileptal)** are particularly useful for the "squeezing" or "bandlike" dysesthesias and for trigeminal neuralgia. **Topiramate (Topamax), lamotrigine (Lamictal), and zonisamide (Zonegran)** are also useful in treatment of neuropathic pain. Low-potency opiate analgesics may be used in combination with non-narcotic analgesics. A continuous-release opiate preparation such as the fentanyl transdermal patch (Duragesic patch, 25 to 75 µg/hr) may be necessary for pain refractory to non-narcotic medications.

Paroxysmal Symptoms

The Lhermitte symptom and tonic spasms respond to treatment with **carbamazepine, oxcarbazepine, gabapentin,** and **acetozolamide (Diamox) 125 mg to 250 mg two to three times daily.** Acetozolamide and **ondansetron (Zofran), 4 mg to 8 mg twice a day,** can be useful for intermittent central vertigo. Meclizine (Antivert) is rarely of benefit in central vertigo. Nocturnal flexor spasms respond well to antispasmodic agents such as **baclofen** or **tizanidine**.

Bladder Dysfunction

Bladder spasticity is treated with anticholinergic agents such as **oxybutinin (Ditropan) 5 mg three or four times daily** or **tolteradine (Detrol) 2 mg twice daily.** Long-acting formulations and an oxybutinin transdermal patch applied twice weekly are available. The denervated bladder is treated by intermittent self-catheterization, and patients should be taught this technique as soon as urinary retention is diagnosed. Sphincter dyssynergia can be treated with **terazosin (Hytrin) 1 to 5 mg at** night in combination with **an** anticholinergic and, in some cases, intermittent catheterization.

Bowel Dysfunction

Bowel dysfunction is often undertreated in MS. Constipation can be treated with a combination of fiber (e.g., **Metamucil, 1 teaspoon three times a day with meals), a** stool softener **(docusate sodium, 100 mg three times daily with meals),** and a stimulant **(e.g., senna, two tablets at night).** Enemas, suppositories, and digital stimulation may be necessary. Urge incontinence can be treated with a bowel regimen to trigger voiding at a convenient time each day.

TABLE 20–5 Non-narcotic Medications Commonly Used to Treat Neuropathic Pain in MS

Medication	Dosage Range	Serious Adverse Reactions	Common Adverse Reactions	Laboratory Monitoring
Amitriptyline (Elavil)	50-150 mg/day	Seizures, myocardial infarction, stroke, bone marrow suppression	Dry mouth, drowsiness, dizziness, constipation, urinary retention, confusion	CBC
Carbamazepine (Tegretol)	200-1200 mg/day	Hypersensitivity, cardiac arrhythmias, bone marrow suppression, cutaneous eruptions, hyponatremia	Dizziness, drowsiness, ataxia, blurred vision, allergic rash	CBC, Na
Gabapentin (Neurontin)	900-3600 mg/day	Leucopenia	Drowsiness, lightheadedness, ataxia, fatigue, weight gain	
Lamotrigine (Lamictal)	50-200 mg/day	Cutaneous eruptions, bone marrow suppression, hepatic failure, pancreatitis	Fatigue, dizziness, headache, rash, cognitive dysfunction	CBC, LFTs
Oxcarbazepine (Trileptal)	600-2400 mg/day	Angioedema, bone marrow suppression, cutaneous eruptions, hyponatremia	Dizziness, drowsiness, diplopia, fatigue, acne, alopecia, elevated LFTs	CBC, Na, LFTs

TABLE 20–5 cont.

Topiramate (Topamax)	50-200 mg/day	Metabolic acidosis, nephrolithiasis, bone loss, angle closure glaucoma, bone marrow suppression, cutaneous eruptions	Metabolic acidosis, dizziness, somnolence, cognitive disturbance, visual disturbance, weight loss, agitation	CBC
Tramadol (Ultram)	50-400 mg/day	Seizures, respiratory depression, angioedema, cutaneous eruptions, serotonin syndrome, orthostatic hypotension, hallucinations, withdrawal symptoms	Dizziness, nausea, constipation, headache, somnolence, psychiatric disturbance, urinary retention	
Zonisamide (Zonegran)	100-600 mg/day	Cutaneous eruptions, bone marrow suppression, heat stroke, nephrolithiasis, pancreatitis, psychiatric disturbance, withdrawal seizures	Somnolence, dizziness, psychiatric disturbance, weight loss, constipation	CBC

Medications used to treat neuropathic pain are listed with typical dosage range, adverse event, and laboratory studies for monitoring adverse reactions. See the manufacturer's package inserts for complete information. Not all known adverse events are listed.
CBC, complete blood count; Na, serum sodium; LFTs, liver function tests.

Sexual Dysfunction

Male erectile dysfunction can be treated with **sildenafil (Viagra) 50 to 100 mg, vardenafil (Levitra) 5 to 20 mg,** or **tadalafil (Cialis) 5 to 20 mg before intercourse.** Alprostadil (Edex) 2.5 to 40 µg injected intracavernously is used for nonresponders to oral preparations. Diminished vaginal lubrication causes dyspareunia and can be treated with water-based lubrication. Vaginismus may respond to antispasmodic medications.

MS VARIANTS

Acute Transverse Myelitis (ATM)

ATM is inflammation of the spinal cord that results in bilateral lower extremity weakness, a sensory level, and sphincter impairment. ATM is the presenting manifestation in approximately 2% of MS cases and occurs in many MS patients during the course of the disease. Nevertheless, there are many other potential causes of ATM (Table 20–6), and 75% to 90% of cases not associated with MS follow a

TABLE 20–6 **Differential Diagnosis of Acute Transverse Myelitis**

V (vascular): spinal dural arteriovenous malformation, stroke
I (infectious): viral: herpetoviridae (varicella zoster virus, herpes simplex 1 and 2, Epstein-Barr virus, cytomegalovirus), group B arboviruses (West Nile and Dengue), exanthemas (measles, mumps, rubella), rare causes (enteroviruses, hepatitis A, B, C, lymphocytic choriomeningitis virus) Mycobacterial and bacterial: *Mycobacterium tuberculsis* (tuberculosis), *Mycoplasma pneumoniae, Chlamydia pneumoniae, Borrelia burgdorferi* (Lyme disease), *Treponema pallidum* (syphilis), *Brucella melitensis* (brucellosis), *Bartonella henselae* (cat-scratch disease), bacterial meningitis, intraparenchymal abscess, and epidural abscess
Parasitic: *Schistosoma haematobium, Schistosoma mansonii, Schistosoma japonicum, Toxocara species*
T (trauma): cord compression secondary to trauma, herniated disc, or extradural mass lesion (metastatic disease to the spine, epidural abscess, Pott's disease)
A (autoimmune): Sjögren syndrome, systemic lupus erythematosus, mixed connective tissue disease, anticardiolipin autoantibodies, primary angiitis of the central nervous system, p-ANCA autoantibodies, Hashimoto's encephalopathy (myelopathy), linear scleroderma, sarcoidosis
M (metabolic/toxic): chemotherapy
I (idiopathic/hereditary): multiple sclerosis, acute disseminated encephalomyelitis (postvaccination), neuromyelitis optica
N (neoplastic): lymphoma, leukemia, and other infiltrating tumors
Paraneoplastic: Hodgkin's lymphoma, other tumors
S (psychiatric): conversion disorder

monophasic course. Patients presenting with ATM should undergo spinal cord imaging to exclude compressive etiologies, tumors, and arteriovenous malformations. Brain imaging is also indicated to look for evidence of disseminated demyelination. Cerebrospinal fluid analysis is used to detect infectious etiologies, and blood studies can reveal evidence of systemic inflammation. In severe or rapidly progressive cases, empiric treatment includes administration of **high-dose glucocorticoids** and **intravenous acyclovir** while definitive diagnostic tests are pending. Plasma exchange is indicated in cases that are glucocorticoid-nonresponsive.

Neuromyelitis Optica

The co-occurrence of ATM with optic neuritis, a normal brain MRI study at onset, and spinal cord lesions spanning three or more vertebral segments of the cord are the hallmarks of neuromyelitis optica (NMO or Devic's disease), a rare demyelinating disease. NMO is a syndrome with several etiologies including collagen vascular diseases (systemic lupus erythematosus, Sjögren syndrome, mixed connective tissue disease, p-ANCA autoantibodies, anticardiolipin autoantibodies) and infections (varicella zoster virus, Epstein-Barr virus, HIV, tuberculosis, brucellosis). The idiopathic form can be either monophasic or polyphasic. Although patients recover poorly from the monophasic form, patients with polyphasic disease are at high risk for respiratory compromise from recurrent cervical cord lesions. An immunohistochemical assay with 75% sensitivity and 91% specificity is available for idiopathic NMO. Acute attacks are treated with a combination of **glucocorticoids** and **plasma exchange.** There are no FDA-approved treatments that alter the course of the disease.

Acute MS

Acute MS, or Marburg variant MS, is a rare fulminant demyelinating disease. Brain MRI shows large edematous contrast-enhancing lesions with mass effect, similar to a brain tumor, and many patients undergo brain biopsy. Historically, acute MS was a fatal disease, with death occurring within a year of onset, often secondary to extensive brain stem demyelination. Treatment recommendations, based on anecdotes, include **plasma exchange** in conjunction with high-dose **glucocorticoids** (e.g., 1 to 2 g/day of methylprednisolone for 10 days followed by a slow taper). For patients who survive the acute attack, follow-up treatments include immunosuppression (monthly mitoxantrone or cyclophosphamide) either alone or in combination with IFN beta or GA.

Acute Disseminated Encephalomyelitis

ADEM is a monophasic illness characterized by multifocal inflammation and demyelination and is most common in children. ADEM can be associated with recent rabies or smallpox vaccination (post-vaccination encephalomyelitis) and recent infection (postinfectious encephalomyelitis). Common antecedent infections include childhood exanthemas such as measles and varicella (chickenpox) as well as *M. pneumoniae*, mononucleosis, rubella, mumps influenza, and parainfluenza. Acute hemorrhagic leukoencephalitis (Hurst's disease) is a fulminant and devastating form of ADEM associated with microvascular hemorrhagic lesions. ADEM is distinguished from MS by a history of antecedent vaccination or infection, a rapid onset, and multifocal symptomatic involvement of the cerebrum, brain stem, cerebellum, and spinal cord. Alterations in consciousness and seizures are common in ADEM. Brain MRI in ADEM shows multiple areas of abnormal signal change that are acute and often enhance with gadolinium-DPTA. Cerebrospinal fluid findings are similar to MS. Treatment consists of **high-dose glucocorticoids.** When patients do not respond to glucocorticoids, **plasma exchange** (1.5 to 2 volumes) or **IVIG** is used. In children, behavioral disorders, learning disorders, and epilepsy may be sequelae.

SYSTEMIC INFLAMMATORY DISORDERS WITH CNS MANIFESTATIONS

Sarcoidosis

Sarcoidosis is a systemic chronic inflammatory condition disease characterized histopathologically by multiple noncaseating granulomas affecting one or more organ systems. The condition is idiopathic but may reflect a granulomatous reaction to an as of yet unidentified pathogen. It most commonly affects the lungs, mediastinal lymph nodes, and skin. Systemic features include fever, malaise, lassitude, erythema nodosa, polyarthralgia, mediastinal hilar lymphadenopathy, uveoparotid fever (Heerfordt's syndrome: parotitis, uveitis, and facial palsy), keratoconjunctivitis sicca, hepatosplenomegaly, anemia, cardiac conduction defects, phalangeal bone cysts, and hypercalcemia.

Sarcoidosis affects the nervous system in 10% of patients, primarily the leptomeninges, producing a syndrome consistent with chronic meningitis. The clinical presentation relates to the site of involvement and may include headache, vertigo, impaired vision, isolated cranial nerve lesions (e.g., bilateral facial palsy), intracranial mass lesions, hemiparesis, ataxia, paresthesias, diabetes insipidus, or hypotestosteronism (from pituitary and hypothalamic dysfunction), seizures, encephalopathy, psychosis, dementia, hydrocephalus, polyradiculopathy, peripheral neuropathy, or myopathy. Rarely the spinal cord is involved. Sarcoidosis is five times more common in women. The median age of onset of sarcoidosis is 25 to 30 years; however, the range is broad.

Diagnosis

Laboratory investigations in sarcoidosis may reveal hypercalcemia, hyperuricemia, a raised serum globulin level, and increased serum angiotensin-converting enzyme (ACE). The CSF ACE is positive in 55% of patients with neurosarcoidosis. The CSF may be abnormal, with raised pressure, a slight pleocytosis, markedly raised protein, and hypoglycorrhachia in 20% to 30% of patients. An elevated IgG index is found in 33% of patients. MRI with gadolinium classically shows nodular leptomeningeal enhancement and parenchymal lesions. The diagnosis is made clinically and confirmed by a biopsy of a suitable granuloma revealing a focal collection of epithelioid histiocytes surrounded by a rim of lymphocytes, endothelial cells, and giant cells (Langhans' type) without organisms or caseation. Isolated neurosarcoidosis, seen in only 2% to 3% of patients with CNS involvement, is a difficult diagnosis to make. Meningeal and brain biopsy is necessary to confirm the diagnosis.

Management

Corticosteroids **(prednisone 100 mg daily)** and azathioprine **(1 to 3 mg/kg/day)** are the first-line treatments for CNS sarcoidosis, but many patients do poorly despite therapy.

Behçet's Disease

Behçet's disease is an inflammatory disorder of unknown etiology characterized by a relapsing iritis and uveitis associated with oral (100%) and genital (75%) aphthous ulceration. Systemic features include recurrent fevers, keratoconjunctivitis, hypopyon, migrating superficial thrombophlebitis (25%) that may present as deep venous thrombosis, erythema nodosum (65%), furunculosis, intestinal ulceration, epididymitis, systemic and pulmonary arterial aneurysms, and arthralgia of large joints (60%).

Neurologic manifestations, including abrupt onset of recurrent meningoencephalitis and cranial nerve palsies, occur in 5% to 30% of patients with Behçet's disease. Papilledema, venous sinus occlusion, hemiparesis, quadriparesis, pseudobulbar palsy, and involvement of the basal ganglia, cerebellum, or spinal cord involvement can occur. It is more common and more severe in men, and the peak age of onset is in the twenties.

Diagnosis

The diagnosis is chiefly clinical and is based on the occurrence of a meningoencephalitis in combination with the characteristic cutaneous and ocular lesions. It may mimic MS or strokes, with transient or persistent multifocal involvement of the nervous system. There is no single confirmatory test, but an ESR over 50 mm/hr is common. CSF studies show a mild pleocytosis with a moderate increase in protein. Brain imaging may show infarction (25%), hypodense/hypointense enhancing lesions, and leptomeningeal enhancement. Pathologically, inflammatory changes are found in the iris, choroid, retina, optic nerve, and meninges and in the perivascular spaces (vasculitis) of the brain.

Management

Treatment may include analgesics, anticoagulants, colchicine, dapsone, levamisole, thalidomide, glucocorticoids, and immunosuppression (azathioprine, chlorambucil, cyclophosphamide). Posterior uveal tract and neurologic lesions, if untreated, may lead to blindness or death.

Central Pontine Myelinolysis

This condition is characterized by symmetric destruction of the pontine white matter. Rapid correction of hyponatremia is associated with the onset of CPM in most cases. CPM occurs more frequently in patients with a history of alcoholism, malnutrition, and multiorgan failure. The lesion destroys the myelin sheath, sparing neurons and axons. It presents as a rapidly progressing spastic quadriplegia with facial, glottal, and pharyngeal paralysis in a debilitated patient suffering from an acute illness. When the pons alone is involved, the patient may become "locked-in," mute and paralyzed. In more severe cases, demyelination also involves white matter tracts in the basal ganglia, a condition termed *extrapontine myelinolysis*. MRI is the imaging modality of choice. Recovery from even the most severe cases is possible but may take 4 to 12 months. The disease is

TABLE 20–7 **Formula for Correcting Hyponatremia***

Change in serum Na^+ =	$\dfrac{\text{infusate } Na^+ - \text{serum } Na^+}{\text{total body water} + 1}$

Infusates:	
3% saline	513 mEq/L
0.9% saline	154 mEq/L
Ringer's lactate	130 mEq/L
0.45% saline	77 mEq/L

*Equation yields the effect of 1 L of infusate on serum Na^+ concentration in milliequivalents per liter. The rate of the infusion should be adjusted to correct the serum Na^+ no faster than 8 to 12 mEq/L per day. The suggested target Na^+ concentration is 130 mmol/L. Total body water in liters is estimated as a fraction of body weight in kilograms; the fraction is 0.6 in men and 0.5 in women.

Adapted from Adrogue HJ, Madias NE: Hyponatremia. N Engl J Med 2000;342: 1581-1589.

rarely directly fatal, but the mortality rate can be high as a result of secondary complications.

CPM is best avoided in severely hyponatremic patients by slowly correcting the serum sodium no faster than 0.5 mEq/L per hour (12 mEq/L per day), to a maximum level of 130 mEq/L (Table 20–7).

Infections of the Central Nervous System

Infections of the CNS can be life threatening. Prompt diagnosis and treatment are essential to prevent death or permanent neurologic disability. **The combination of fever, headache, and neurologic signs or symptoms must be treated as a CNS infection until proven otherwise.** A management algorithm (Fig. 21–1) should be followed for suspected cases of bacterial meningitis. Empirical treatment for bacterial causes is outlined in Table 21–1. Based on presentation and risk factors, antiviral (e.g., acyclovir) and antifungal agents should be included in the empirical treatment. Definitive treatment will later be based on the results of cultures or other diagnostic tests.

APPROACH TO THE PATIENT WITH SUSPECTED CNS INFECTION

History and Examination

1. Ascertain the acuity and tempo of symptoms.
2. Identify any predisposing risk factors:
   - **Immunosuppression:** diabetes, alcoholism, malignancy, steroids, chemotherapy, HIV infection
   - **Head trauma**
   - **Otological or neurosurgical procedures**
   - **Unusual Exposures:** foreign travel, wooded areas, sick contacts, animals, or insects
3. Check for the following symptoms: fever, headache or neck pain, change in mental status, focal weakness, or back pain.
4. Check for evidence of infection elsewhere in the body: sinusitis, endocarditis, pneumonia, osteomyelitis, urinary tract infection, skin eruption.
5. Always be sure to check for the following signs: papilledema, meningismus, exanthem, sinus tenderness, otitis media, or spine tenderness.

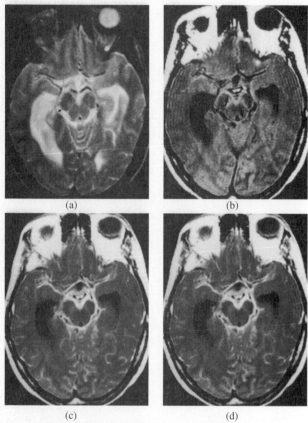

(a)   (b)

(c)   (d)

Figure 21–1 MRI findings of tuberculous meningitis. (a) T2- and (b) precontrast T1-weighted images show hydrocephalus. (c) Precontrast T1-weighted magnetization transfer (MT) image shows thick basal meninges as hyperintense signal around the brain stem (small arrows), not seen on T1-weighted image (b). (d) Postcontrast T1 image demonstrates thick enhancement of the basal meninges and exudates. (Reproduced with permission from Kapra P, et al: Infectious meningitis: Prospective evaluation with magnetization transfer MRI. Br J Radiol 2004;77:387-394.)

Lumbar Puncture

LP is the most important test to confirm a CNS infection and identify the causative organism. The technique for performing LP is covered in Chapter 3. **If CNS infection is suspected, when deciding whether to perform an LP, the following clinical rule may be helpful:**

TABLE 21–1 Cerebrospinal Fluid Findings in Selected Infections of the Central Nervous System

	No. of White Blood Cells (per mm³)	Cell Type	Concentration of Protein (mg/dl)	Concentration of Glucose (mg/dl)	CSF Pressure (cm H₂O)
Normal	≤5	Lymphocytes and monocytes only	15 to 45	45 to 80	80 to 180
Bacterial meningitis	5 to 10,000	Polymorphonuclear leukocytes	Increased	Decreased	Increased
Viral meningitis	5 to 1000	Lymphocytes	Increased	Normal	Normal, occasionally increased
Tubercular meningitis	5 to 500	Lymphocytes	Increased	Decreased	Increased
Cryptococcal meningitis	5 to 100	Lymphocytes	Increased	Normal, occasionally decreased	Increased
Active neurosyphilis	5 to 500	Lymphocytes	Increased	Normal, occasionally decreased	Normal

1. Fever
2. Headache ⎫ **Any 2 of these 3 require LP**
3. Change in mental status ⎭

Because herniation is a serious but rare complication of LP, **CT scan** may be **required prior to LP** (see Fig. 21–1).

ACUTE MENINGITIS

Acute Bacterial Meningitis

Bacterial meningitis typically presents as the classic triad of *fever, headache, and stiff neck*. The presentation is usually dramatic but may be less obvious at the extremes of age (in infants and in the elderly), in whom change in mental status is often the only symptom. Seeding of the leptomeninges usually occurs from hematogenous spread of the infecting organism (e.g., pneumococcal pneumonia complicated by meningitis), but it can also result from a parameningeal infection (e.g., otitis media) or following trauma, cochlear implants, or neurosurgery (e.g., CSF leak). *Streptococcus pneumoniae* (50% of cases) and *Neisseria meningiditis* (25% of cases) are the most common causes of bacterial meningitis. Mortality is approximately 20%.

Diagnosis

The diagnosis is established by abnormal CSF indices including polymorphonuclear pleocytosis, elevated protein level, and reduced glucose level (Table 21–1). The organism is identified by CSF cultures. However, when CSF is sterile, for example, in cases in which antibiotics are given prior to LP, blood cultures often identify the causative organism. Interpreting CSF profiles in neurosurgical patients with recently placed ventricular drains can be difficult. A rising white blood cell (WBC) count and falling glucose level suggests an infection. Because of impaired CSF circulation in shunted patients, CSF should be sampled from the drain or shunt when possible.

Treatment

The prognosis in bacterial meningitis depends on the interval between onset of disease and initiation of therapy. Selection of empirical antibiotics depends on age and risk factors, as shown in Table 21–1. Most adults with suspected community-acquired bacterial meningitis should be treated with **dexamethasone 6 mg IV every 6 hours for 4 days** (first dose given 15 minutes prior to antibiotics), and **ceftriaxone and vancomycin** until cultures provide for a definite diagnosis and antibiotic sensitivity. Treatment with dexamethasone blunts the acute inflammatory response and results in a 50% reduction in mortality; efficacy is greatest with *pneumococcal* meningitis. In neonates and older or immunosuppressed patients, **ampicillin** should be added as well to cover *Listeria monocytogenes* infection. Recently placed shunts or intracranial hardware should be removed.

Viral (Aseptic) Meningitis

Viral meningitis is a self-limited illness seen most frequently in children and young adults. The presentation is similar to bacterial meningitis, except that neurologic dysfunction (e.g., change in mental status, neurologic focality) does not occur. The diagnosis is suggested by lymphocytic pleocytosis with a normal glucose level in the CSF (see Table 21–1) and negative CSF and blood bacterial cultures. In some cases of viral meningitis, the virus can be cultured or amplified (PCR) from CSF, blood, nasal pharyngeal secretions, or fecal material. The presence of intrathecal production of virus-specific IgG antibodies acquired weeks after the onset of symptoms can establish a retrospective diagnosis (for West Nile virus, IgM can be found as early as 1 week after onset of symptoms). The most common causes of viral meningitis include enteroviruses, arthropod-borne viruses (especially West Nile virus), herpes simplex virus-2, lymphocytic choriomeningitis virus, and infection with HIV during the acute conversion period. Medications can cause aseptic meningitis simulating viral meningitis. The usual culprits include NSAIDs, metronidazole, carbamazepine, trimethoprim/sulfamethoxazole, and IVIG. Treatment is supportive. Prognosis is excellent.

CHRONIC MENINGITIS

Chronic meningitis refers to a more indolent infection that by definition develops over a period of 2 weeks or more.

Tuberculosis Meningitis

Tuberculosis meningitis, caused by the bacterium *Mycobacterium tuberculosis*, typically evolves over weeks to months, but the diagnosis is often overlooked until a fulminant syndrome develops. *Cranial nerve palsies, vasculitic small-vessel infarctions, and obstructive hydrocephalus* occur frequently and result from severe granulomatous inflammation of the basal meninges (see Fig. 21–1). Tuberculosis can *cause focal abscess formation*, which can evolve into space-occupying mass lesions *(tuberculoma)*, even without meningitis. Patients who are chronically exposed, immunosuppressed (AIDS or alcoholic patients), or at the extremes of age are particularly at risk. Morbidity and mortality are high unless treated early. *Hydrocephalus, seizures, and cognitive impairment* are frequent late complications.

Diagnosis

The CSF shows lymphocytic pleocytosis, elevated protein level, and moderately reduced glucose level (see Table 21–1). The diagnosis is established by observing *acid-fast* mycobacteria in the CSF; the yield exceeds 50% when multiple large-volume taps (10 to 25 ml) are examined. *M. tuberculosis* can also be *cultured* from the CSF, but the yield is low, and up to 6 weeks are needed for the organism to grow. *PCR* testing can establish the diagnosis by amplifying small amounts of tubercle bacillus DNA, but sensitivity is variable depending on the quantity of nucleic acid circulating in the CSF. Evidence of active pulmonary disease is found in only 30% of the cases; purified protein derivative (PPD) testing is too unreliable to be a useful diagnostic tool in working up TB meningitis.

Treatment

Initial treatment consists of the four-drug regimen of **isoniazid 300 mg per day** (also give **pyridoxine 50 mg per day**), **rifampin 600 mg per day, pyrazinamide 15 to 30 mg/kg per day,** and **ethambutol 15 to 20 mg/kg per day**. Cotreatment with **dexamethasone 6 mg IV every 6 hours** may also be used in severe cases (with depressed level of consciousness, focal deficits, or multiple cranial nerve palsies) to inhibit the inflammatory response and limit damage. An infectious disease specialist should be consulted, given possible drug resistance and the high rate of unacceptable drug toxicity arising from these agents.

Neurosyphilis

Syphilis is a chronic systemic infection caused by the spirochete *Treponema pallidum*. **Primary infection** is characterized by a chancre (firm, painless, genital ulcer). A **secondary bacteremic stage** may occur 2 to 12 weeks later, resulting in generalized mucocutaneous lesions (palmar and plantar rash) and lymphadenopathy. In up to 60% of cases, the CNS is seeded during the bacteremic stage; 10% of these patients will develop symptomatic early neurosyphilis (meningitis, meningovasculitis, cranial neuritis). Mild inflammatory CSF changes (elevation of cells and protein) can be detected at this stage.

Following a latent period of 15 to 20 years, **tertiary syphilis** manifests as a slowly progressive, systemic inflammatory disease of the skin (gummas), heart (aortitis), eyes (chorioretinitis), or CNS. *Tertiary neurosyphilis* develops in 5% of patients with untreated primary syphilis. The classic manifestations include the following:

1. **General paresis**

    This condition results from chronic, diffuse encephalitis and manifests as dementia with prominent psychiatric features and bilateral upper motor neuron signs.

2. **Tabes dorsalis**

    Tabes dorsalis results from chronic spinal polyradiculitis with secondary dorsal root and column degeneration. Symptoms may include neuropathic shooting pains in the lower extremities, loss of posterior column sensation, and areflexia.

3. Argyll Robertson pupils

These are small irregular pupils that react to accommodation but not to light and reflect chronic optic neuritis. Optic atrophy and blindness may also occur.

In **HIV patients** the course of syphilis is often accelerated, and the early symptomatic forms of secondary syphilis (meningitis and meningovasculitis) predominate. Symptoms may occur during any stage of HIV infection.

Diagnosis

LP is required to rule out neurosyphilis in patients with a serum nontreponemal antibody (RPR or VDRL) titer = 1:32, or in any patient with a positive serologic test and neurologic symptoms, no prior treatment, concurrent systemic tertiary syphilis, or HIV infection.

Standard CSF laboratory criteria to diagnose neurosyphilis do not exist. A positive CSF VDRL test is highly specific but only 50% sensitive. Many advocate routine testing of CSF FTA-ABS, which is highly sensitive but not specific. A negative CSF FTA-ABS and CSF VDRL virtually exclude the diagnosis of neurosyphilis. Some advocate treating if the CSF FTA-ABS is positive and there is either a CSF pleocytosis or elevated protein level.

In HIV patients laboratory diagnosis is more difficult because treponemal and nontreponemal tests are less reliable, and CSF indices can be difficult to interpret depending on the stage of HIV infection. Some advocate a positive CSF FTA-ABS along with a CSF pleocytosis as grounds for treating as neurosyphilis.

Treatment

Neurosyphilis, whether latent or active, is treated with **penicillin G 3 to 4 million U IV every 4 hours for 10 to 14 days.**

Lyme Disease

Lyme disease is caused by the spirochete *Borrelia burgdorferi,* which is inoculated into humans by the bite of an infected deer tick *(Ixodes dammini).* A characteristic expanding erythematous "target" lesion, erythema chronicum migrans, develops at the site of the tick bite. Acute, chronic, and relapsing dermatologic, immunologic, rheumatologic, cardiac, and neurologic complications may occur. Both the peripheral and central nervous systems can be involved, either by direct effects of the infection or by immune-mediated processes, and are usually divided into early or late manifestations (Table 21–2).

Diagnosis

To diagnose CNS Lyme disease, there must be evidence of intrathecal production of IgG antibody (IgM during acute phase) to *Borrelia* using an enzyme-linked immunosorbent assay (ELISA) or Western blot. A PCR test for *Borrelia* DNA in CSF is also available but is less

TABLE 21–2 **Neurologic Manifestations of Lyme Disease**

Early (Less Than 6 Month after Infection)

Mild meningitis or meningoencephalitis
Cranial neuropathy (particularly unilateral or bilateral facial nerve and
optic nerve)
Myelitis
Radiculoneuritis
Mononeuritis multiplex
Acute polyneuropathy (resembles Guillain-Barré syndrome)

Chronic (Months to Years after Infection)

Lyme encephalopathy (immune-mediated)
Recurrent or chronic meningoencephalitis
Chronic myelitis
Chronic axonal polyneuropathy

sensitive than antibody testing. A lymphocytic pleocytosis with
mildly elevated protein is found is menigitic forms or Lyme
disease.

Treatment

Patients with CNS Lyme disease should receive **ceftriaxone 2 g IV
per day or penicillin G 4 million U IV every 4 hours** for 2 to 4
weeks. Isolated facial palsy with normal CSF can be treated with
doxycycline 100 mg PO two times a day or **amoxicillin 50 mg PO
three times a day** for 7 to 21 days.

Fungal Meningitis

Fungal infection of the CNS is usually opportunistic, occurring in
hosts with impaired cellular immunity (HIV/AIDS, organ transplant,
malignancy, immunosuppressive therapy, diabetes, or alcoholism).
Cryptococcus neoformans accounts for most cases in the United States;
other causes include *Coccidioides immitis* (southwestern United
States), *Candida albicans, Histoplasma capsulatum,* and *Blastomyces*
species. *Aspergillus* and *Mucor* species are unique in their tendency
to invade local tissues and cause vasculitic infarction.

Diagnosis

The most consistent CSF abnormality is an elevated protein level. A
lymphocytic pleocytosis and low glucose level are variably present.
Diagnosis is based on demonstrating the organism by wet smear or
culture. *Cryptococcus* infection is most rapidly diagnosed using the
India ink stain or by detecting capsular antigen in the CSF.

Treatment

All forms of fungal meningitis are treated with **fluconazole 400 to
800 mg PO daily** for mild cases or **amphotericin B 0.5 to 1.5 mg/kg**

per day IV for severe cases. Treatment should continue for 2 to 4 weeks. Non-HIV cryptococcal meningitis is treated with the combination of **amphotericin B** and **flucytosine (5-FC) 37.5 mg/kg PO every 6 hours** with dose adjustment to maintain a peak (70 to 80 mg/L) and trough (30 to 40 mg/L) levels. In the most severe cases, amphotericin B (0.1 to 0.3 mg daily) can be given intrathecally via a reservoir. Elevated ICP may respond to acetazolamide, but severe cases mandate frequent therapeutic lumbar punctures and, if refractory, lumbar or ventricular shunting.

BRAIN ABSCESS AND PARAMENINGEAL INFECTIONS

Bacterial Abscess

Brain abscess most commonly presents with subacute progression of headache (in 75% of patients), altered mental status (in 50% of patients), focal neurologic signs (in 50% of patients), and fever (in 50% of patients). The infection usually begins as a focus of cerebritis, which develops into a localized collection of pus with a surrounding fibrovascular capsule. Most abscesses are formed by contiguous spread from a parameningeal infection (otitis media, osteomyelitis, sinusitis) or by hematogenous spread in patients with endocarditis, bronchiectasis, congenital cyanotic heart disease, or pulmonary arteriovenous malformations. The most common organisms encountered are streptococci, *Staphylococcus aureus*, Enterobacteriacae, and anaerobes such as *Bacteroides fragilis*. Polymicrobial infections are common.

Diagnosis

The diagnosis is suggested by a ring-enhancing lesion (Fig. 21–2) in the brain on CT or MRI. The CSF may be normal or may show a mild pleocytosis; a pathogen is isolated from CSF cultures in less than 10% of cases. Blood cultures, echocardiography, chest x-ray, HIV testing, and a dedicated skull CT scan (to rule out sinusitis, otitis, or tooth abscess) should be performed in addition to LP in all patients with brain abscess of unknown etiology. Cultures of pus obtained from a surgical drainage procedure are often the only way to establish the diagnosis, but even these cultures are negative in 20% of cases.

Treatment

For broad-spectrum empiric coverage of suspected bacterial abscess, treat with (1) **penicillin G 4 million U IV every 4 hours** or **ceftriaxone 2 g IV every 12 hours** AND (2) **metronidazole 15 mg/kg IV every 12 hours.** For postsurgical or posttraumatic cases or if *S. aureas* is a consideration (positive blood culture), **vancomycin** should be added until sensitivities are known. When the pathogen underlying

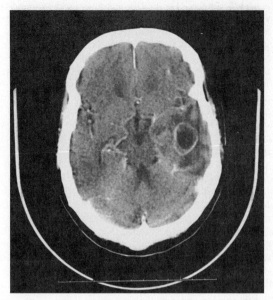

Figure 21–2 Ring-enhancing lesion on CT scan, characteristic of bacterial abscess.

the abscess is in doubt, one must consider broadening coverage to include tuberculosis (see TB meningitis), fungus (amphotericin B), and toxoplasmosis (see HIV section below). Aggressive organisms can cause the abscess to quickly expand, leading to rapid neurologic deterioration and herniation. Therefore neurosurgical consult is mandatory for possible emergent drainage and decompression. Patients with depressed level of consciousness should also be treated with **dexamethasone 4 to 10 mg IV every 6 hours** for 4 to 6 days to reduce edema.

Subdural Empyema

Subdural empyema is a closed-space infection between the dura and arachnoid, usually over the hemispheric convexity. In adults, spread of infection from a contiguous source (e.g., sinusitis or otitis) is the cause in most cases, whereas in children, subdural empyema often occurs as a complication of meningitis. The organisms most often cultured are similar to those for brain abscess, and empirical antibiotic coverage is the same. Surgical drainage at the earliest opportunity is essential for successful treatment.

Cranial and Spinal Epidural Abscess

Epidural CNS infection almost always results from infection from a contiguous source and is often seen in combination with osteomyelitis. The CSF often shows mild signs of inflammation (elevated WBC and protein levels) but is sterile.

Cranial epidural abscess usually presents with localized pain and tenderness and can lead to cranial nerve deficits. For example, infection of the petrous temporal bone (Gradenigo's syndrome) often results in CN 5 and CN 6 deficits. Common infecting organisms are the same as for brain abscess, and empirical antibiotic treatment is the same.

Spinal epidural abscess is most common in the thoracic region and often occurs in diabetics and intravenous drug users. Symptoms may include intense local pain and tenderness, local root irritation with referred pain, and cord compression, which is a neurologic emergency. *S. aureus* and streptococci account for 75% of the infections, and gram-negative organisms account for 20%; unusual causes include *M. tuberculosis* (Pott's disease) and fungi. MRI of the spine is the diagnostic technique of choice. Treatment with high-dose steroids **(dexamethasone 60 to 100 mg IVP, followed by 10 to 20 mg IV every 6 hours)** and **surgical drainage** should be performed immediately to prevent cord compression. **Vancomycin** and **ceftriaxone** usually provide adequate empirical antibiotic coverage for bacterial infection (Table 21–3).

Cysticercosis

Cysticercosis is the most common parasitic CNS infection worldwide and typically presents with seizures. Ova shed by the intestinal tapeworm *Taenia solium* in human feces can contaminate food ingested by the host or others, which leads to hematogenous dissemination of encysted larvae throughout the body, including the CNS. Most cases occur in Latin America (e.g., Mexico) and Southeast Asia.

Diagnosis

CT and MRI scans are usually highly characteristic. *Uninflamed cysts* appear as small (less than 1 cm) fluid-filled cysts. *Active, inflamed cysts* occur when the larvae are dying and are identified by the presence of contrast enhancement. *Inactive cysts* result once the inflammatory reaction to a dying larval cyst has resolved; they appear as small, punctuate, calcified lesions. In the *racemic form,* cystic membranes fill the ventricles and the subarachnoid space, resulting in hydrocephalus. Detection of *serum antibody titers* to *Cysticercus* can confirm the diagnosis, but sensitivity is less than 100% in patients with inactive disease or with a single enhancing lesion. Patients and family members should undergo stool examinations for ova and parasites, because treatment can prevent reinfection.

Treatment

Patients with inactive (calcified) neurocysticercosis or with few viable or degenerating cysts and minimal symptoms (e.g., seizures

TABLE 21-3 Empirical Antibiotic Therapy for Bacterial Meningitis

Risk Group	Pathogen	Empiric Therapy
Neonates (<1 month)	Group B streptococci, E. coli, Listeria monocytogenes, Klebsiella	Cefotaxime or gentamycin + ampicillin
Infants to young adults (1 month-50 years)	S. pneumoniae, N. meningitides	Ceftriaxone or cefotaxime + vancomycin
Adults >50 years old	S. pneumoniae, L. monocytogenes, gram-negative bacilli	Ceftriaxone + vancomycin + ampicillin
Postneurosurgical, head Trauma/skull fracture, cochlear implant	S. pneumoniae, P. aeruginosa, S. aureas S. epidermidis, Enterobacteriacae	Cefepime or ceftazidime or meropenem + vancomycin
Shunt-related ventriculitis or meningitis	S. aureas, S. epidermidis, P. acnes, Enterobacteriacae	Cefepime or ceftazidime or meropenem + vancomycin

Adult Dosages
  Ampicillin 2.0 g IV every 4 hours
  Cefepime 2 g IV every 8 hours
  Cefotaxime 2 g IV every 6 hours
  Ceftazidime 2 g IV every 8 hours
  Ceftriaxone 2 g IV every 12 hours
  Merapenem 2 g IV every 8 hours
  Vancomycin 1 g IV every 8 hours
  Dexamethasone 0.15 mg/kg IV every 6 hours

controlled with anticonvulsants and a nonfocal examination) do not require antimicrobial treatment. In the latter case, follow-up neuro-imaging 6 to 10 weeks later usually shows progression of the enhancing lesion to a small, calcified nodule. For those with many cysts, giant cyst(s), or intraventricular/ subarachnoid cysts, give **praziquantel 25 mg/kg PO three times daily** or **albendazole 7.5 mg/kg PO twice daily, for 14 days.** For patients undergoing treatment with a large lesion burden, give **dexamethasone 4 to 6 mg PO every 6 hours for 5 days** to attenuate the inflammatory reaction and an antiseizure medication (e.g., **phenytoin 300 PO daily**) to minimize symptoms related to the inflammatory response caused by dying cysts. Surgical resection is often more effective than ventriculoperitoneal shunting for treating intraventricular cysticercosis resulting in hydrocephalus.

VIRAL ENCEPHALITIS

Herpes Simplex Encephalitis

Herpes simplex virus type 1 (HSV-1) encephalitis is the most common cause of sporadic viral encephalitis and is fatal in up to 70% of untreated patients. Patients present with fever, altered mental status, headache, and seizures. The disease results from reactivation of dormant HSV-1 within the trigeminal ganglion, with viral spread via sensory pathways into the brain, rather than the more common picture of retrograde viral expression leading to perioral herpetic lesions.

Diagnosis

The CSF may show mild lymphocytic pleocytosis, increased red blood cells, and increased protein, but it may be normal, particularly early in the disease. A positive CSF HSV PCR confirms the diagnosis, but false-negative results occur, particularly if CSF is acquired after acyclovir use. The presence of intrathecal HSV antibody (IgM or IgG) from CSF acquired at least 1 week after onset of symptoms assists in making a retrospective diagnosis. CSF cultures usually do not yield the virus. Focal necrotizing lesions of the inferior frontal and temporal lobes are highly characteristic and are best seen with contrast MRI. An EEG often shows periodic lateralized epileptiform discharges, consistent with structural temporal lobe lesions. Definitive diagnosis is made by brain biopsy, which demonstrates eosinophilic intracellular (Cowdry type I) inclusions but is rarely necessary when the clinical, radiologic, and EEG findings are highly characteristic.

Treatment

All patients with suspected viral encephalitis should be treated empirically with **acyclovir 10 mg/kg IV every 8 hours for 14 to 21**

days. *Because efficacy depends on early treatment, acyclovir should be started as soon as possible and should never be withheld pending the results of diagnostic studies.* Anticonvulsants (e.g., **phenytoin**) should be given to all critically ill patients and discontinued after 2 weeks if no seizures occur. Continuous EEG monitoring to rule out nonconvulsive seizure activity is recommended in patients with abnormal mental status.

West Nile Virus Infection

West Nile virus (WNV), an arthropod-borne virus transmitted by the bite of the *Culix* mosquito, is the most common cause of epidemic encephalitis in the United States. Disease activity is now concentrated in the western United States, with outbreaks occurring predominately in the summer and fall months when mosquito activity is highest. Transmission has been reported via blood transfusion, organ transplantation, and breast-feeding; of those infected, only 20% become symptomatic and less than 1% develop neurologic complications (neuroinvasive WNV). The majority of neuroinvasive cases manifest as *meningoencephalitis* (60% to 75%), characterized by altered mental status, focal neurologic deficits, and tremor, or *meningitis* (25% to 30%), characterized by headache, neck pain, and occasionally cranial nerve palsy's (facial nerve particularly). Less commonly *myelitis and polyradiculitis* occur, characterized by the acute onset of asymmetric limb weakness, the absence of sensory less, and lower motor neuron signs.

Diagnosis

Neuroinvasive West Nile virus is a diagnosis based on clinical suspicion (risk of exposure and suggestive signs and symptoms) and the presence of West Nile virus IgM in the blood or CSF. A negative WNV IgM antibody test should be repeated in 7 days to allow for seroconversion after an acute infection. Serum WNV IgM antibody, which does not cross the blood-brain barrier, should also be present, and a fourfold change in acute to convalescent titers indicates a recent infection. Both serum and CSF IgM antibody can persist for months, and therefore a single positive test does not necessarily imply recent infection. False-positives can also occur when antibodies to St. Louis encephalitis virus and Japanese encephalitis virus are present. CSF typically shows a mild pleocytosis, elevated protein level, and normal glucose level. West Nile poliomyelitis should be considered in cases of rapidly ascending paralysis with an inflammatory CSF profile. Isolation (culture) or amplification (PCR) techniques have a low sensitivity.

Treatment

Treatment remains supportive, but clinical trials with IVIG and interferon alpha are in progress.

Other Causes of Encephalitis

Causes of viral encephalitis other than HSV-1 and WNV are listed below. PCR testing on CSF is available for most viruses, but the sensitivity of most assays, when utilized in a clinical setting, is unknown. Virus-specific antibody testing on CSF is the most reliable method of making a diagnosis, albeit retrospectively.

1. **Enteroviruses**

   This group includes **coxsackievirus, echovirus,** and **poliovirus**. Outbreaks of meningitis and to a lesser extent encephalitis occur during the fall/winter months. The course is usually mild. CSF viral cultures and PCR are sensitive.

2. **Arboviruses (arthropod-borne viruses)**

   These viruses are transmitted to humans and a variety of vectors including mosquitoes and ticks and are restricted by geography and season

   - **Eastern equine virus** (Gulf and Atlantic coast) causes a severe encephalitis with high morbidity and mortality.
   - **Western equine virus** (western United States) causes a mild meningoencephalitis.
   - **St. Louis encephalitis virus** (entire United States) causes a severe encephalitis with occasional epidemics.
   - **California encephalitis virus** (eastern and central United States) may simulate HSV-1 encephalitis.
   - **Colorado tick fever virus** (Rocky Mountains) is transmitted from the bite from a *Dermacentor andersoni* tick.
   - **Powassan virus** (Northeast United States) is transmitted from *Ixodes cookie,* or woodchuck tick.
   - **Japanese encephalitis virus** (Asia), transmitted by the *Culex* mosquito, is the most common cause of encephalitis worldwide and is not endemic to the United States. The mortality rate is approximately 30%.

3. **Herpes family viruses**

   - **HSV-2** is a common cause of encephalitis in neonates and meningitis in children and adults.
   - **Epstein Barr virus (EBV)** is typically associated with polyradiculitis or cerebellitis.
   - **Varicella-zoster virus (VZV)** can cause encephalitis in association with a systemic primary infection (chickenpox), or a focal granulomatous vasculitis of the brain or spinal cord following a zoster eruption in the corresponding vascular territory.
   - **Cytomegalovirus (CMV)**-related neurologic complications are seen only in those with impaired cellular immunity (see HIV section).
   - **Human herpes virus 6 (HHV-6)** can cause severe encephalitis in patients on immunosuppressive treatment.

4. **Measles virus**

Besides causing acute encephalitis 1 to 14 days after a viral exanthem (rubeola), measles virus can cause (1) a relentlessly progressive subacute encephalitis in immunosuppressed patients, (2) postinfectious immune-mediated demyelinating encephalomyelitis, and (3) *subacute sclerosing panencephalitis (SSPE)*, a "slow" viral infection characterized by progressive dementia, ataxia, myoclonus, periodic sharp waves on EEG, elevated titers of antimeasles virus antibodies in the CSF, and pathologic intracellular viral inclusion bodies.

5. **Rabies virus**

Rabies is spread by the bite of an infected (rabid) animal. After a variable incubation period (1 to 3 months), rabies encephalomyelitis invariably leads to delirium, seizures, paralysis, and death. After inoculation, the virus travels to the CNS via retrograde axonal transport. Negri bodies and dark intracellular viral inclusions are the characteristic pathologic lesion.

VIRAL MYELITIS

Acute Viral Myelitis

Acute myelitis, a relatively rare disease, may occur in isolation or concomitant with meningitis or encephalitis. Herpes family viruses (e.g., HSV-2, EBV, CMV, VZV), enteroviruses, and West Nile virus are the most common causes. It presents with acute onset of weakness, sensory loss, and autonomic (particularly bladder) dysfunction. West Nile virus and poliovirus are exceptional in that they infect motor neurons, causing asymmetric flaccid weakness (poliomyelitis). Clinically discriminating viral from autoimmune causes of acute myelitis can be difficult, but as a general rule viral myelitis is more likely to affect only one spinal cord level.

Diagnosis

CSF typically reveals a mild lymphocytic pleocytosis with an elevated protein level. Many of the viruses can be amplified by virus-specific PCR assays, although the sensitivity of the assays in clinical practice is unproven. The presence of virus-specific antibody in CSF acquired weeks after the onset confirms the diagnosis. MRI typically shows focal area of increased T2-weighted signal that enhances with contrast.

Treatment

Antiviral treatment needs to be tailored to the specific causative virus, when known. EBV, VZV, or HSV type 1 or 2 is treated with **acyclovir 10 mg/kg IV every 8 hours,** and CMV is treated with

ganciclovir 5 mg/kg IV every 12 hours and/or **foscarnet 90 to 120 mg/kg/day.** Corticosteroids are not indicated for viral myelitis but should be given when immune-mediated causes are a diagnostic consideration. Particular attention must be paid to bladder and bowel dysfunction.

Chronic Viral Myelopathy

Human T-cell lymphotropic virus type 1 or 2 (HTLV-1/2) and HIV, and less commonly HSV-2 and VZV, are recognized causes of chronic viral myelopathy. HTLV infection, which causes a myelopathy formerly known as tropical spastic pararesis, is endemic in the Caribbean basin, Brazil, Japan, and parts of Africa. Symptoms include subacute to insidious onset of spastic paresis, sensory loss, and autonomic (erectile, urinary, and bowel) dysfunction.

Diagnosis

CSF may show mild nonspecific abnormalities including a lymphocytic pleocytosis and elevated protein level. HSV-2 and VZV infection can be confirmed by virus-specific PCR or IgG antibody in the CSF. HTLV-1/2 is confirmed by the presence of IgG antibody in the CSF. HIV myelopathy is a clinical diagnosis.

Treatment

Acyclovir 10 mg/kg IV every 8 hours should be given for HSV or VZV myelopathy. HIV myelopathy may respond to virologic control with highly active antiretroviral therapy (HAART). Otherwise, treatment is supportive, and particular attention must be paid to bladder and bowel dysfunction.

NEUROLOGIC COMPLICATIONS OF AIDS

Both the peripheral and central nervous systems are vulnerable to HIV-related complications. The risk for *opportunistic infection* is greatest in those with CD4+ T helper lymphocyte counts less than 200/mm^3, whereas *immune-mediated conditions* and *medication-related toxicities* can occur at any time. *Patients with AIDS are at risk for multiple, simultaneous, opportunistic infections.*

Opportunistic Infections

1. **CNS toxoplasmosis**
   Toxoplasmosis, the most common cause of a space-occupying mass lesion in HIV patients, usually presents with fever, subacute encephalopathy, focal neurologic deficits, and seizures. A presumed diagnosis is based on brain imaging showing one or more ring-enhancing mass lesions that respond to antitoxoplasmosis treatment within 2 weeks.

Ocular and spinal cord abscesses may occur; meningoencephalitis from a ruptured abscess is rare. The presence of serum toxoplasma IgG antibody at presentation raises the probability of the diagnosis. CSF analysis does not assist in making the diagnosis but may help exclude others.

Patients with suspected toxoplasmosis should be treated empirically with **sulfadiazine 25 mg/kg PO every 6 hours** and **pyrimethamine 200 mg PO on day 1, followed by 75 to 100 mg per day for 6 to 8 weeks.** Folinic acid 10 to 20 mg PO every day should also be given to minimize hematologic toxicity. **Clindamycin 600 mg IV or PO four times a day** can be used instead of sulfadiazine in patients who are allergic to sulfa drugs. **Dexamethasone 6 mg IV every 6 hours** should be restricted to patients with large mass lesions with impending herniation, as its use may obscure the diagnosis. Repeat imaging, preferably MRI, with contrast should be performed 10 to 14 days after initiation of treatment. Nonresponders require a biopsy for definitive diagnosis and differentiation from malignant (e.g., CNS lymphoma) or other infectious (e.g., tuberculosis, bacterial) lesions.

2. **Cryptococcus meningitis**

This diagnosis should be considered in any AIDS patient with a headache. Because this is a systemic infection, the presence of serum cryptococcal antigen is a sensitive (95%) but not specific screening test for meningitis. The diagnosis can be easily made or excluded with CSF analysis for cryptococcal antigen or fungal culture. CSF WBC count may be normal or minimally elevated. All HIV patients should undergo brain imaging before LP to rule out a space-occupying mass lesion. Treatment depends on the severity of infection. *Mild cases* (normal neurologic exam, CSF cryptococcal antigen <1:1024) can be treated with **fluconazole 400 mg PO each day for 8 to 10 weeks.** *More severe cases* require **amphotericin B 0.7 to 1.0 mg/kg per day IV for 2 weeks or until the CSF is sterile** followed by **fluconazole 400 mg PO every day** to complete a treatment course of at least 10 weeks. **5-FC, 25 mg/kg PO every 6 hours for 2 weeks,** may be added, but this requires drug level monitoring (peak 70 to 80 mg/L, trough 30 to 40 mg/L) and is associated with bone marrow toxicity.

3. **Progressive multifocal leukoencephalopathy (PML)**

PML is a demyelinating disorder caused by JC virus and presents with subacute onset of focal neurologic deficits and dementia; the peripheral nervous system is spared. MRI typically shows striking white matter hyperintensities on T2-weighted images. CSF profile is often normal. PCR for JC virus in CSF is not a sensitive test but can help confirm the diagnosis. The most important treatment is HAART to reconstitute the immune system.

4. **CMV infection**

CMV can affect both the central and peripheral nervous system. CMV retinitis, which presents with slowly progressive, painless visual loss, is the most common neurologic complication. Other complications are rare and usually occur in very advanced AIDS (CD4 <50). *Ventriculoencephalitis* presents with rapidly progressive cognitive and behavioral changes; *myelitis* with acute onset of weakness, urinary dysfunction, and a sensory level; *polyradiculitis* with acute onset of back pain, asymmetric flaccid paresis of legs, paresthesia (often in a "saddle" distribution), and urinary dysfunction; and *mononeuritis multiplex* with asymmetric motor and sensory deficits conforming to a peripheral nerve distribution. CNS infection is accompanied by CSF pleocytosis (often in the 1000s and with polymorphonuclear predominance), elevated protein level, and low glucose level. CMV PCR is highly sensitive for both systemic (blood) and CNS (CSF) infection. MRI typically shows inflammation and enhancement of affected areas, including a distinctive pattern of ependymal enhancement. CMV infections involving the CNS can rapidly progress; suspected cases require immediate treatment with **ganciclovir 5 mg/kg IV every 12 hours,** although efficacy is variable. **Foscarnet 60 mg/kg IV every 8 hours for 14 days** can be used as a second-line agent.

5. **Primary CNS lymphoma (PCNSL)**

PCNSL lymphoma is caused by EBV and presents with subacute focal neurologic and cognitive deficits. Brain imaging shows one or more enhancing mass lesions, simulating toxoplasmosis abscesses. If not contraindicated, LP can help establish the diagnosis with the presence of amplifiable EBV by PCR. Thallium SPECT showing increased local uptake ("hot" spot) or positron emission tomography (PET) imaging revealing a hypermetabolic lesion can also help discriminate PCNSL from an abscess such as toxoplasmosis. In most patients, however, the diagnosis is established by biopsy after failure to respond to empirical treatment for toxoplasmosis. Because malignancies and abscesses alike may respond favorably to steroids, **dexamethasone should be withheld** unless absolutely necessary until a definite diagnosis is ascertained. Whole-brain radiation, methotrexate, and HAART are the mainstays of treatment. Prognosis is variable from months to years, often depending on the patient's response to HAART.

6. **Herpes zoster (shingles)**

Herpes zoster radiculitis/ganglionitis, caused by the reactivation of VZV, is a common HIV-related complication. Multiple dermatomes are often involved. In contrast to other infections, zoster may occur when the CD4 count is well above 200. VZV also causes a CNS vasculopathy, presenting with strokelike syndromes or myelopathy and often heralded by a zoster eruption Uncomplicated zoster can be treated with **acyclovir (800 mg PO five times daily)** or **valacyclovir (1000 mg PO three times daily)** along with analgesics. If CNS vasculopathy is suspected or multiple dermatomes are affected, then further workup with lumbar puncture and MRI is warranted, and **IV treatment (acyclovir 10 to 12.5 mg/kg every 8 hours)** should be given.

7. **Syphilis**

The course of syphilis is often accelerated in HIV-infected patients, and the early symptomatic forms of secondary syphilis (meningitis and meningovasculitis) predominate. Symptoms may occur during any stage of HIV infection. There is a higher rate of both false-positive and false-negative treponemal and nontreponemal tests in HIV patients. Treatment may require a more prolonged course of **penicillin G** (>10 days) than in immunocompetent patients.

8. **HIV (aseptic) meningitis**

HIV frequently causes a self-limited meningitis, rarely meningoencephalitis, during primary viremia. CSF may show a mild pleocytosis, and HIV is readily amplifiable with PCR. Only symptomatic treatment is necessary.

Nonopportunistic Nervous System Complications of AIDS

1. **Distal sensory polyneuropathy (DSP)**

DSP is the most common HIV-related neurologic complication and is caused by immune-mediated pathways or antiretroviral toxicity (ddI, ddC, and d4T). Symmetric, painful paresthesias, sensory loss, allodynia in a stocking and glove distribution, and loss of ankle jerks are the clinical features. Antiretroviral (ARV) toxicity tends to have a more abrupt onset, occurring shortly after initiation or dose escalation. Treatment of the neuropathic pain is symptomatic (see Chapter 17); the mainstay of treatment is improved virologic control with HAART. ARV-mediated DSP usually improves with cessation of the offending agent.

2. **HIV-associated dementia**

HIV invades the CNS and infects non-neuronal cells shortly after primary viremia. Years later, in the setting of immune failure (CD4 <200) and dysregulation, a chronic encephalitis ensues, manifesting with insidious onset of cognitive impairment (executive function), motor slowing, and behavioral changes (depression, apathy) resembling a subcortical dementia. The diagnosis is clinical. MRI typically shows central atrophy and leukopathy, and the CSF may show a mild pleocytosis. Virologic control with HAART can arrest and in some cases reverse the dementing process (see Chapter 27).

3. **HIV-associated myelopathy**

This uncommon disorder occurs in the advanced stages of HIV (CD4 <200). It is characterized by an insidious onset of spastic paraparesis, sensory ataxia (posterior column dysfunction), and bowel, bladder, and erectile dysfunction. The syndrome resembles that seen with B_{12} deficiency. Infections (e.g., HTLV-1 CMV, HSV, TB, toxoplasma, bacterial abscess) and malignancies should be considered in the differential diagnosis. MRI of the spine may show atrophy and abnormal signal in the posterior columns but is usually normal. Somatosensory-evoked potentials are typically prolonged. Virologic control with HAART and symptomatic management is the only treatment available.

5. **HIV-associated myopathy**

Despite its myriad causes (infectious agents, immune-mediated processes, or AZT toxicity), HIV-related myopathy is rare. Subacute onset of proximal muscle weakness, CK elevation, and myalgias characterize most cases. Diagnosis but not etiology can be confirmed by EMG. Treatment depends on the cause.

6. **HIV-associated neuromuscular weakness syndrome**

A severe sensorimotor neuropathy can develop in the setting of nucleoside reverse transcriptase use, particularly d4T. The syndrome is characterized by rapidly progressive weakness, simulating a Guillain-Barré syndrome, and constitutional symptoms (fever, general malaise, nausea, headache). Serum lactate levels are almost always elevated. CSF may show nonspecific abnormalities but is indicated to rule out other infectious causes (e.g., CMV). Electrophysiology studies typically show both axonal and demyelinating pathology, and muscle biopsy may show a myopathy suggestive of mitochondrial disease. Treatment consists of withdrawal of all nucleoside antiretrovirals and supportive care.

7. **Acute demyelinating polyneuropathy (AIDP)**

This complication is clinically indistinguishable from Guillain-Barré syndrome (see Chapter 15) and occurs shortly after HIV seroconversion. CSF is characterized by a lymphocytic pleocytosis, in contrast to the acellular CSF seen with seronegatives with AIPD, and an elevated protein level. CMV polyradiculitis should be ruled out with PCR. Treatment consists of **intravenous immunoglobulin (0.4 mg/kg every day for 5 days)** or **plasmapheresis** and supportive care in a monitored setting.

Neuro-Oncology

Most brain tumors are diagnosed when CT or MRI shows an enhancing intracranial mass lesion in a patient with new progressive neurologic symptoms that have developed over weeks to months. Many brain tumors are known to arise in particular locations within the CNS, and the differential diagnosis of a suspected brain tumor is greatly influenced by considering age and location. Figure 22–1 lists the most common primary CNS neoplasms in adults by location. Except in patients with known systemic cancer and presumed metastases, tissue biopsy is mandatory for establishing the diagnosis.

Dexamethasone, 4 to 10 mg IV or PO every 6 hours, is a potent glucocorticoid that can dramatically reduce vasogenic peritumoral edema associated with CNS neoplasms. It is indicated in all patients who are symptomatic from mass effect related to a brain tumor, but it should be withheld prior to biopsy if possible if primary CNS lymphoma is a consideration because of its tendency to produce nondiagnostic results. Apart from dexamethasone, which is a mainstay of treatment for CNS neoplasms, diagnostic and management considerations for specific tumors are provided here.

GLIOMAS

Gliomas are the most common type of primary brain tumor, secondary in incidence only to metastases. In the United States approximately 13,000 new gliomas are diagnosed each year, and their incidence seems to be on the rise. These tumors arise from glial cells and are classified according to their oncogenic precursors as astrocytoma, oligodendroglioma, and ependymoma.

Astrocytoma

Astrocytomas are the most common type of glioma (approximately 80% of all gliomas). They are highly infiltrative tumors; in their early stages, astrocytomas can infiltrate between neurons without affecting their function. They are heterogeneous, with different areas of the tumor harboring cells of different histologic and malignant characteristics. Astrocytoma cells also have the potential to mutate, becoming more malignant as time passes.

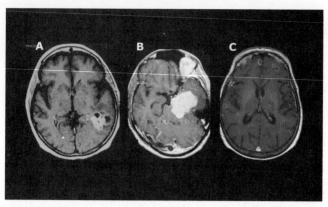

Figure 22–1 MR images of brain tumors. *A*, Gadolinium-enhanced T1 image of a left posterior temporal glioblastoma multiforme with heterogenous enhancement. *B*, Densely enhancing left skull base meningioma, extending into the left temporal lobe, with significant mass effect on the left pons. *C*, Multiple small ring-enhancing metastases with characteristic location at the gray-white junction in a woman with small cell lung cancer.

Glioblastoma Multiforme

Glioblastoma multiforme tumors (GBMs) (grade IV astrocytoma) are the most malignant and common form of astrocytoma. They are rapidly growing and infiltrative, with cells reaching several centimeters beyond the gross margins of the tumor.

Epidemiology. GBMs represent approximately 50% of all gliomas. The peak incidence of GBM is between ages 50 and 60, and the incidence is slightly higher in men than women.

Pathology. The main histologic features of GBM are hypercellularity, nuclear atypia with multiple mitotic figures, endothelial proliferation, and necrosis. This development leads to a pattern of necrotic tissue surrounded by ribbons of hypercellularity, a phenomenon termed "pseudopalisading."

Presentation. Patients present most often with headache (80%), mental status changes (50%), and focal motor deficits (40%). Seizures are less common, occurring at presentation in fewer than 30% of patients.

Diagnosis. The imaging test of choice is gadolinium-enhanced MRI, which typically reveals a mass of irregularly enhancing tissue surrounding a nonenhancing necrotic center (Fig. 22–2). This appearance has been described as a "ring-enhancing lesion." GBMs can also be seen to grow along white matter tracts, such as the corpus

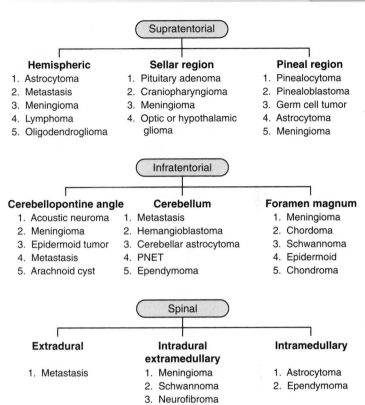

Figure 22–2 Radiographic differential diagnosis of solitary CNS neoplasms in the adult patient, by location. PNET, primitive neuroectodermal tumor.

callosum, giving rise to the pathognomonic butterfly glioma. The tumor mass is poorly demarcated and is surrounded by variable amounts of cerebral edema that shows as areas of hypointensity on T1-weighted and hyperintensity on T2-weighted or flare images.

Treatment. *Surgical resection* is the most effective means to achieve substantial tumor load reduction (debulking) and should be performed whenever feasible. Extent of resection has been shown to positively correlate with survival. Biopsy or subtotal resection is reserved for cases in which the tumor is inaccessible or in which more complete removal is deemed likely to result in severe neurologic deficit. *External beam radiation* directed with wide margins is effective in temporarily curbing tumor growth. A dose of up to 60 Gy (6000 rads) in 30 fractions is administered. *Chemotherapy* may be used in conjunction with radiation or in patients in whom tumor recurs after initial therapy. Adjuvant chemotherapy with **temozolide (75 mg/m² daily throughout radiation treatment, followed by 150 to 200 mg/m² daily orally for 5 days every 28 days for 6 cycles)** has been shown to improve mean survival from 12 to 14 months and increases the 2-year survival rate from 10% to 27%. Most of the benefit of this agent occurs in patients who express "silencing" of the methylguanine methyltransferase (MGMT) gene, which can be demonstrated by PCR analysis of tumor specimens obtained at surgery. The MGMT gene codes for molecules that repair the O6-methylation induced by temozolomide and other alkylating agents. Thus, absence of this gene confers a high degree of chemosensitivity and a vastly improved clinical response: 2-year survival with temozolomide is a remarkable 46% among MGMT-silent patients compared with those who possess this gene. Given the highly refractory nature of GBM to conventional chemotherapeutic agents such as the nitrosoureas (**BCNU, CCNU**) and a regimen called PCV (**procarbazine, CCNU, vincristine**), temozolide represents a therapeutic breakthrough for this disease and is currently considered the new standard of care.

Even after gross total resection, and even despite aggressive radiation and chemotherapy GBM is inevitably fatal. The tumor will invariably recur, and two thirds of the time it recurs within the margin of the previous resection. In patients with good neurologic performance status, reoperation should always be considered. Experimental treatments are in various stages of development and include brachytherapy (placement of radioactive seeds within the tumor), local delivery of chemotherapy by placing BCNU-impregnated (Gliadel) wafers into the resection cavity at the time of surgery, gene therapy, therapy with immune modulators, and high-dose chemotherapy with bone marrow rescue.

Prognosis. The prognosis for this tumor is poor, with approximately one half of the patients dying within a year and historically only 10% or less surviving more than 2 years. Poor prognosis is associated with advanced age, poor performance status, and tumor location within eloquent brain, precluding aggressive surgical resection. With multimodality therapy the median survival improves incrementally (Box 22–1).

Anaplastic Astrocytoma

Anaplastic astrocytomas (grade III astrocytoma) are gliomas of intermediate malignancy between GBM and low-grade astrocytoma.

Epidemiology. Anaplastic astrocytoma accounts for approximately 30% of gliomas. The peak incidence is between ages 40 and 50.

Pathology. These are hypercellular tumors, with variable amounts of nuclear pleomorphism and mitoses. As in GBM, there may be

---

BOX 22–1 **Prognosis for GBM with Multiple Therapies**

Therapy	Survival Time
Corticosteroids alone	<3 months
Surgery	16-20 weeks
Surgery plus radiation	45-50 weeks
Surgery plus radiation plus chemotherapy	55-60 weeks

---

neovascular proliferation, but endothelial proliferation is rare, and necrosis is distinctly absent.

Presentation. The average duration of symptoms at the time of diagnosis is 15 months compared with 5 months for GBM. Seizures are the most common presentation, occurring in at least 50% of cases. Headache and focal neurologic deficit are also common.

Diagnosis. Gadolinium-enhanced MRI is the imaging test of choice. The tumor may or may not enhance with contrast material, and the borders of the tumor are generally poorly defined. Biopsy is required to make the diagnosis.

Treatment. Treatment strategy is identical to that for its more malignant counterpart, the GBM, including gross total resection, fractionated radiation therapy, and temozolomide.

Prognosis. Median survival time with multimodality treatment is approximately 2 years.

Low-Grade Astrocytoma

Low-grade astrocytomas (grades I to II astrocytoma) are slow-growing tumors. These cells often infiltrate areas of brain without destroying them or interfering with their normal function. Over time, these tumors have the potential to dedifferentiate into more malignant forms of glioma; approximately 85% of low-grade astrocytomas will eventually degenerate into a GBM. This change usually occurs within 8 to 10 years from the time of diagnosis.

Incidence. Low-grade astrocytomas constitute approximately 20% of all gliomas. They occur primarily in young adults.

Pathology. These tumors have mild hypercellularity but completely lack mitotic figures, nuclear atypia, endothelial proliferation, and necrosis. Astrocytoma cells may resemble reactive astrocytes. This benign histologic feature has caused these tumors on occasion to be confused with simple glial scars.

Presentation. The presentation is typically indolent and of long duration. The most common presentation is seizures (65%), which in many cases may be present years prior to the diagnosis. Headache occurs in nearly half of patients. Focal deficits are rare.

Diagnosis. MRI is the imaging test of choice. The tumor does not enhance with gadolinium. It appears as areas of hypointensity on T1-weighted images and hyperintensity on T2-weighted images. There is no surrounding edema, and despite the occasionally large size of these lesions, there is remarkably little mass effect. Biopsy is required for confirmation.

Treatment. Because of the lack of good prospective data, the treatment of low-grade astrocytomas is a topic of intense controversy. Some authorities advocate aggressive surgical resection and radiation, whereas others advise mere follow-up. Several retrospective studies suggest that aggressive treatment may ameliorate symptoms (particularly seizures) and lower the incidence of malignant transformation. Because as many as 75% of these tumors may include areas of perfectly functioning brain within them, surgery is an option only when the tumor is located within noneloquent areas of brain.

Prognosis. Median survival is 8 to 10 years. Older age, change in mental status, and focality on neurologic examination are poor prognostic factors.

Oligodendroglioma

These uncommon tumors arise from oligodendrocytes, the cells that form axonal myelin sheaths within the CNS.

Epidemiology. Oligodendrogliomas represent approximately 5% of all gliomas and occur with peak incidence from ages 40 to 50.

Pathology. The tumor cells have a characteristic "fried egg" appearance, with an area of clear cytoplasm surrounding the nucleus. They are frequently observed histologically to invade the cerebral cortex. Anaplastic features such as hypercellularity, nuclear pleomorphism, and abundant mitoses may or may not be present. Depending on the degree of histologic anaplasia, they can be classified as low-grade or anaplastic oligodendrogliomas, but their histologic appearance does not correlate well with the degree of biologic malignancy.

Presentation. Seizures are the most common presenting problem (~60%); headaches are also common (~20%). Because these tumors are highly infiltrative, they often cause subtle behavioral or cognitive problems that can be detected only with formal neuropsychologic testing. Focal neurologic deficits are uncommon even when the tumor has attained a large size.

Diagnosis. MRI reveals a tumor with indistinct margins and variable amounts of contrast enhancement. Calcification is present in nearly 75% of these tumors. Gene expression profiling using gene arrays on tissue obtained at surgery is now allowing the separation of oligo-dendrogliomas into specific subsets that vary according to histology, tumor grade, and prognosis. The best characterized of these variants is combined loss of the long arm of chromosome 1 (1p) and the short arm of chromosome 19, which is associated with an MRI appearance of indistinct tumor margins and mixed signal intensity on T2-weighted images, and very high sensitivity to chemotherapy.

Treatment. Low-grade nonenhancing oligodendrogliomas may simply be followed unless they are highly symptomatic or until there is evidence of clinical or radiographic progression of the tumor. Traditionally anaplastic oligodendrogliomas have been treated with surgical resection, followed by whole brain fractionated radiation. Oligodendrogliomas are fortunately often exquisitely sensitive to chemotherapy. The traditional chemotherapeutic regimen is combined **procarbazine, CCNU,** and **vincristine** (PCV). **Temozolomide** is a reasonable alternative because it appears to work with similar efficacy and is better tolerated. Chemotherapy can be started either at the time of diagnosis or at the time of first recurrence if a gross total resection is obtained surgically. With either regimen, approximately 55% of patients experience a clinical response with reduction in tumor burden, and 40% remain free of disease progression at 1 year.

Prognosis. As with all gliomas, this tumor tends to become increasingly malignant over time. Median survival is approximately 3 years. Variables that predict longer survival include lack of enhancement on MRI, presentation with seizures, and age under 40.

Ependymoma

These rare neoplasms arise from ependymal cells and can arise anywhere within the neuraxis.

Epidemiology. Ependymomas account for less than 5% of all gliomas. They are most common in children and young adults, with two peak ages of incidence at 5 and 25 years. They comprise approximately 3% of intracranial gliomas and approximately 60% of spinal cord gliomas.

Pathology. *Papillary ependymomas* are most common, with well-differentiated cuboidal cells that form rosettes (around a central blood vessel) or perivascular pseudorosettes. *Myxopapillary ependymomas* are more benign and occur exclusively in the sacral filum terminale. *Ependymoblastomas* are more malignant and tend to occur in children. *Drop metastases*, which result from seeding via the CSF, occur in approximately 10% of patients.

Presentation. Presentation depends on the location of origin and on the presence of drop metastases. In children, in whom the most common site of origin is the floor of the fourth ventricle, they tend to cause noncommunicating hydrocephalus, giving rise to increased intracranial pressure with headache (~80%), vomiting (~70%), or ataxia (~50%). Less commonly, they present with signs of brain stem dysfunction such as vertigo or cranial nerve deficits.

Diagnosis. MRI is the imaging test of choice. The tumor enhances irregularly with gadolinium, and some degree of calcification is present in more than half of cases. When the tumor arises in the fourth ventricle, it tends to grow to fill and dilate this structure, sometimes extruding itself into the subarachnoid space through the foramina of Luschka and Magendie. Spinal MRI and lumbar puncture for CSF cytologic examination are mandatory for the detection of drop metastases.

Treatment. Surgical resection is indicated to confirm the diagnosis and debulk the tumor. Surgery by itself may relieve hydrocephalus by removing the obstruction to CSF flow at the level of the fourth ventricle; in some cases ventriculoperitoneal shunting may also be considered. Ependymomas are very radiosensitive. **Focal irradiation (40 to 60 Gy)** should be directed postoperatively to the tumor bed. If drop metastases are detected, they are treated with low-dose radiation to the entire neuraxis, with boosts to the lesions themselves.

Prognosis. Even with complete gross total resection, approximately 80% of tumors will recur, most locally. The 5-year survival rate is approximately 40%, and the prognosis tends to be worse in children.

NONGLIAL BRAIN TUMORS

Primitive Neuroectodermal Tumor

This category encompasses several different tumors that seem to have common origin from embryonic remnants of neuroectodermal cells. They are highly malignant and have the propensity to disseminate through the CSF (drop metastases).

Epidemiology. Primitive neuroectodermal tumors (PNETs) occur almost exclusively in children and adolescents. PNETs comprise almost 25% of all brain tumors diagnosed in childhood.

Pathology. PNETs arise from primitive neuroectodermal cells. They are cellular tumors that often exhibit signs of frank malignancy such as nuclear pleomorphism and abundant mitotic figures. Individual cells are small and darkly staining and often show evidence of neuronal differentiation on immunocytochemistry. Subtypes of PNETs include:

Medulloblastoma
The most common malignant brain tumor in children (~20% of all pediatric brain tumors) is usually localized to the cerebellar vermis, where on MRI it appears as a bulky and uniformly

enhancing mass. Because of their tendency to grow, obstructing the fourth ventricle, they most frequently present with hydrocephalus and signs of raised intracranial pressure. Nearly one third of these tumors have given rise to detectable drop metastases by the time they are diagnosed.

Pineoblastoma

These tumors occur in the pineal region and are highly responsive to radiation and chemotherapy. They present with hydrocephalus and Parinaud's syndrome (impaired upward gaze, loss of accommodation, retraction nystagmus).

Neuroblastoma

Neuroblastomas may arise in the cerebral hemispheres or be intrathoracic (sympathetic ganglia), and sometimes they present with paraneoplastic opsoclonus.

Retinoblastoma

This tumor presents as an intraocular mass in infants. It is often bilateral, involving both eyes, and it is associated with an abnormality in the 13th chromosome.

Esthesioneuroblastoma

These tumors arise from the olfactory neuroepithelial tissue in the nasal passages and extend through the cribriform plate into the base of the skull and brain.

Presentation. Symptoms depend on tumor location. Extraneural metastases (to bone, lymph nodes, liver, and lung) occur more often with PNETs than any other CNS neoplasm.

Treatment. Complete *surgical resection* should be performed in all patients, as limited by the eloquence of surrounding brain structures. Most PNETs are responsive to *radiation* (36 Gy), but recurrence is common. Even if seeding of the CSF is not documented, many practitioners advocate prophylactic craniospinal irradiation. Because high-dose radiation can lead to disabling neurocognitive deficits in long-term survivors, newer approaches combining lower dose radiation (24 Gy) with early chemotherapy (vincristine, CCNU, cisplatin) are currently under investigation. *Chemotherapy* for highly advanced disease is rarely successful.

Prognosis. The overall prognosis is poor. Even with surgery, radiation, and chemotherapy, the average survival time is 2 years. Surgery and radiation are sometimes curative with highly localized tumors; patients surviving for a period of time equal to age at diagnosis plus 9 months can be considered cured.

Primary CNS Lymphoma

Epidemiology. Primary CNS lymphoma (PCNSL) accounts for 1% to 2% of all primary brain tumors, but the incidence is rising. Patients who are immunocompromised (e.g., patients with AIDS, organ transplant recipients) are at particularly high risk.

Pathology. PCNSLs are non-Hodgkin's lymphomas, usually of B cell origin, occurring in the absence of systemic lymphoma.

Presentation. There are four distinct clinical presentations of primary CNS lymphoma.

> *Solitary or multiple discrete tumors* are the most common form of presentation; ~50% are multifocal.
>
> *Diffuse infiltrative PCNSL* presents as a widespread infiltrative process throughout the brain, or as carcinomatous meningitis.
>
> *Ocular PCNSL* demonstrates retinal or vitreous infiltration that antedates or follows the development of CNS lesions in 20% of patients.
>
> *Spinal PCNSL* is an isolated intramedullary spinal cord lesion and is rare.

Diagnosis. MRI is the imaging test of choice, because PSNSL may appear isointense on CT. The tumor is often periventricular and usually enhances uniformly with gadolinium, although ring enhancement may occur with larger tumors. The diagnosis is established by biopsy. Because steroids have a strong tumoricidal effect and greatly increase the likelihood of a nondiagnostic biopsy, every attempt should be made to prevent treatment with dexamethasone prior to tissue diagnosis. *Spinal tap* should be performed unless significant mass effect is present; positive CSF cytologic findings may confirm the diagnosis and obviate the need for a biopsy. Spinal tap may also help in detecting CSF dissemination, which occurs in up to 35% of patients. *Slit-lamp examination* is required in all patients to detect ocular involvement. In patients with ocular symptoms, a vitreous biopsy should be performed. HIV testing should be obtained in every patient with documented PCNSL.

Treatment. The role of surgery is limited to tissue diagnosis, and a complete surgical resection should not be attempted. **Dexamethasone 10 mg four times a day** leads to dramatic tumor regression in 40% patients, but recurrence eventually occurs quickly. *Methotrexate-based multiagent chemotherapy* with or without *whole brain radiation* is the mainstay of treatment. A commonly used multimodality regimen consists of five cycles (10 weeks) of preirradiation intravenous methotrexate 2.5 g/m^2, intravenous vincristine 1.4 mg/m^2, oral procarbazine 100 $mg/m^2/day$ for 7 days, intraventricular methotrexate 12 mg, and a dexamethasone taper followed by WBRT 45 Gy and post-WBRT high-dose cytarabine 3 $g/m^2/day$ for two doses. In one study, this regimen was associated with a median regression-free survival of 2 years. Radiotherapy (up to 5000 cGy) may be whole-brain or craniospinal, depending on the extent of dissemination. Chemotherapy without radiation is increasingly being used in patients over the age of 60, who are at higher risk for radiation-induced neurologic toxicity. Intrathecal methotrexate via an Ommaya reservoir is sometimes used to treat patients with diffuse meningeal disease.

Prognosis. Mean survival time with treatment is 1 to 2 years in immunocompetent patients, and much less in immunosuppressed patients. Poor prognostic factors include age >60, poor functional status on diagnosis, elevated serum lactate dehydrogenase (LDH), high CSF protein, and tumor location within the deep regions of the brain (basal ganglia, brain stem, and/or cerebellum). Two-year survival is as high as 85% if none of these risk factors is present, and is only 15% if all are present. Neuraxis dissemination ultimately occurs in 60% and systemic lymphoma in 10% of patients who survive 1 year, suggesting that systemic chemotherapy should be used as a primary treatment for this disease.

Meningioma

Epidemiology. Meningiomas account for 20% of all intracranial tumors and, after gliomas, are the second most common type of brain tumor in adults. They are twice as common in females than in males; peak incidence is between ages 40 and 60.

Pathology. Meningiomas are usually histologically benign tumors that arise from arachnoid cap cells. They do not invade cerebral tissue, and they cause symptoms by compressing surrounding structures. The more benign histologic subtypes (meningothelial, fibroblastic, transitional, psammomatous) are indolent and slowly growing; because of this they can often attain a very large size before becoming symptomatic. The more malignant subtypes (sarcomatous, angioblastic, and hemangiopericytoma) grow more rapidly, tend to be invasive, and have a high tendency to recur even after gross total resection. Meningiomas are described as atypical when increased cellularity, >4 mitoses per 10 HPF, prominent nucleoli, small cell cytology, sheetlike growth, or necrosis are present, and anaplastic when focal or diffuse loss of normal meningothelial differentiation, resembling transformation into carcinoma, is present.

Presentation. The most frequent sites of meningioma in decreasing order are as follows:

> *Hemispheric (parasagittal or convexity)* tumors account for 50% of meningiomas; they usually present with headache, focal symptoms, and seizures.
>
> *Sphenoid wing* tumors present with headache, diplopia (especially when the cavernous sinus is involved), or visual loss. Proptosis may occur if significant hyperostosis of the bony orbit is present.
>
> *Olfactory groove* tumors classically present with dementia, or ipsilateral optic atrophy and contralateral papilledema (Foster-Kennedy syndrome).

Suprasellar tumors present with headache, bitemporal hemianopia, and less frequently, hypothalamic dysfunction.

Posterior fossa (clivus, foramen magnum, cerebellopontine angle) tumors
typically present with cranial nerve deficits (dysphagia, dysarthria, diplopia, tinnitus, vertigo). When large, they can lead to
symptoms of brain stem compression (ataxia, hemiparesis).

Diagnosis. MRI and CT reveal a homogeneous, sharply demarcated
tumor that enhances uniformly with contrast material and has a
broad-based dural attachment (see Fig. 22–2). Enhanced MRI may
show a classic enhancing "dural tail." CT or plain x-rays of the skull
may often show overlying areas of calvarial thickening and sclerosis
(hyperostosis), which may be helpful for differentiating meningiomas from other dura-based tumors.

Treatment. Tumors that are asymptomatic may simply be followed
with serial MRI, definitive treatment being withheld until symptoms
arise or the tumor is seen to enlarge. Definitive treatment for these
tumors is *surgical resection* of the tumor along with its dural attachment. When planning surgery it should be noted that these tumors
cause symptoms only because of their sheer bulk and that they grow
slowly. In many cases, as in the elderly and the infirm, it is not necessary to achieve a total removal, which would add to the surgical
morbidity. The rate of symptomatic recurrence directly correlates
with the degree of resection and can range from 9% to over 30% in
10 years.

Prognosis. Prolonged survival after surgical resection is the rule.
The rate of symptomatic resection directly correlates with the degree
of resection and can range from 9% to over 30% in 10 years.

Acoustic Neuroma

This tumor arises from the Schwann cells of the vestibular division
of the eighth cranial nerve; hence, a more appropriate name is "vestibular schwannoma." This benign tumor arises within the internal
acoustic canal and follows the path of least resistance, growing into
the cerebellopontine angle.

Epidemiology. These tumors account for 8% of all brain tumors
and occur mainly in middle-aged adults. Approximately 5% to 10%
of patients have neurofibromatosis type 2 and may harbor bilateral
acoustic neuromas, cranial or spinal meningiomas, schwannomas,
and gliomas.

Presentation. The most common presenting symptom is unilateral
tinnitus or hearing loss. As the tumor grows it compresses the adja-

cent cranial nerves, including the trigeminal (facial numbness, reduced corneal reflex), facial, and vestibular (vertigo) nerves. Ataxia from compression of the pons and cerebellum is a late sign.

Diagnosis. *Gadolinium-enhanced MRI* can reveal even small intracanalicular tumors. Both *audiography* and *brain stem auditory-evoked potentials* are important for quantifying the extent of damage to the cochlear nerve.

Treatment. *Surgical resection* is curative in most cases, particularly when the tumor is small (<2 cm in diameter). The main difficulty of surgery is preservation of the cochlear and facial nerves, something that becomes progressively difficult with increasing tumor size. Conventionally administered radiation is not effective in the treatment of these tumors, but *stereotactic radiosurgery* (i.e., gamma knife) shows promise in treating patients with small tumors, in which medical comorbidity precludes surgery.

Pituitary Adenoma

Epidemiology. Pituitary adenomas account for approximately 15% of all brain tumors and occur most frequently in young adults (twenties and thirties). They arise from the adenohypophysis within the sella turcica, where they frequently remain. When large they can extend into the suprasellar region through an incompetent diaphragma sella.

Pathology. These histologically benign tumors tend to be slow growing and compress rather than invade surrounding neural tissue. Anatomically, pituitary adenomas can be divided into microadenomas (<10 mm in diameter), macroadenomas (>10 mm in diameter but surrounded by dura), and invasive adenomas (infiltrating dura, bone, or brain). Histologically, cells may appear chromophobic (most common), acidophilic, or basophilic (least common). However, the light microscopic appearance correlates poorly with secretory activity. The majority of pituitary adenomas are nonsecretory or prolactinomas.

Presentation. Pituitary adenomas may present via one of three mechanisms:

Pituitary hormone hypersecretion: Functional or secretory pituitary adenomas may present as (1) Cushing's disease, from ACTH secretion, (2) amenorrhea/galactorrhea, from prolactin secretion, or (3) acromegalic gigantism, from growth hormone secretion. Production of sex hormones (LH, FSH) or TSH by a pituitary adenoma is extremely uncommon. Secreting tumors are most frequently diagnosed when quite small (<1 cm), as severe endocrinologic disturbances bring them to medical attention early.

Mass effect: Nonsecreting tumors rarely cause symptoms until they have attained a large size. They can then cause panhypo-

pituitarism by compressing the normal pituitary, visual disturbances (bitemporal hemianopia) by compressing the optic
apparatus, and headache.

Pituitary apoplexy: This syndrome results from acute infarction or
hemorrhage into a large, highly vascular tumor and can be
life-threatening. Patients present suddenly with headache,
visual loss, ophthalmoparesis, and mental status changes.
Emergency decompression may be required. This mode of presentation is particularly common during pregnancy.

Diagnosis. MRI is more sensitive than CT for detecting microadenomas and is the imaging study of choice. Gadolinium normally causes
enhancement of the pituitary gland, and tumor enhancement can
be variable. Nonetheless, secretory adenomas are sometimes too
small to be seen, even on MRI. In these cases the diagnosis is made
on careful endocrinologic evaluation, which should include the following: T3, T4, TSH, GH, prolactin, LH, FSH, fasting glucose, serum
cortisol, and estradiol (women) or testosterone (men) levels. Formal
ophthalmologic testing should be performed in all cases of
macroadenoma.

Treatment. With the exception of prolactinomas, surgery is generally indicated if signs of mass effect on the optic chiasm or cranial
nerves are present. *Trans-sphenoidal surgery* has the lowest morbidity
and mortality rates and results in visual improvement in approximately 75% of cases. Complication rates including cranial nerve and
chiasmal injury may be further reduced with the use of intraopera-
tive high-field MRI. Adrenal insufficiency or diabetes insipidus may
occur postoperatively but is usually temporary. It is often impossible
to completely remove a tumor with suprasellar extension, and in
these cases the tumor usually recurs. Focused *radiation* (40 to 60 Gy
over 4 to 6 weeks) reduces the postoperative recurrence rate and is
indicated if the tumor could not be completely removed.

Medical therapy with a dopamine agonist is the treatment of
choice for prolactinomas. **Bromocriptine 2.5 to 5 mg three times
a day,** a synthetic dopamine agonist that inhibits pituitary secretion
of prolactin, is the first line of treatment for prolactinomas regardless
of size. The ultralong-acting D2-receptor agonist **cabergoline, given
as 1.5 mg once a week,** appears to be as effective as bromocriptine
and is better tolerated, but is not currently FDA-approved for this
indication. In approximately 80% of cases, prolactinomas shrink
dramatically with dopamine agonist therapy, with resolution of
visual field and endocrine disturbances. If significant deficits persist,
surgery may then be performed with the added benefit of bromocriptine pretreatment.

Prognosis. The overall recurrence rate following surgical resection
of pituitary adenoma is approximately 12%, with most tumors

recurring after 4 years. In patients treated surgically for Cushing's disease, a positive dexamethasone suppression test during the first week after surgery (AM serum cortisol <3 µg/dl following 1 mg of dexamethasone PO given the night before) predicts a >90% chance of remaining disease-free after 5 years.

Craniopharyngioma

These tumors arise from squamous cell nests in the region of the pituitary stalk, and they present as suprasellar lesions.

Epidemiology. Craniopharyngiomas occur both in childhood and adulthood and represent 3% of all brain tumors. They are slightly more common in males.

Pathology. They are biologically and histologically benign but have the tendency to recur if incompletely resected.

Presentation. As with other suprasellar tumors, craniopharyngiomas cause symptoms by compressing the optic tracts, depressing hypothalamic or pituitary function, or increasing ICP.

Diagnosis. The tumor is often irregular and well demarcated from surrounding structures. Enhancement with contrast material is irregular, and many tumors are cystic. A common characteristic is of calcification (40% to 80%), which is best appreciated by CT.

Treatment. Most authorities advocate complete *surgical resection* whenever feasible. Subtotal resection carries a rate of recurrence of over 75% without adjuvant treatment. Postoperative *radiation* may substantially reduce or delay tumor recurrence.

Pineal Region Tumors

Epidemiology. Pinealomas represent 1% of intracranial tumors in adults and 3% to 8% of brain tumors in children. The average age at presentation is 13 years.

Pathology. Pinealomas may arise from germ cells or from pineal parenchymal cells.

> *Germ cell tumors:* The most common type of pineal tumor, these tumors are histologically indistinguishable from systemic germ cell tumors. There are two types: *germinomas* and *nongerminomatous germ cell tumors*. The latter secrete ß-HCG and/or α-fetoprotein (AFP) in serum, CSF, or both. Elevation of these markers is associated with a more aggressive behavior; serial measurements are useful both for diagnosis and for monitoring response to therapy.

> *Pineal parenchymal tumors:* These tumors arise from the pineal gland and surrounding tissue. *Pinealoblastomas* are more aggressive and tend to seed the CSF. *Pineocytomas* are less aggressive and tend to present during adolescence.

Presentation. Common symptoms include nausea and vomiting caused by aqueductal compression, and headaches and mental status changes related to obstructive hydrocephalus. Compression of the superior colliculus can result in Parinaud's syndrome (forced downgaze, impaired pupillary reactivity, and retractory nystagmus). Pseudoprecocious puberty caused by ß-HCG can be observed with germ cell tumors.

Diagnosis. Evaluation of patients with a pineal-region tumor should include (1) MRI of the head and entire spine with gadolinium, (2) serum and CSF germ cell markers (ß-HCG and AFP), (3) CSF cytologic examination, (4) evaluation of pituitary function if endocrine abnormalities are suspected, and (5) a visual field examination if suprasellar extension of tumor is noted on MRI.

Treatment. Initial management is directed at treating hydrocephalus and establishing a diagnosis. Further therapy is based on tumor pathology. *Surgery* is reserved for tumors with significant mass effect; small germinomas can often be successfully treated with chemotherapy and radiation alone. *Chemotherapy* with cisplatin is particularly useful for germinomas. *Radiation* (400 to 6000 cGy) may be delivered to the whole brain and to the spinal axis if drop metastases are present. Prophylactic spinal irradiation is controversial.

Prognosis. Because germinomas are very sensitive to chemotherapy and radiation, the long-term survival rate is higher than 90%. Nongerminomatous germ cell tumors have a 30% to 40% 5-year survival rate with radiation therapy alone. Pineal region tumors can recur more than 5 years after diagnosis; lifelong follow-up is mandatory. MRI scans should be obtained periodically, as well as tumor markers for patients with germ cell tumors, even if these were normal at diagnosis.

METASTATIC DISEASE

Brain metastases occur in up to 25% of patients with cancer, and the incidence seems to be increasing. Metastases represent the most common form of intracranial neoplasms. Systemic cancers can spread to the CNS either hematogenously or by direct invasion. Systemic cancer can also affect the nervous system through the remote effects of cancer, which are known as paraneoplastic syndromes (Table 22–1).

Brain Metastases

Epidemiology. Approximately 40% of patients have a *solitary metastasis*. Gastrointestinal (e.g., colon) and gynecologic (e.g., ovarian, endometrial, and cervical) malignancies are the most common sources of a solitary metastasis. *Multiple metastases* are encountered

TABLE 22–1 **Paraneoplastic Syndromes**

Clinical Syndrome	Associated Tumor(s)	Autoantibodies
Multifocal encephalomyelitis/ Sensory neuronopathy	Small cell lung carcinoma	Anti-Hu (ANNA-1), anti-CV2 (CRMP-5), anti-amphiphysin, ANNA-3
	Various carcinomas	Anti-Ma, anti-Hu, anti-CV2
Cerebellar degeneration	Breast, ovarian, others	Anti-Yo, anti-Ma, anti-Ri (ANNA-2)
	Lung, others	Anti-Hu, anti-CV2, PCA-2, ANNA-3, anti-Ri, anti-VGCC, anti-Zic4
	Hodgkin's lymphoma	Anti-Tr, anti-mGluR1
Limbic encephalitis	Small cell lung carcinoma	Anti-Hu, anti-CV2, PCA-2, ANNA-3, anti-amphiphysin, anti-VGKC, anti-Zic4
	Testicular, breast	Anti-Ma2
	Thymoma	Anti-VGKC, anti-CV2
Opsoclonus-myoclonus	Breast, ovarian	Anti-Ri, anti-Yo
	Small cell lung carcinoma	Anti-Hu, anti-amphiphysin
	Neuroblastoma	Anti-Hu
	Testicular, others	Anti-Ma2
Extrapyramidal syndrome	Small cell lung carcinoma	Anti-CV2, anti-Hu
Brain stem encephalitis	Lung carcinoma	Anti-Hu, anti-Ri, anti-Ma
	Breast	Anti-Ri
	Testicular, others	Anti-Ma2
Stiff person syndrome	Breast, small cell lung	Anti-amphiphysin
	Breast	Anti-GAD
Optic neuritis	Small cell lung	Anti-CV2
Retinal degeneration	Small cell lung, others	Anti-recoverin
	Melanoma	Anti-bipolar cell
Neuromyotonia	Thymoma	Anti-VGKC
Sensorimotor polyneuropathy	Small cell lung carcinoma, others	Anti-Hu, anti-CV2, ANNA-3
Autonomic insufficiency	Small cell lung carcinoma	Anti-Hu
Lambert-Eaton myasthenic syndrome	Small cell lung carcinoma	Anti-VGCC

Only the most frequent associations are listed. For each of the clinical syndromes a number of other tumor types may be associated. A varying proportion of patients with each of the syndromes is "antibody negative," or has one or more autoantibody specificities that do not fit the well-characterized patterns listed.

GAD, glutamic acid decarboxylase; mGlu, glutamate receptor; VGCC, voltage-gated calcium channel; VGKC, voltage-gated potassium channel. (Reproduced with permission from Dropcho EJ: Curr Op Neurol 2005;18:331-336.)

radiographically in approximately 60% of cases, particularly with lung and breast cancer and, especially with melanoma.

Pathology. Brain metastases are typically well demarcated and surrounded by extensive brain edema. Although they can occur anywhere in the brain, they are most commonly located at the *gray-white junction*. Because of their frequent occurrence near the cerebral surface, they are usually amenable to surgical resection.

Presentation. Symptoms usually develop over weeks to months. Headache (60%), motor weakness (60%), and mental status changes (35%) are the most common presenting complaints. *Seizures* occur in approximately 20% of patients and are most commonly seen with multiple lesions and with melanoma. An acute, strokelike presentation can occur with sudden hemorrhage into the tumor. This is most common in highly vascular metastases, such as melanoma or renal cell carcinoma.

Diagnosis. Contrast-enhanced CT and MRI with gadolinium can show metastases to the brain (see Fig. 22–2). Because of its higher sensitivity, however, MRI is the test of choice. These lesions show as uniform or ring-enhancing lesions surrounded by extensive peritumoral edema. A comprehensive evaluation should be performed to identify the primary neoplasm and the extent of spread whenever brain metastasis is suspected. This may include CT scans of the chest, abdomen, and pelvis, a rectal examination or colonoscopy, mammography, a radionuclide bone scan, or whole body PET.

Treatment. Left untreated, median survival among all patients presenting with one or more brain metastases is 1 to 2 months; with aggressive therapy, median survival increases to 6 to 12 months. Dexamethasone 4 to10 mg q6h should be given to stabilize patients who are acutely symptomatic from edema and mass effect. *Surgical resection followed by whole brain radiation therapy (WBRT)* is the gold standard for the treatment of solitary brain metastases. Surgery is generally contraindicated in patients with multiple metastases, unless one of the lesions is imminently life-threatening because of its size or location. Surgery may also be necessary to obtain tissue for histologic diagnosis in cases of metastases from an unknown primary tumor or in cases in which the primary disease has been well controlled for a long period of time. Surgical resection may also be required in cases in which the cellular type of the tumor is known to be relatively radioresistant (e.g., melanoma, renal cell carcinoma).

Radiation is recommended for patients with multiple metastases and for patients with solitary metastases in whom the location of the tumor or medical comorbidity precludes craniotomy. A total dose of approximately 30 Gy is typically divided in fractions over 10 to 14 days. Concomitant administration of corticosteroids lowers the cerebral toxicity of radiation. Radiation leads to neurologic improvement in approximately 60% of cases, with complete disappearance of the lesion in up to 25% and reduction in size in another 35% of patients. Sarcoma, melanoma, and renal cell carcinoma are resistant to fractionated radiotherapy, but this can be overcome with stereotactic radiosurgery.

Stereotaxic radiosurgery (e.g., linear accelerator, gamma knife) is a newer modality in the treatment of brain metastases. Current trials are comparing it to surgery for the treatment of solitary lesions. Its greatest advantage is that it is a noninvasive, ambulatory procedure that is able to eradicate or significantly shrink the lesion in more than 75% of cases. Its main disadvantages compared with surgery are that it may take 3 to 6 months for the lesion to respond and that its rate of success inversely correlates with the size of the lesion. It is generally not recommended for lesions >3 cm in greatest diameter. *Chemotherapy* has generally yielded disappointing results. It has been used with limited success for patients who have asymptomatic brain disease and who are responding favorably to systemic drugs.

Prognosis. Poor prognosis is indicated by poor baseline functional status, age >60, and metastases to sites other than the brain.

Leptomeningeal Metastases

Epidemiology. This condition is also known as *meningeal carcinomatosis* or *carcinomatous meningitis*. Leptomeningeal spread is most common with carcinoma from the breast or lung, non-Hodgkin's lymphoma, and malignant melanoma.

Pathology. Malignant cells reach the leptomeninges via hematogenous spread. Once established, tumor cells can be carried by the CSF throughout the neuraxis and can invade structures traversing the subarachnoid space, such as cranial nerves and nerve roots. Cells can also enter the Virchow-Robin perivascular spaces, causing venous thrombosis and widespread microinfarctions of the brain. Malignant cells can also obstruct CSF flow, causing hydrocephalus.

Presentation. Leptomeningeal metastases classically present with multiple cranial neuropathies or spinal radiculopathies. Numbness in the distribution of the mental nerve *(numb chin syndrome)* can be a hallmark. Headache is extremely common, and in advanced cases there can be changes in mental status and seizures.

Diagnosis. *Lumbar puncture* for analysis of the CSF is the mainstay of diagnosis. The CSF reveals pleocytosis (mostly lymphocytic), elevated protein, and low glucose. CSF cytologic examination reveals neoplastic cells and confirms the diagnosis. Because there is a high rate of false-negative cytologic findings, up to three spinal taps may be necessary to confirm the diagnosis. *MRI* may reveal leptomeningeal enhancement or nodules of disease throughout the leptomeninges, particularly along the surface of the spinal cord. When MRI is

unavailable or contraindicated, *myelography* may be helpful for identifying spinal deposits of tumor.

Treatment. The prognosis of patients with leptomeningeal metastasis is dismal, with median survival ranging from 3 to 6 months.
Chemotherapy is given intrathecally via lumbar puncture or preferably
via an Ommaya reservoir. The most commonly used agents are **methotrexate (12 mg biweekly)** and **ara-C (50 mg biweekly)**. These drugs
are given twice weekly at first, then less frequently as the CSF begins
to clear. *Craniospinal radiation* (40 Gy to brain, 30 Gy to spine) may
also be offered in an attempt to reduce the tumor burden but may
not be feasible in patients who have already received whole-brain
radiation or in patients receiving concurrent chemotherapy due to
the high risk of pancytopenia from bone marrow suppression.

Skull Metastases

Epidemiology. Tumors arising from the paranasal sinuses and
nasopharynx can involve the CNS. They can do so either by directly
invading and eroding through the skull base or by insinuating themselves through one of its multiple foramina. Hematogenous spread
of tumor to the skull is rare. The most common tumors to reach the
skull in this fashion are carcinomas of the breast and prostate.

Pathology. Skull base metastases can cause symptoms via one or
more of the following mechanisms: compression of cranial nerves,
invasion and erosion of the meninges, and increased brain compression with intracranial pressure when the tumor grows into a large
bulky mass.

Presentation. The most common symptoms are localized pain
from direct invasion of the dura mater and cranial nerve deficits.
Five typical clinical syndromes have been described. *Orbital syndrome*
presents with dull supraorbital pain, blurred vision, and diplopia.
Examination may reveal proptosis, ophthalmoplegia, and decreased
sensation along V1. *Parasellar syndrome* presents with frontal headache and ophthalmoparesis, but usually not proptosis. *Middle cranial
fossa syndrome* presents as numbness along the distribution of V2 and
V3 (numb chin syndrome). *Jugular foramen syndrome* is caused by
tumor compressing CN 9, CN 10, and CN 11 as they exit the skull
through the jugular foramen. This entity presents with unilateral
occipital or glossopharyngeal pain, followed by hoarseness and dysphagia. *Occipital condyle syndrome* presents with orbital pain that
worsens with neck flexion. On examination, patients tend to hold
the neck stiffly, have tenderness on palpation over the occiput, and
may have a CN 12 palsy.

Diagnosis. Optimal workup should include gadolinium-enhanced
MRI and noncontrast CT. The former can better visualize the extent
of the tumor, while the CT gives better detail of bony erosion/
invasion.

Treatment. Surgical resection followed by focal radiation is the preferred mode of treatment. Good patient selection, however, is key as some of the surgical procedures required involve major reconstructive work on the base of the skull and carry a significant morbidity rate. Patients who are not candidates for surgery should be treated with focal radiation.

Spinal Metastases

Pathology. Metastases may reach the vertebral spine and spinal cord via *Batson's vertebral venous plexus,* a preferred drainage site for pelvic, abdominal, and thoracic organs. Blood vessel concentration in the *vertebral body* exceeds other parts of the vertebra and makes it vulnerable. Epidural cord compression usually results from direct extension of tumor from the vertebral column or from paravertebral metastases that grow through the neural foramina.

Presentation. The thoracic spine is the most common site of involvement. Pain is the first symptom in 95% of patients with cord compression. Features that help differentiate metastatic from musculoskeletal back pain include thoracic level pain and aggravation by lying supine.

Diagnosis. *Radiographs* are abnormal in 85% of patients with cord compression; loss of the vertebral pedicles is the first sign. *Noncontrast MRI* is preferred for detecting epidural tumor. Twenty-five percent of patients with focal signs show *multiple sites* of compression, so MRI should include the entire spine.

Treatment. The goals of treatment are preservation of neurologic function and alleviation of pain. *Radiation* usually includes two vertebral bodies above and two below the lesion. *Surgery* is considered for cord compression, neurologic deterioration despite radiotherapy and steroids, spinal instability, and radioresistant tumors. Prognosis depends on the patient's condition at the time of treatment; up to 80% of ambulatory patients remain ambulatory, whereas only 10% of those with paralysis will walk again.

NEUROLOGIC COMPLICATIONS OF CANCER TREATMENT

Radiation Toxicity

Delayed injury to the brain or spinal cord may occur weeks to years after radiation therapy. Radiation can also affect peripheral and cranial nerves.

1. **Acute toxicity (1 to 6 weeks after radiation)** may include headache, nausea, and vomiting; this type of toxicity occurs more frequently when large doses are given per fraction or elevated intracranial pressure is present. MRI shows localized

brain swelling without enhancement. Steroids may reduce symptoms. Otitis can follow radiation therapy to the posterior fossa.

2. **Early-delayed toxicity (3 weeks to several months)** presents as somnolence and headache; it is seen most commonly in children receiving prophylactic whole-brain radiation for leukemia. Spontaneous recovery is the rule. *Rhombencephalopathy* with ataxia, dysarthria, and nystagmus may follow radiation to the middle ear area or for glomus jugulare tumors. Radiation myelopathy often takes the form of Lhermitte's sign.

3. **Late-delayed toxicity (months to years)** can take several forms.
   * *Radiation necrosis* occurs in approximately 5% of patients given total doses above 5000 cGy with daily fraction sizes over 200 cGy. Median time for development is 14 months after treatment. Radiation necrosis may simulate the original tumor and can be difficult to differentiate from tumor recurrence on MRI. An enhancing mass lesion and diffuse white matter changes are the most common MRI abnormalities. Positron emission tomography may help distinguish tumor recurrence from radiation necrosis, because the latter is hypometabolic. Biopsy is often needed to establish the diagnosis. Steroids can lead to clinical stabilization, but when there is marked mass effect, surgical resection may be needed.
   * *Cognitive impairment* is common in long-term survivors. Children under 5 years old are particularly susceptible. Memory is typically most severely affected. A syndrome of ataxia, cognitive disturbances, and urinary incontinence, sometimes ameliorated by ventriculoperitoneal shunting, has been described in adults.
   * *Radiation myelopathy* develops within 3 years; the average latency period is 12 months. It is observed in 5% of patients who receive >4500 cGy at fractions of over 180 cGy. Symptoms include painless subacute numbness and paresthesias, a spastic gait disorder, and sphincter symptoms. MRI may be normal or may show cord swelling or atrophy. The diagnosis is made by exclusion. Steroids may improve symptoms.
   * *Radiation-induced vasculopathy* can affect both the intracranial and extracranial vessels. Most patients have had neck irradiation for head and neck cancer or for optic nerve or suprasellar tumors. Clinically, stroke occurs in the setting of occlusive large-artery disease.
   * *Endocrine dysfunction* can take several forms. Growth hormone deficiency is the most common; growth arrest occurs in children, whereas adults have a decrease in muscle mass and an increase in adipose tissue. Gonadotropin defi-

ciencies manifest in children as failure to enter puberty and amenorrhea; adults have infertility, sexual dysfunction, and decreased libido. Thyrotropin deficiency manifests as weight gain and lethargy. ACTH deficiency presents with lethargy and decreased stamina.

- *Radiation optic neuropathy* follows treatment to the orbit, sinuses, pituitary, or intracranial tumors. Painless visual loss occurs within 3 years of treatment. Approximately half of the patients improve. Steroids are ineffective. Measures to shield the optic nerve from the radiation portals may reduce the incidence of this complication.
- *Brachial plexopathy* resulting from radiation is described in Chapter 19.

4. **Secondary tumors** are an uncommon late complication of radiation therapy. *Peripheral nerve tumors* occur within the port of radiation in up to 9% of patients, especially those treated for breast cancer or lymphoma. Clinical presentation is an enlarging painful mass with progressive neurologic deficits. The mean interval is 16 years. *Meningiomas* may follow radiation for CNS tumors or for tinea capitis. The mean latency period is 37 years if low-dose irradiation is given, and 18 months for doses >2000 cGy. Compared with spontaneously arising meningiomas, radiation-induced meningiomas are more likely to recur and undergo malignant degeneration.

Cancer Chemotherapy Toxicity

Antitumor chemotherapy may be toxic to both the peripheral and central nervous systems. The incidence of neurotoxicity may depend on the dosage, route, and schedule of administration, the age of the patient, and whether additional chemotherapy or radiation was given.

Antineoplastic drugs can cause a wide variety of neurotoxic effects (Table 22–2). *Peripheral nervous system toxicity* is most common with vincristine and vinblastine. Cisplatin causes a sensory polyneuropathy. The taxanes paclitaxel (Taxol) and docetaxel (Taxotere) cause a sensorimotor neuropathy. *Autonomic neuropathy* predominantly affects the GI tract with abdominal pain and constipation. 5-Fluorouracil causes a rare (5%) but characteristic acute *cerebellar syndrome.* A delayed *leukoencephalopathy* is associated with IV high-dose or intrathecal methotrexate.

Bone Marrow Transplantation

Bone marrow transplantation (BMT) from an HLA-matched donor often results in *graft-versus-host disease* (GVHD). Neurologic disorders include polymyositis, myasthenia gravis, sensorimotor neuropathy, aseptic meningitis, and leukoencephalopathy. Remission of neurologic toxicity has been reported with successful treatment of GVHD. *Neurologic complications* in patients who undergo alloge-

TABLE 22–2 **Neurotoxicity of Antineoplastic Drugs**

Neurologic Disorder	Drugs
Peripheral neuropathy	Carboplatin, cisplatin, cytarabine, etoposide, fludarabine, oxaliplatin, procarbazine, suramin, taxol, taxotere, vinblastine, vinorelbine
Cranial neuropathy	Carmustine, cisplatin, 5-fluorouracil, ifosfamide, vinblastine, vincristine
Autonomic neuropathy	Cisplatin, procarbazine, taxol, vinblastine, vincristine, vinorelbine
Encephalopathy	L-Asparaginase, busulfan, carmustine, cisplatin, cytarabine, 5-fluorouracil, fludarabine, ifosfamide, methotrexate, procarbazine
Cerebellar syndrome	Cytarabine, 5-fluorouracil, procarbazine
Acute myelopathy	Cytarabine, methotrexate, thiotepa

neic or autologous bone marrow transplant are cerebral hemorrhage (4%), metabolic encephalopathy (3%), and CNS infections (2%). Hemorrhages are mostly subdural and correlate with platelet dysfunction. Post-BMT leukoencephalopathy and a rare acute Parkinsonian syndrome have also been described. Progressive multifocal leukoencephalopathy may occur in immunocompromised patients after either autologous or allogeneic bone marrow transplantation for chronic myelogenous leukemia.

Immunosuppressant drugs are used for BMT. *Cyclosporine* neurotoxicity may include tremor, paresthesias, lethargy, ataxia, and a reversible leukoencephalopathy that can lead to seizures and coma. White matter lesions are seen on CT and MRI. *FK-506* toxicity presents as tremors, headache, and paresthesias. *OKT3* toxicity presents as confusion, seizures, and lethargy.

Cerebrovascular Disease

Cerebrovascular disease includes a wide spectrum of disorders, all sharing an acquired or inherited pathology of the cerebral vasculature. Stroke syndromes range in scope from a minor hemisensory loss in a single limb to hemiplegia, cognitive changes, and coma. The onset of deficits usually occurs in seconds to minutes. The **physical examination** can give an impression of the size and a fair estimate of the location of the infarct and can thus guide the urgency of subsequent management steps. **Brain imaging** is necessary in almost all evaluations of stroke. MRI should identify all but the smallest lesions and is superior to CT for brain stem and small, deep infarcts. CT is the equal of MRI in detecting acute hemorrhage and is superior for assessing bony abnormalities. Whereas CT may miss an infarct within the first several hours of onset, MR DWI can show ischemia within minutes of onset. The brain can tolerate only a few hours of ischemia before becoming irreversibly infarcted. The window of opportunity for acute intervention therefore is narrow. This chapter focuses on the presentation of acute stroke, with attention to the pathophysiologic mechanisms that drive the management decisions discussed in Chapter 6.

CLASSIFICATION

Acute stroke comprises three broad categories: **subarachnoid hemorrhage (SAH)**, **ischemic stroke**, and **intracerebral hemorrhage (ICH)**. The clinical presentations may be similar, yet the pathophysiology and consequent management algorithms are distinct.

Subarachnoid Hemorrhage

Clinical Presentation

Sudden, severe ("thunderclap") headache is the classic presentation of SAH from a ruptured cerebral aneurysm. When asked, patients usually classify the headache as the worst they have ever had or rate it a 10 on a scale of 1 to 10. Stiff neck and photophobia are often present, requiring a consideration of acute bacterial meningitis in the differential diagnosis. Preceding minor headache may occur from a sentinel bleed as a preamble to a major hemorrhage. Trauma is a more common cause of hemorrhage in the subarachnoid space, but the clinical presentation is then usually obvious. The most common neurologic finding in SAH is altered mental status. If focal signs or symptoms appear, it is often because of the presence of a local, intracerebral clot or because of direct compression of the aneurysm on a cranial nerve (causing, for example, a CN 3 palsy).

Missing the diagnosis of SAH can be disastrous. Untreated SAH may be fatal in up to 50% of patients. A large percentage of the deaths may be an immediate consequence of the hemorrhage, but secondary vasospasm, rerupture of the aneurysm, and obstructive hydrocephalus can add significantly to the morbidity and mortality. The rate of rerupture is 4% within the first 24 hours and 1% to 2% per day for the first 2 weeks. Early diagnosis and surgical clipping or endovascular embolization of the aneurysm are therefore essential.

Diagnosis

1. **A CT or MRI should be obtained as soon as possible.**

   Both CT and MRI are good at detecting acute hemorrhage. CT hyperdensity in the sulci, major fissures, or around the brain stem is diagnostic. Particular attention should be paid to the basal cisterns. Subarachnoid blood pooling in the quadrigeminal plate cistern, for example, may appear only as a subtle hyperdensity in this space and may even appear isodense with brain if the blood is 5 to 7 days old. Figure 6-1 shows an example of SAH on CT. Other causes of SAH that may be detectable on CT or MRI include vascular malformation, venous thrombosis, and tumor.

2. **A negative CT or MRI scan does not rule out the diagnosis of SAH.**

   If there is clinical suspicion, and if CT or MRI is negative, a lumbar puncture should be performed. Cerebrospinal fluid will show greater than 1000 red blood cells (RBCs) per mm^3 that do not clear in later tubes. Pathognomonic for SAH is *xanthochromia*, a straw-colored appearance of the CSF supernatant after centrifugation. Lumbar puncture can also rule out a diagnosis of bacterial meningitis.

3. **Patients should be classified according to the SAH grading scale of Hunt and Hess** (Table 23–1).

   Grading SAH patients not only will help monitor the clinical course but also will allow more accurate determination of prognosis and will guide management decisions. SAH of Hunt and Hess grades 1 and 2 has a good prognosis. Patients with grades 3 and 4 have a worse prognosis, and grade 5 patients are moribund. Aggressive, early intervention can yield good results even in poor grade patients.

TABLE 23–1 **Hunt and Hess Grading Scale for Aneurysmal SAH**

Grade	Clinical Findings	Hospital Mortality (%)*	
		1968	*2002*
I	Asymptomatic or mild headache	11	7
II	Moderate to severe headache, or oculomotor palsy	26	2
III	Confused, drowsy, or mild focal signs	37	10
IV	Stupor (localizes to pain)	71	35
V	Coma (posturing or no motor response to pain)	100	65
TOTAL		**35**	**20**

*Data from 275 patients reported by Hunt and Hess in 1968, and 404 patients treated at Columbia University Medical Center between 2000 and 2002. Reproduced with permission from Mayer SA, Bernardini GL, Solomon RA, Brust JCM: Subarachnoid hemorrhage. In: Rowland LP [ed]: *Merritt's Textbook of Neurology*, 11th Ed. Baltimore: Lippincott Williams & Wilkins, 2005:328-338.

4. **Once a diagnosis of SAH is made, a four-vessel cerebral angiogram should be performed as soon as possible.**

MR or CT angiography is an option if emergency surgery is planned to evacuate a massive hematoma, but these tests have lower sensitivity than catheter angiography, particularly for small aneurysms. Thus, whether or not an MR or CT angiogram is positive, a conventional angiogram will still be necessary at some point to rule out a second unruptured aneurysm, which is present in 15% of cases. The most common sites for aneurysm formation are at vascular branching points around the circle of Willis (Fig. 23–1) (see Box 23–1 for management of unruptured aneurysms). Nonaneurysmal causes for SAH that may be detectable on angiogram include arteriovenous malformation (AVM), angiopathies such as vasculitis and fibromuscular dysplasia, vertebral artery dissection, and venous thrombosis.

5. **If both MRI and angiogram are negative, the SAH may have arisen from a venous rupture around the midbrain (perimesencephalic SAH).**

A coagulation profile and toxicology screen for cocaine should also be obtained if the diagnosis is still unclear. Cervical MRI may reveal a dural AVM, but this is rare. All patients with a negative initial angiogram require follow-up angiography within 2 weeks unless the patient is grade 1 or 2 and the initial CT shows a classic perimesencephalic pattern.

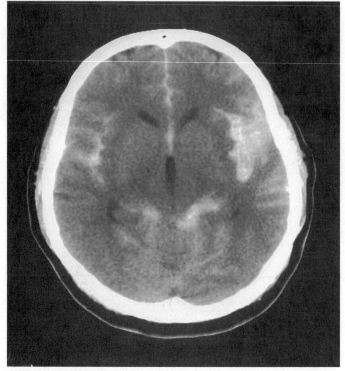

Figure 23–1 Subarachnoid hemorrhage on CT.

Management

For patients with aneurysm identified by angiography, management is two-pronged. First, early intervention by clipping or coiling the aneurysm (see below) will improve short- and long-term morbidity and mortality. Because the rerupture rate is as high as 20% in the first 2 weeks, treating a ruptured aneurysm acutely will remove a substantial secondary risk. Many centers have adopted a policy of early antifibrinolytic therapy (Table 23–2) with **epsilon aminoca-proic acid** (U.S.) or **tranexamic acid** (Europe) to prevent early rebleeding prior to aneurysm repair, or until 72 hours after onset. The second major aspect of management is the prevention of delayed ischemic deficits from vasospasm, which affects 20% to 30% of patients. Fluid and blood pressure management are crucial both preoperatively and postoperatively to maintain adequate cerebral blood flow in the presence of cerebral ischemia from vasospasm (see Table 23–2).

BOX 23–1 **Unruptured Intracranial Aneurysms**

Intracranial aneurysms are uncommon in children but occur with a frequency of 2% in adults, suggesting that approximately 2 to 3 million Americans have an aneurysm. Unruptured intracranial aneurysms (IUAs) may be discovered incidentally or detected in patients who present with another symptomatic aneurysm (e.g., SAH cranial nerve compression, headache, seizure). Because surgical or endovascular aneurysm repair carries a 2% to 5% risk of stroke or death, the management of these aneurysms (which in most cases remain asymptomatic throughout life) is controversial. The annual risk of rupture of an IUA is approximately 0.7%, but this risk is higher in patients with large aneurysms (>10 mm), prior SAH, cigarette use, a family history of cerebral aneurysm, or a midline aneurysm (anterior communicating or basilar apex). Generally, treatment is strongly recommended for all patients with symptomatic IUAs or prior SAH and in young patients (<50) with large aneurysms. In light of their low risk of bleeding, incidental small IUAs (<10 mm) should be managed conservatively and followed with serial imaging, although treatment should be considered in younger patients with a larger (6 to 9 mm) midline aneurysm, a positive family history, or evidence of aneurysm growth. In addition, all patients should be counseled to avoid cigarette smoking.

1. **Surgery**

   Surgical clipping of the aneurysm is generally done as early as possible after the hemorrhage, but it cannot be done without substantial risk if cerebral vasospasm is present. Vasospasm is rare in the first 3 days, and it peaks around day 7. If, within the first 5 days after hemorrhage, an angiogram shows the aneurysm clearly and shows no vasospasm, surgery should be done within the following 24 hours. Transcranial Doppler ultrasonography (TCD) is an important means of monitoring vasospasm both preoperatively and postoperatively, checking for increases in flow velocity in the major vessels around the circle of Willis. Identification of impaired cerebral vasoreactivity with TCD by a blunted vasodilatory response to inhaled CO_2 may be an early marker of impending symptomatic vasospasm.

2. **Endovascular embolization**

   An alternative to surgical clipping, packing the aneurysm with Guglielmi detachable coils (GDC), is an effective way to prevent rebleeding In a large trial of predominantly good-grade patients with small anterior circulation aneurysms, coil embolization was found to be associated with better 1-year outcomes compared with clipping, presumably because it is associated with fewer complications. In this procedure, the tiny coils are delivered to the aneurysm by superselective

TABLE 23-2 **Emergency Department and Intensive Care Unit Management Protocol for Acute SAH**

Blood pressure	• Control elevated blood pressure during the preoperative phase (systolic BP <160 mm Hg) with IV labetolol or nicardipine to prevent rebleeding
Antifibrinolytic therapy IV drip	• Epsilon aminocaproic acid (Aimcar) 4g IV upon diagnosis, then 1 g/hr until aneurysm repair, or a maximum of 72 hours after onset
IV hydration	• Preoperative: normal (0.9%) saline at 80-100 ml/hr • Postoperative: normal (0.9%) saline at 80-100 ml/hr, and 250 ml 5% albumin every 2 hours if the CVP is ≤5 mm Hg
Laboratory testing	• Periodically check complete blood count; transfuse for hematocrit <24% in stable patients, or <30% in patients with symptomatic vasospasm • Periodically check electrolytes to detect hyponatremia • Obtain serial ECGs and check admission cardiac troponin I (cTI) level to evaluate for cardiac injury; perform echocardiography in patients with abnormal ECG findings or cTI elevation
Seizure prophylaxis	• Fosphenytoin or phenytoin IV load (15-20 mg/kg); discontinue on postoperative day 2 unless patient has seized or is unstable
Vasospasm prophylaxis	• Nimodipine 60 mg PO every 4 hours for 21 days
Physiologic homeostasis	• Cooling blankets to maintain T ≤37.5° C • Insulin drip to maintain glucose ≤120 mg/dl
Ventricular drainage	• Begin trials of clamping external ventricular drain and monitoring ICP on day 3 after placement
Vasospasm diagnosis	• Transcranial Doppler sonography every 1 to 2 days until the eighth day after SAH • CT perfusion on day 4-8 after SAH if high risk
Therapy for symptomatic vasospasm	• Place patient in Trendelenberg (head down) position • Infuse 500 ml 5% albumin over 15 minutes • If the deficit persists, raise the systolic BP with phenylephrine or dopamine until the deficit resolves, up to a maximum of 180-220 mm Hg • 250 ml 5% albumin solution every 2 hours if the CVP is ≤8 mm Hg or the PADP is ≤14 mm Hg • If refractory, place pulmonary artery catheter and add dobutamine to maintain cardiac index ≥4.0 L/min/m² • Emergency angiogram for possible cerebral angioplasty unless the patient responds well to the above measures

Adapted with permission from Mayer SA, Bernardini GL, Solomon RA, Brust JCM: Subarachnoid hemorrhage. In: Rowland LP (ed): *Merritt's Textbook of Neurology*, 11th Ed. Baltimore: Lippincott Williams & Wilkins, 2005:328-338.

angiography catheterization. Thrombosis of the aneurysm is induced by the presence of the coils.

3. **Medical management**

    Patients with SAH are best managed in an intensive care unit. Abnormalities of fluid and sodium homeostasis after SAH favor free-water retention and sodium loss. The emphasis on fluid management is therefore on maintaining normal or increased intravascular volume using isotonic fluids and on avoiding all potential sources of free water. A central venous or pulmonary artery catheter may be helpful in assessing volume status, particularly when there is symptomatic vasospasm (see Table 23–2). **Nimodipine 60 mg PO 60 mg q4h** should be given for 21 days following SAH.

4. **Treatment of vasospasm**

    Angiographic vasospasm affects 70% of patients with SAH, and 20% to 30% will experience delayed focal or global neurologic deficits related to cerebral ischemia resulting from this process. The risk of developing symptomatic vasospasm can be predicted by the modified Fisher CT rating Scale (Table 23–3), with the highest risk occurring in patients with both thick cisternal clot and significant intraventricular hemorrhage. In addition to hypertensive hypervolemic therapy (see Table 23–2), which results in some degree of clinical improvement in approximately 70% of patients, angioplasty of intracranial vessels that are narrowed by vasospasm is becoming an important treatment modality in centers with appropriate interventional neuroradiologic expertise. Angioplasty is increasingly being performed as a first-line intervention for acute symptomatic vasospasm, rather than as salvage therapy for medically refractory cases; the best outcomes occur when angioplasty is performed within 2 hours of the onset of a new significant neurologic deficit.

Ischemic Stroke

Clinical Presentation and Diagnosis

Unlike SAH, both ischemic stroke and ICH typically present with focal signs. The syndrome produced by infarction depends on the location of the lesion. Pain of any kind is uncommon, although headache may occur with larger stroke or hematoma. One of the most difficult aspects of managing acute stroke patients is that focal symptoms, particularly minor ones, are often attributed by the patient to some non-neurologic cause and ignored. Visual changes may be interpreted as a need for new glasses. Sensory loss or weakness in an extremity may be brushed off as the result of lifting a heavy package or bumping into the door the day before. Transient symptoms (i.e., TIA) may portend stroke but may be identified as important only retrospectively (Box 23–2). Delay in treatment

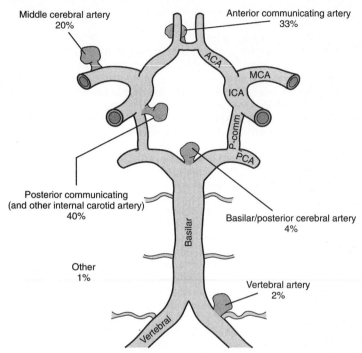

Figure 23–2 Most common sites for aneurysms. ACA, Anterior communicating artery; ICA, internal carotid artery; MCA, middle cerebral artery; PCA, posterior cerebral artery; P-comm, posterior communicating artery.

beyond the first several hours can result in a missed opportunity for acute intervention with a thrombolytic or neuroprotective agent. Despite an overlap in clinical syndromes among the various pathophysiologic etiologies, one should try to identify the stroke subtype. The management algorithm for secondary prevention depends on the stroke mechanism. Four major categories of stroke mechanism are discussed.

CARDIOEMBOLIC STROKE

Fifteen to 30% of strokes are embolic from a cardiac cause such as atrial fibrillation or valvular disease. The classic clinical presentation of cardioembolic stroke is of sudden deficit, maximal at onset. Syndromes more likely to be embolic include hemianopia without hemiparesis, pure Wernicke's aphasia, and top-of-the-basilar syndrome (ocular dysmotility, altered mental status, visual impairment). Hemiparesis and forced gaze deviation suggest a large hemispheric (eyes look away from the side of weakness) or critical

TABLE 23–3 **Modified Fisher CT Rating Scale for the Prediction of Symptomatic Vasospasm**

Grade	Criteria	Percentage of Patients	DCI	Frequency of Infarction
0	No SAH or IVH	5%	0%	0%
1	Minimal/thin SAH, no biventricular IVH	30%	12%	6%
2	Minimal/thin SAH, *with* biventricular IVH	5%	21%	14%
3	Thick SAH, no biventricular IVH	43%	19%	12%
4	Thick SAH, *with* biventricular IVH	17%	40%	28%
	All patients	100%	20%	12%

Thick SAH refers to subarachnoid clot >5 mm in width completely fills at least one cistern or fissure.

DCI, delayed cerebral ischemia (defined as symptomatic deterioration, cerebral infarction, or both resulting from vasospasm).

Data are based on a prospectively studied cohort of 276 patients at Columbia University Medical Center. From Claassen J, et al: Stroke 2001;32:2012-2020, with permission.

BOX 23–2 **Transient Ischemic Attacks**

Transient ischemic attacks (TIAs) are defined as transient symptoms of vascular etiology that do not result in infarction. Although the standard clinical definition includes symptoms lasting up to 24 hours, most TIAs last from minutes to a few hours. Deficits lasting longer than 1 to 2 hours may show a lesion on MRI, even if the symptoms resolve completely by 24 hours. The definition of TIA and stroke is further complicated by recent advances in brain imaging, which may identify a small infarction even when the stroke symptoms resolve within a day. **The clinical importance of TIA is highlighted by the high incidence of subsequent strokes.** Up to 50% of patients with TIA proceed to have an infarction within 5 years, if they are untreated, with 10% occurring in the first 90 days. *Age greater than 60 years, diabetes mellitus, symptoms lasting longer than 10 minutes,* and the *symptoms of weakness or speech impairment* all raise the likelihood of subsequent stroke. The most important etiology of TIA is high-grade carotid stenosis, producing hemodynamic failure or microemboli in the territory of the affected artery. Transient monocular blindness (TMB, amaurosis fugax) or a hemispheric syndrome such as unilateral weakness or sensory changes is a common presentation. Although TIAs may also arise from cardiac embolism or, rarely, from lacunar disease, the most important initial management step is to evaluate the internal carotid arteries, either with duplex Doppler ultrasonography or MR angiography. If stenosis greater than 70% is found, the patient should be considered for carotid endarterectomy or stenting. If no large-vessel stenosis is identified, the algorithm for investigating etiology of ischemic stroke should be followed. If no carotid stenosis or cardioembolic source is identified, **ASA 81 mg or 325 mg per day** is the first line of treatment.

brain stem (eyes look toward the side of weakness) lesion, particularly if these signs are accompanied by decreased level of consciousness. Behavioral abnormalities such as aphasia or hemineglect without a gaze preference or altered level of consciousness suggest smaller hemispheric lesions. CT and MRI scans that show a single cortical branch territory infarct are also consistent with an embolic source, because atheroma rarely extends into the surface vessels. Main stem branch occlusions are also often embolic, but local atherostenosis is also a possibility in such a setting. A potentially misleading scenario is one in which the initial CT scan shows a deep-lying lucency involving the internal capsule and basal ganglia approximately 2 to 3 cm in size, apparently sparing cortex, which can be misidentified as a large lacune. Often such instances are of embolic origin, involving several lenticulostriate branches of the middle cerebral artery after occlusion of the middle cerebral stem. Rapid collateralization from anterior or posterior cerebral branches or recanalization of the occlusion with distal migration of the embolus reperfuses the cortex, sparing it from infarction. A right-to-left shunt, usually a patent cardiac foramen ovale, can be inferred when transcranial Doppler ultrasonography shows microbubbles in the intracranial vessels after injection of 10 ml of agitated saline in the antecubital vein. Contrast transesophageal echocardiography can usually locate the defect in the cardiac atrial wall. If atrial fibrillation is suspected but is not apparent on routine ECG, Holter monitoring may be useful.

LARGE-VESSEL STENOSIS

In 15% of cases, severe large-vessel atherosclerosis is present and appears to be responsible for the stroke, particularly when there is severe extracranial internal carotid artery stenosis or occlusion and a "distal field" lesion is imaged on CT or MRI as an infarct high over the convexity, spreading caudally from the border zone between arterial territories. The most common clinical profile of this type of infarct is fractional weakness (the shoulder weaker than the hand, hip weaker than ankle). Male gender, hypertension, and diabetes mellitus appear significantly more frequently in this group than in patients with cardioembolic stroke. Intracranial atherosclerosis is more prevalent in non-Caucasian populations, whereas extracranial disease is more prevalent in Caucasians. Duplex Doppler ultrasonography readily delineates the severity of the internal carotid stenosis and shows high-velocity, turbulent flow. TCD ultrasonography often shows dampened pulsatility in the ipsilateral middle cerebral artery. Cerebral vasoreactivity as measured by a blunted TCD response to inhaled CO_2 is usually impaired. Focal stenoses in the intracranial ICA or other major intracranial vessels may also be documented by transcranial Doppler ultrasonography or MR angiography. Noninvasive imaging with gadolinium-enhanced MR angiography or computerized tomographic angiography can now approach the resolution of the more invasive traditional cut-film angiography.

In another 15% of all stroke patients, significant large-vessel atherosclerosis is detected when, radiographically, the infarct appears embolic. In such a setting, embolic fragments may have arisen from atherosclerotic lesions in the ICA. Distinguishing interarterial embolism from a possible cardioembolic etiology may be difficult. The former usually produces a smaller cortical infarct, however, and the latter is more often associated with a decreased level of consciousness and an abnormal initial CT scan.

Small, deep lesions in the subcortical white matter, the thalamus, the basal ganglia, or the pons accompanied by an appropriate clinical syndrome suggest lacunar disease, accounting for 15% to 20% of all strokes. Arteriolar wall lipohyalinosis with fibrinoid necrosis is the most common pathologic finding, although microatheroma, or even microemboli, may produce small infarcts. Although more than 70 syndromes have been reported with small, deep infarcts, the classic lacunar syndromes are *clumsy hand dysarthria, pure motor hemiparesis, ataxic hemiparesis, sensorimotor syndrome,* and *pure hemisensory loss.* All are typically characterized by an absence of cortical signs or symptoms. CT scanning is positive in only 50% of lacunar stroke patients, with MRI increasing the yield substantially, especially in the hyperacute period with DWI. Asymptomatic lacunes (silent strokes) occur in up to 20% of patients over age 65. Hypertension is the risk factor most associated with lacunar infarction.

Despite efforts to arrive at a diagnosis, the cause of infarction in up to 40% of cases remains undetermined after the standard workup is completed. This may result from an inability to perform appropriate laboratory studies because of the patient's advanced age or comorbidity or because of unwillingness on the part of the physician or patient. It may also result from improper timing of tests, such as an angiogram performed after an embolus has cleared or CT done before the infarction appears. In many cases, however, appropriate testing done at the proper time produces normal or ambiguous findings. Some of these cases may be explained by *hypercoagulable states* from protein C or protein S deficiency, abnormal fibrinogen levels, genetic mutations such as factor V Leiden or factor II prothrombin (G20210A), or by lupus anticoagulant or anticardiolipin antibodies. Other patients may have had emboli from *aortic arch atherosclerosis* that is >4 mm in thickness or ulcerated. Pain in the neck, side of face, teeth, jaw, or retro-orbital area may indicate *vertebral or carotid artery dissection,* even without a history of neck trauma. Migraine, meningitis, arteritis, or inherited metabolic abnormality may explain

BOX 23-3 **Cerebral Vasculitis**

Vasculitis is a rare cause of ischemic stroke. Infrequently appearing in the setting of a systemic collagen vascular disease such as polyarteritis nodosa, temporal arteritis, or Takayasu syndrome (aortic arch disease, pulseless disease), stroke may occasionally result from autoimmune disease restricted to the central nervous system. **Granulomatous angitis of the brain** is a rare condition that produces multiple small infarctions in the cortex and deep structures. The clinical presentation is usually one of fluctuating or stepwise progression of mental obtundation, with or without focal signs. CSF protein is elevated above 100 mg/dl, and a pleocytosis of up to 500 mononuclear cells per mm^3 is common. The typical arteriographic appearance is of multiple segmental areas of arterial narrowing, often giving a "beaded" look. Clinical and radiographic data can be compelling in any given patient, but it is recommended that a brain and leptomeningeal biopsy specimen be obtained before embarking on the necessarily aggressive treatment regimen. The diagnosis is secured if there are multinucleated giant cells infiltrating arterial walls. Because of the multifocal nature of the disease, however, biopsy results may be negative in up to 50% of cases. Progression of encephalopathy or new focal signs in combination with new areas of arterial narrowing on angiography may be sufficient to begin treatment if the biopsy yields negative results initially. The usual treatment regimen includes high-dose steroids and pulse doses of an immunosuppressive agent such as cyclophosphamide for more than a year. The prognosis is poor overall, but occasionally there is functional restoration approximating previous levels.

rare cases. For the purposes of management, cases that cannot be categorized under one of the first four etiologies should be called "cryptogenic stroke." Additional diagnostic studies may be needed to secure a final diagnosis. Because of its grave prognosis, vasculitis of the central nervous system should not be missed (Box 23-3).

Management

1. All patients with suspected stroke in which a deficit persists for more than 1 hour should undergo a CT or MRI head scan.
2. All patients with stroke symptoms of less than 3 hours duration should be considered for acute treatment with intravenous recombinant tissue plasminogen activator (rt-PA). If CT scan shows no hemorrhage, mass effect, or edema and if the patient meets inclusion and exclusion criteria guidelines, **IV rt-PA 0.9 mg/kg** should be given according to protocol (Box 23-4).
3. If the patient's stroke symptoms are of 3 to 6 hours duration, intra-arterial thrombolysis may be performed, provided that interventional radiologic expertise and experience are avail-

BOX 23–4 **American Heart Association Guidelines for Use of Intravenous rt-PA**

Inclusion Criteria

1. Symptoms are consistent with acute ischemic stroke.
2. Timing of onset is clear; start rt-PA within 3 hours of symptom onset.
3. CT is negative or shows only early signs of ischemic stroke (blurring of gray-white junction, minor hypodensity). If sulcal effacement, mass effect, or edema is present, rt-PA should not be given. CT should be read by an experienced neurologist, neurosurgeon, or neuroradiologist.
4. Appropriate facilities must be available to handle bleeding complications should they occur (e.g., neurologic intensive care unit or stroke unit).

Exclusion Criteria

1. Current use of oral anticoagulants, PT >15 seconds or INR >1.7
2. Use of IV heparin or IM low-molecular-weight heparin within 24 hours or prolonged partial thromboplastin time
3. Platelet count <100,000/mm^3
4. Large stroke or serious head injury within the past 3 months
5. Major surgery within the past 14 days
6. Pretreatment SBP >185 mm Hg or DBP >110 mm Hg
7. Blood glucose <50 mg/dl or >400 mg/dl
8. Gastrointestinal or urinary bleeding within the preceding 21 days
9. Recent myocardial infarction
10. Neurologic signs that are rapidly improving
11. Isolated, minor neurologic deficits (e.g., pure sensory loss, isolated dysarthria, isolated ataxia)
12. Seizure at onset of stroke

Administration of rt-PA

1. Intravenous rt-PA (0.9 mg/kg, maximum 90 mg) with 10% of the dose given as a bolus followed by an infusion lasting 60 minutes
2. No anticoagulants or antiplatelet agents to be given within the first 24 hours after administration of rt-PA
3. Blood pressure elevation to be treated by IV labetalol 10 to 150 mg (for SBP = 180 to 230 mm Hg or DBP = 105 to 120 mm Hg) or IV nitroprusside 0.5 to 10 µg/kg per minute (for SBP >230 mm Hg or DBP >120 mm Hg)

able. Newer MRI algorithms can identify an area of hypoperfusion significantly larger than the area of infarction.

4. Patients whose symptoms are less than 8 hours old or who have a contraindication to thrombolytic therapy may be eligible for mechanical clot extraction, performed by a neuro-

interventional radiologist with special training with this technique (see Figure 23–3).

5. If the clinical picture and CT or MRI appearances are consistent with a small or moderate-sized ischemic stroke, and the suspected etiology is cardioembolic or large-vessel stenosis, intravenous **heparin may be administered** until the stroke subtype is confirmed, maintaining a PTT of 1.5 to 2 times control. IV heparin has no proven efficacy in preventing early recurrent stroke or stroke progression but may be used as a bridge to long-term anticoagulation. Anticoagulation may be given if there is hemorrhagic infarction on brain imaging, *but only if the infarction is minor.*

6. If the stroke is large and disabling, there is greater risk of *hemorrhagic transformation;* brain imaging should be repeated 48 to 72 hours after stroke onset, and anticoagulation should be started only if hemorrhagic conversion has not occurred. If the clinical and imaging diagnosis is of intracranial hemorrhage, anticoagulants and antiplatelet agents should not be given.

7. *Investigation of stroke etiology* should focus first on cardioembolic sources and large-vessel atherothrombosis. Transthoracic echocardiography, carotid duplex Doppler ultrasonography, and transcranial Doppler ultrasonography should be performed in nearly all cases. MR angiography and transesophageal echocardiography may deliver a diagnosis when the aforementioned studies are inconclusive.

8. Stroke patients with recent myocardial infarction, atrial fibrillation, valvular disease, or intracardiac thrombus should be given **oral anticoagulants such as warfarin** for at least 1 year. Patients with a patent foramen ovale or severe atherosclerosis of the aortic arch may be anticoagulated as well, although the efficacy of warfarin for these two conditions has not been proven. The INR of the PT should be targeted at 2.0 to 3.0. If there is atrial fibrillation, warfarin should be continued indefinitely, provided that reliable monitoring is available. Anticoagulation with **enoxaparin (Lovenox) 1mg/ kg SC bid** is an alternative to oral anticoagulation for those unable to swallow or in pregnant women to avoid teratogenicity of warfarin.

9. If the stroke is small, the heart is normal, and a duplex Doppler sonogram shows significant carotid stenosis (greater than 70%), a revascularization procedure should be considered. **Intravenous heparin, ASA 325 mg PO qd, or clopidogrel 75 mg PO qd** should be continued until the exact degree of stenosis has been determined by MR angiography or CT angiography. Digital subtraction or cut-film angiography may be used in instances in which MR or CT angiography is unavailable or noninvasive angiography results are

equivocal. Prophylactic revascularization by *endarterectomy* (CEA) or *carotid artery stent angioplasty* (CAS) for patients with greater than 70% stenosis should be undertaken as soon as possible. CAS is indicated for cases of restenosis or radiation-induced stenosis where surgery is more risky. Efficacy and procedural risk are otherwise similar for CEA and CAS, although comparisons of long-term durability and subtle differences in risk between the procedures are yet to be established. For stenting, interventionalists generally prefer patients to be on **clopidogrel 75 mg PO qd** for 3 days prior to the procedure, although a single loading dose of **clopidogrel 300 mg PO** may be used the day before the procedure. For patients with 50% to 69% stenosis, the benefit of surgery is lower compared with medical treatment, but may still be considered. Doppler monitoring should be undertaken at intervals of 3 to 12 months to document those patients whose stenosis increases to greater than 70%. Patients in whom asymptomatic carotid stenosis greater than 60% is identified should be considered for endarterectomy or stenting as well, provided the operation is done at a center at which the perioperative morbidity and mortality is less than 3%. The benefit from endarterectomy compared with medical therapy is a 6% versus an 11% chance of stroke in 5 years for the asymptomatic carotid stenosis group, and a 9% versus 26% chance of stroke in 2 years for the >70% symptomatic group.

10. If no cardioembolic source or operable carotid stenosis is identified, and if the patient is not considered at risk for hemorrhage, antiplatelet treatment with **aspirin 81 mg to 325 mg daily** should be given as chronic outpatient therapy. **Aspirin 25 mg/extended-release dipyridamole 200 mg twice a day** or **clopidogrel 75 mg PO once a day** may also be used, particularly if aspirin therapy has failed. Clopidogrel is often preferred when there is coronary artery disease or peripheral vascular disease. Some patients develop headache from ASA/extended-release dipyridamole, although its efficacy appears to be overall better than ASA.

Intracerebral Hemorrhage

Clinical Presentation

Primary ICH is defined as nontraumatic bleeding into the parenchyma of the brain. ICH accounts for approximately 15% of all strokes. Except for a higher frequency of headache and severe hypertension, the presentation of ICH may be identical to that for ischemic stroke occurring in the same location. Coma occurs with greater frequency, particularly when the hemorrhage is of larger volume or involves the brain stem. Patients with hematoma volumes less than

---

BOX 23–5 **Cerebral Amyloid Angiopathy**

Cerebral amyloid angiopathy (CAA) results from the pathologic deposition of an amorphous eosinophilic amyloid material (that stains with Congo red) in small blood vessels of the cerebral neocortex and adjacent leptomeninges. CAA causes lobar hemorrhage in elderly adults with a mean age of 72. Recurrent hemorrhages are common. The amyloid protein precursor is a gene product from chromosome 21, stimulating interest about the role of amyloid in Down syndrome and Alzheimer's disease. The disease may occur as a familial trait or sporadically. More than 40% of patients with CAA have some degree of dementia. Hemorrhages are most common in the frontal and parietal lobes. MRI, particularly gradient echo sequences, will usually demonstrate several old hemorrhages that may have been asymptomatic. No definitive treatment is currently available.

---

20 ml have an excellent prognosis, whereas those with volumes greater than 80 ml are usually fatal. Chronic hypertension is the most common cause of ICH and is presumed to result from rupture of the smallest penetrating arteries that have undergone degenerative changes such as lipohyalinosis, fibrinoid necrosis, and microaneurysm formation. Acute hypertension is present in 90% of the cases. Hypertension from sympathomimetics such as pseudoephedrine, amphetamines, or cocaine may also be seen. Hypertensive bleeds occur most commonly in the territory of small penetrating arteries, in the basal ganglia or thalamus (70%), in the brain stem (13%), or in the cerebellum (9%). In the 10% of cerebral hemorrhages that occur in the hemispheres, other causes must be suspected. The differential diagnosis of lobar ICH includes cerebral amyloid angiopathy (Box 23–5), primary or metastatic tumors (melanoma, choriocarcinoma, bronchiogenic carcinoma, or renal cell carcinoma), coagulopathies (disseminated intravascular coagulation, hemophilia, leukemia, thrombocytopenia, overdose of anticoagulant therapy), and vascular malformations.

Diagnosis

The cornerstone for diagnosis of ICH is neuroimaging. Both CT and MRI can detect fresh parenchymal blood in the hyperacute stage. Because the clinical presentation may be indistinguishable from ischemic stroke but the treatment strategies are quite different, any patient presenting with suspected ICH must undergo CT or MRI as soon as possible. In a patient under 60 years of age with a lobar hemorrhage of unclear etiology, an MRI with and without contrast material may disclose tumor or the abnormal vessels of a vascular malformation. For an arteriovenous malformation, cut-film angiography would then be necessary to make a definitive diagnosis and plan for treatment.

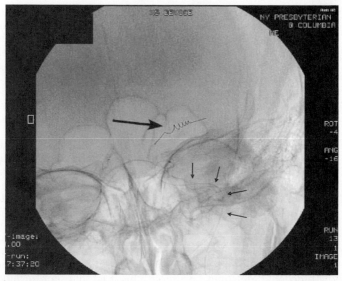

Figure 23–3 X-ray of head showing a catheter *(small arrows)* threaded into a middle cerebral artery with a clot extraction device *(large arrow)* imbedded in the thrombus.

Distinguishing between ICH and ischemic infarction with hemorrhagic conversion may present a challenge. ICH tends to have a denser, homogeneous appearance, whereas the hemorrhagic infarction is usually spotted or mottled. The location of ICH is more often subcortical, often in the deep gray matter, whereas hemorrhagic infarction, most often occurring in the setting of embolic arterial occlusion, usually involves the cortex and follows a branch artery territory. Intraventricular blood may be seen with ICH, particularly if the hemorrhage is in the thalamus or basal ganglia. Ventricular hemorrhage from embolic infarction does not occur. Significant mass effect may be present from the outset in ICH, whereas the mass effect from hemorrhagic infarction results from secondary edema formation, which peaks after 48 hours. The appearance of the hematoma on MRI follows a characteristic course from the acute to the subacute to the chronic stage (see Chapter 3). Coagulation studies (PT/PTT, platelet count) should be obtained at the time of diagnosis to rule out coagulopathy as a cause for the hemorrhage. Liver function tests should be obtained.

Management

1. **Correction of a coagulopathy** with administration of **fresh frozen plasma** may be necessary to terminate active bleeding in a patient with a coagulation disorder.

2. **Active control of blood pressure** to systolic levels of 160 to 180 mm Hg should be attempted with oral or intravenous antihypertensives. Unlike in ischemic infarction in which reduction of blood pressure may result in decreased cerebral blood flow and consequent extension of infarction, reducing blood pressure in ICH may help prevent recurrent bleeding.

3. **Control of increased intracranial pressure** with pharmacologic measures and hyperventilation may allow the patient to pass through a critical phase until the hematoma begins to resolve (see Chapter 12).

4. **Placement of an intraventricular drain** may be necessary because intraventricular blood or direct compression of the cerebral aqueduct by a brain stem hematoma may cause obstructive hydrocephalus. If there is any clinical deterioration, a CT or MRI scan should be obtained to distinguish between hydrocephalus and worsening as a result of extension of the hemorrhage or edema.

5. In 2005 the landmark STICH Trial established that for the vast majority of patients with supratentorial ICH, **surgical hematoma evacuation** confers no benefit in terms of survival or functional outcome. However, this trial did not include patients who have traditionally been considered strong candidates for surgery, particularly younger patients with large (>30 ml) lobar hemorrhages and early deterioration due to symptomatic mass effect. Surgical hematoma evacuation should still be strongly considered in these patients, as well as in patients with cerebellar hematomas greater than 3 cm in diameter. For patients presenting in coma or for those with a stable neurologic deficit, surgery is unlikely to help.

24

Movement Disorders

Movement disorders may be defined simply as *abnormal involuntary movements.* These movements are not the result of weakness or sensory deficits. Rather, they are the result of dysfunction of what may be defined anatomically as either the basal ganglia or cerebellum and functionally as the extrapyramidal motor system.

The diversity of movement disorders can be overwhelming, with movements including those that are commonly known (tremors, tics) and those that are less familiar (dystonia, chorea, and hemiballismus). Despite this diversity, movement disorders may be conveniently categorized into two types:

1. *Hyperkinesias* are characterized by an excess of movement.
2. *Hypokinesias* are characterized by a paucity of movement. Some basic principles should be kept in mind when first approaching a patient with a movement disorder.

BASIC PRINCIPLES

1. Take time to **observe** the patient. Some movements may be quite elaborate. At this point, do not make interpretations or think about treatment.
2. **Describe** what you see. Do not label anything yet. For example, note that "the eyes seem to be intermittently squeezing closed" or that "there are jerking movements of the left arm every 5 seconds."
3. **Classify** the movement as a hyperkinesia or a hypokinesia, as defined earlier.
4. **Give the movement a name** (e.g., tremor, chorea). The list of different types of abnormal movements (see Step 4 in the following paragraphs) provides a glossary of terms. Read each term and its definition and try to decide which of these terms best describes what you have seen.
5. **Diagnose a specific disease** after naming the movement. For example, both tremor and bradykinesia are features of Parkinson's disease.

6. Finally, think about the appropriate **treatment.** Table 24–1 lists the medications and dosages for treatment of movement disorders.

The most common error is for students to skip straight to diagnosis and treatment. It is important first to **observe, describe, classify, and name.**

The remainder of this chapter will follow the preceding six-step outline.

Step 1: Observe

Inform the patient that you are going to watch his or her movements and then *just observe the patient.* Some patients may be self-conscious and may try to inhibit their movements, particularly if these are embarrassing. If this is the case, ask the patient to allow the body to behave naturally and not stop any movements. Sometimes, you may need to ask the patient to perform certain maneuvers that will bring out the movement (e.g., writing may bring out a tremor, walking may bring out a dystonic foot movement). Some movements may be elaborate, and the period of observation may be lengthy before you get a sense of a pattern or before you can fully describe what you see.

Step 2: Describe

Try to describe the movements. This is not easy. In fact, neurologists sometimes find it easier to use gestures, rather than words, when describing a movement.

Some descriptions may be straightforward. For example, you might describe Mr. H.'s movements in the following way: "The right side of Mr. H.'s face twitches every 5 seconds." Other descriptions may be elaborate. For example, you might describe Mrs. R.'s movements as follows: "Mrs. R.'s neck remains completely hyperextended, and once every minute, there is a rapid, violent movement in the opposite direction, so that the head is completely anteroflexed for a brief moment."

Avoid describing Mr. H. as having hemifacial spasm and Mrs. R. as having torticollis. These statements are not descriptions; they are diagnoses.

Step 3: Classify

It is important to classify the movement as a hyperkinesia or a hypokinesia. This is the easiest step. One caveat is that some patients may simultaneously exhibit both types of movements. For example, a patient with Parkinson's disease may have a tremor (hyperkinesia) as well as bradykinesia (hypokinesia).

Step 4: Give the Movement a Name

The following is a list of different types of abnormal movements. Movements in **bold** letters are the hypokinesias; all others are hyperkinesias. The essential element of each movement is *italicized.*

TABLE 24–1 Movement Disorder Medications and Dosages

Medication	Dose	Condition Treated
Alprazolom (Xanax)	0.75 to 2 mg per day (two to three times a day)	Essential tremor
Amantadine (Symmetrel)	100 to 300 mg per day (two to three times a day)	Parkinson's disease, chorea
Baclofen (Lioresal)	10 to 80 mg per day (three times a day)	Dystonia
Bromocriptine (Parlodel)	7.5 to 30 mg per day (three to four times a day)	Parkinson's disease or
	0.75 mg qhs	Restless leg syndrome
Carbamazepine (Tegretol)	300 to 1200 mg per day (three to four times a day)	Dystonia
Clonazepam (Klonopin)	1 to 10 mg per day (two to three times a day)	Tics or
	1 to 4 mg qhs	Restless leg syndrome
Clonidine (Catapres)	0.2 to 1.0 mg per day, divided	Tics
Clozapine (Clozaril)	12.5 to 100 mg per day (two to three times a day)	Essential tremor
Diazepam (Valium)	2 to 10 mg per day, divided (two to three times a day)	Dystonia
Entacapone (Comtan)	200 to 600 mg per day divided	Parkinson's disease
Gabapentin (Neurontin)	1200 to 3600 mg per day (three times a day)	Essential tremor or
	300 to 1200 mg qhs	Restless leg syndrome
Haloperidol (Haldol)	1 to 10 mg per day (two to three times a day)	Tics, chorea
Levodopa/carbidopa (Sinemet)	100 to 2000 mg per day, divided	Parkinson's disease or
	100 to 200 mg qhs	Restless leg syndrome
Metyrosine (Demser)	250 to 1000 mg per day (three to four times a day)	Chorea
Olanzapine (Zyprexa)	5 to 20 mg per day (once a day)	Tics
Oxycodone (Oxycontin)	10 to 40 mg qhs	Restless leg syndrome
Penicillamine (Cuprimine)	250 to 1000 mg per day	Wilson's disease
Pergolide (Permax)	0.75 to 3.0 mg per day (three to four times a day)	Parkinson's disease, tics or
	0.25 to 1 mg qhs	Restless leg syndrome

TABLE 24–1 Movement Disorder Medications and Dosages—cont'd

Medication	Dose	Condition Treated
Pimozide (Orap)	2 to 10 mg per day, divided	Tics
Pramipexole (Mirapex)	1.5 to 4.5 mg per day (three times a day)	Parkinson's disease **or**
	0.375 to 0.75 mg qhs	Restless leg syndrome
Primidone (Mysoline)	62.5 to 1000 mg per day (three to four times a day)	Essential tremor
Propoxyphene (Darvon)	65 mg qhs	Restless leg syndrome
Propranolol (Inderal)	40 to 320 mg per day (three to four times a day)	Essential tremor
Reserpine	0.5 to 8 mg per day (three to four times a day)	Tics, chorea
Risperidone (Risperdal)	0.5 to 6 mg per day (two times a day)	Tics
Ropinirole (Requip)	0.75 to 3.0 mg per day (three times a day)	Parkinson's disease **or**
	0.25 to 1.25 mg qhs	Restless leg syndrome
Selegiline (Eldepryl)	5 to 10 mg per day (two times a day)	Parkinson's disease
Tizanidine (Zanaflex)	8 to 24 mg per day (three times a day)	Dystonia
Tolcapone (Tasmar)	300 to 600 mg per day, divided	Parkinson's disease
Topiramate (Topamax)	200 to 400 mg per day (two to three times a day)	Essential tremor
Trientine (Syprine)	750 to 1250 mg per day (two to four times a day)	Wilson's disease
Trihexyphenidyl (Artane)	1 to 10 mg per day (three to four times a day)	Parkinson's disease **or** Dystonia
	1 to 100 mg per day (three to four times a day)	
Zinc acetate (Galzin)	150 mg per day (three times a day)	Wilson's disease

Name of Movement	Definition or Description
Akathisia	A subjective *feeling of inner restlessness* that is relieved by movement. The movements are stereotypic and complex and convey restlessness (e.g., squirming, crossing and uncrossing legs, rocking back and forth, and pacing).
Asterixis	Sudden periods of *cessation of muscle contraction* best seen when the patient's arms are extended in front of their body, as if stopping traffic
Athetosis	Slow, *sinuous, writhing* movements, usually of the distal parts of the limbs
Ballismus	Wild *flinging, flailing* movements of a limb or limbs that represent large-amplitude proximal choreiform movements. Ballismus is often unilateral (hemiballismus).
Bradykinesia	Movements that are either *slow* or of *diminished amplitude*
Chorea	*Semipurposeful flowing* movements that fit from one part of the body to another in a continuous and random pattern
Dyskinesia	A general term for any excessive movement. The term dyskinesia is often used more specifically as an abbreviation for "tardive dyskinesia" (repetitive oral movements often seen in patients taking certain psychiatric medications).
Dystonia	*Twisting* movements or movements that are often *sustained* for variable periods of time
Freezing	Brief episodes (usually lasting several seconds) during which a motor act is temporarily blocked or halted. Walking is the motor act that is most commonly affected.
Myoclonus	Sudden, brief, shocklike *jerks*
Myokymia	*Quivering* or rippling of muscle
Rigidity	Muscle tone that is increased on passive motion. Distinct from spasticity, it is present equally in all directions of movement (i.e., both in flexors and in extensors).
Tachykinesia	Movements or speech characterized by *continuous acceleration* or loss of amplitude

Name of Movement	Definition or Description (*cont.*)
Tics	*Repetitive, stereotypic movements or sounds* that are suppressible and that relieve a feeling of inner tension
Tremor	*Rhythmic, oscillatory movements* that may be present at rest or with action. An intention tremor occurs when the patient's limb approaches a target during purposeful movements (e.g., finger-to-nose maneuver).

Step 5: Diagnose a Specific Disease

Parkinson's Disease

Parkinson's disease was first described by James Parkinson in 1817.

TYPES OF MOVEMENTS

The types of movements involved in this disease are tremor, rigidity, bradykinesia, freezing, and tachykinesia. The *tremor* of Parkinson's disease is most commonly a *rest tremor*. This means that the tremor is present when the arms are resting in the patient's lap side (while standing or walking), or present while lying down. Many patients with Parkinson's disease also have an *action tremor*, which is present when their arms are outstretched in front of their body *(postural tremor)* or when they are using their hands for purposeful movement *(kinetic tremor)*. The *rigidity* is often called *cogwheel* rigidity because it may have a ratchet-like quality. The *bradykinesia* is characterized by a decrease in the frequency of movements (diminished blink frequency, few facial expressions, or *masked facies*) and by slowness of movement, with loss of amplitude. *Postural reflexes*, lost later in the disease, may be tested by performing the *pull test*. Stand behind the patient and pull him or her backward. A normal response is for the patient to take one or two steps back without falling. Always stand behind the patient in the event that you need to catch him or her! *Freezing* is most commonly seen as *start hesitation* or *turning hesitation*. Walking in narrow, cramped quarters may bring on freezing. *Tachykinesia* may take the form of rapid accelerating speech *(tachyphemia)* or rapid accelerated walking *(festination)*.

DIAGNOSTIC TESTS

Parkinson's disease is a clinical diagnosis. The cardinal features are tremor, rigidity, bradykinesia, and loss of postural reflexes. LP, EEG, CT, and MRI are nonspecific. The deoxyglucose PET scan may show increased uptake in the region of the basal ganglia, and the fluorodopa PET scan may show diminished dopa uptake in the basal ganglia.

TREATMENT

Levodopa-carbidopa (Sinemet) 100 to 2000 mg per day of levodopa, with administration of individual doses ranging from every 2 to 3 hours to two times a day

Bromocriptine (Parlodel) 7.5 to 30 mg per day, divided, three to four times a day

Pergolide (Permax) 0.75 to 3.0 mg per day, divided, three to four times a day

Pramipexole (Mirapex) 1.5 to 4.5 mg per day, divided, three times a day

Ropinirole (Requip) 0.75 to 3.0 mg per day, divided, three times a day

Amantadine (Symmetrel) 100 to 300 mg per day, divided, two to three times a day

Trihexyphenidyl (Artane) 1 to 10 mg per day, divided, three to four times a day

Tolcapone (Tasmar) 300 to 600 mg per day, divided, as an adjunct to levodopa-carbidopa

Entacapone (Comtan) 200 to 600 mg per day, divided, as an adjunct to levodopa-carbidopa

Selegiline (Eldepryl) 5 to 10 mg per day, divided, two times a day

Stimulation of the globus pallidus interna following implantation of *deep brain stimulation* electrodes improves bradykinesia, rigidity, rest tremor, impaired balance, and medication-induced dyskinesia and motor fluctuations in the limb contralateral to the electrode; however, it has been supplanted by stimulation of the subthalamic nucleus.

Stereotactic thalamotomy has been shown to decrease the severity of parkinsonian tremor and allow for reductions in dosages of levodopa. However, this procedure has largely been supplanted by electrical stimulation of the ventral intermediate nucleus of the thalamus following implantation of deep brain stimulation electrodes. The procedure is beneficial for the treatment of contralateral parkinsonian tremor or essential tremor.

Essential Tremor

One of the earliest reports of essential tremor was that of Charles Dana in 1887.

TYPES OF MOVEMENTS

The characteristic movement in this disease is tremor. The tremor of essential tremor is most commonly an *action tremor* of the arms. It is present when the patient holds his or her arms extended in front of the body and is often present with tasks such as writing, pouring water, and touching the finger to the nose. Many patients with essential tremor have an *intention tremor* of the arms. The tremor may also involve the head and voice in some patients. In cases of severe essential tremor, a tremor at rest may be present in the arms.

DIAGNOSTIC TESTS

Essential tremor is diagnosed on the basis of the clinical features described above. Other causes of similar tremor, including hyperthyroidism and certain medications (e.g., lithium or valproate), should be ruled out. The diagnosis may be confirmed by computerized tremor analysis with accelerometry.

TREATMENT

Propranolol (Inderal) 40 to 320 mg per day, divided, three to four times a day

Primidone (Mysoline) 62.5 to 1000 mg per day, divided, three to four times a day

Topiramate (Topamax) 200 to 400 mg per day, divided, two to three times per day

Gabapentin (Neurontin) 1200 to 3600 mg per day, divided, three times a day

Alprazalom (Xanax) 0.75 to 2 mg per day, divided, two to three times per day

Clozapine (Clozaril) 12.5 to 100 mg per day, divided, two to three times a day

Huntington's Disease

Huntington's disease was first described by George Huntington in 1872.

TYPES OF MOVEMENTS

Chorea and dystonia are common features of the disease. The *chorea* of Huntington's disease may involve the face, tongue, limbs, or trunk. It is often exacerbated by anxiety or stress and may be brought on by asking the patient to close the eyes, hold the arms extended in front of the body, and count backward or perform simple arithmetic. *Dystonia* and *tics* may also be present. The dystonia may take the form of fist clenching, shoulder elevation, or foot inversion during walking. Another feature of Huntington's disease is *motor impersistence* (inhibitory pauses occurring during voluntary motion that account for the "milkmaid grips" seen when hand grasp is tested). In addition to involuntary movements, patients with Huntington's disease often have psychiatric manifestations (depression, psychosis) as well as cognitive problems, changes in personality, and prominent disinhibition.

DIAGNOSTIC TESTS

Because the disease is transmitted in an autosomal dominant manner, a family history is an important feature of the diagnosis. One should rule out other causes of chorea including hyperthyroidism, use of anticonvulsants, and Sydenham's chorea. The abnormal gene, on the short arm of chromosome 4, consists of an abnormally long CAG repeat fragment. The CT or MRI scan may show atrophy of the caudate nuclei.

MANAGEMENT

In many cases, the movements are not bothersome to the patient, and the psychiatric manifestations are often the focus of treatment. However, treatment for the movements might consist of the following:

Haloperidol (Haldol) 1 to 10 mg per day, divided, two to three times a day

Olanzapine (Zyprexa) 5 to 20 mg per day

Amantadine (Symmetrel) 100 to 300 mg per day, divided, two to three times a day

Reserpine 0.5 to 8 mg per day, divided, three to four times a day

Metyrosine (Demser) 250 to 1000 mg per day, divided, three to four times a day

Idiopathic Torsion Dystonia (Dystonia Musculorum Deformans)

This illness is characterized by twisting dystonic movements and occasional tremor.

TYPES OF MOVEMENTS

The illness usually begins in childhood and has a progressive course. The *dystonia* often initially involves the foot and is most apparent with certain actions but not with others (e.g., intermittent spasmodic inversion of the foot while walking but not while running or walking backward). Eventually, involvement of other limbs and neck often occurs. Although the dystonia initially consists of twisting *movements* with action, sustained dystonic *postures* at rest become apparent eventually. Limbs with dystonia may also exhibit an irregular *dystonic tremor* that resembles the action tremor seen in patients with essential tremor.

DIAGNOSTIC TESTS

The diagnosis is based on clinical history and examination. It should be distinguished from other secondary or symptomatic causes of dystonia (e.g., Wilson's disease) and from adult-onset dystonia. The latter usually runs a more benign course and begins in adulthood with involvement of the neck, eyes, or hand, but it rarely involves the leg. A common gene for idiopathic torsion dystonia, the *DYT1* gene, is located on the long arm of chromosome 9 and is inherited in an autosomal dominant manner with a penetrance as low as 30%.

MANAGEMENT

Trihexyphenidyl (Artane) 1 to 100 mg per day, divided, three to four times a day

Baclofen (Lioresal) 10 to 80 mg per day, divided, three times a day

Diazepam (Valium) 2 to 10 mg per day, divided, two to three times a day

Tizanidine (Zanaflex) 8 to 24 mg per day, divided, three times a day

Carbamazepine (Tegretol) 300 to 1200 mg per day, divided, three to four times a day

Botulinum toxin (Botox) injected into selected muscles several times per year

Tourette's Syndrome

Tourette's syndrome was first definitively described by Gilles de la Tourette in 1885.

TYPES OF MOVEMENTS

This syndrome is characterized by multiple chronic motor and vocal tics that wax and wane over time. The tics may be *simple motor tics* (eye blinking, eyebrow raising), *complex motor tics* (head shaking, wrist shaking), *simple phonic tics* (throat clearing, grunting), or *complex phonic tics* (uttering words). *Coprolalia* (uttering obscenities) and *echolalia* (repeating sounds or words) are examples of the latter. As with most tics, these are voluntarily suppressible for brief periods and may vary in intensity over time. In addition to these motor features, patients with Tourette's syndrome often have psychiatric manifestations including attention deficit hyperactivity disorder and obsessive compulsive disorder.

DIAGNOSTIC TESTS

The diagnosis is clinical. This disorder usually begins in childhood with both motor and phonic tics. Coprolalia is not an essential feature of the diagnosis.

MANAGEMENT

Clonazepam (Klonopin) 1 to 10 mg per day, divided, two to three times a day

Risperidone (Risperdal) 0.5 to 6 mg per day, divided into two doses

Olanzapine (Zyprexa) 5 to 20 mg per day

Pergolide (Permax) 0.75 to 3.0 mg per day, divided, three to four times a day

Reserpine 0.5 to 8 mg, divided, three to four times a day

Clonidine (Catapres) 0.2 to 1.0 mg per day, divided

Pimozide (Orap) 1 to 10 mg per day, divided

Haloperidol (Haldol) 1 to 10 mg per day, divided, two to three times a day

Wilson's Disease

Wilson's disease was first described by Samuel Alexander Kinnier Wilson in 1912.

TYPES OF MOVEMENTS

The movements are protean. Tremor, rigidity, bradykinesia, dystonia, and chorea are all seen in this disease, and one or more of these movements may be present. A *parkinsonian form* of the illness may be characterized by rest tremor, rigidity, or bradykinesia. A *pseudosclerotic* form of the illness is associated with a *wing-beating tremor* (a large-amplitude, flapping, violent tremor that is present when the shoulders are abducted, elbows are flexed, and fingers are facing each other). *Dystonia* and *chorea* may also be present. Dysarthria occurs frequently and may progress to anarthria. Psychiatric manifestations (anxiety, depression, psychosis) are a common feature of the illness.

DIAGNOSTIC TESTS
The diagnosis is based on clinical history and examination and is supported by the presence of Kayser-Fleischer rings (ring-shaped copper deposits in the cornea), low serum ceruloplasmin level, abnormalities in liver function tests, or hepatitis. Lesions in the basal ganglia may be seen on an MRI scan. The gene *pWD* is located on the long arm of chromosome 13.

MANAGEMENT
Penicillamine (Cuprimine) 125 to 1000 mg per day
Trientine (Syprine) 750 to 1250 mg per day, divided, two to four times a day
Zinc acetate (Galzin) 150 mg per day, divided, three times a day

Restless Leg Syndrome

The syndrome is characterized by feelings of discomfort and restless-ness in the legs and occasionally in the arms. These feelings, which occur primarily in the evening hours, are often relieved by move-ment (e.g., moving the legs in bed or getting out of bed to pace).

TYPES OF MOVEMENTS
The movements involved are fidgeting, kicking, or writhing move-ments of the legs and pacing the floor.

The discomfort is deep-seated and is often described as feelings of stretching, itching, crawling, or creeping in the bones, muscles, or tendons. These symptoms are most common when the patient first lies down in bed at night. The feelings may cause writhing movements in the legs, fidgeting, or kicking. Some patients need to pace the floor for temporary relief. Unlike akathisia, which also causes discomfort with a desire to move, restless leg syndrome occurs primarily at night.

DIAGNOSTIC TESTS
Restless leg syndrome is a clinical syndrome that is diagnosed based on the clinical features described. Akathisia can resemble restless leg syndrome but is typically constant throughout the day, has a more generalized distribution (i.e., not just localized leg discomfort), and is confined to patients taking neuroleptic medications or patients with Parkinson's disease.

TREATMENT
Pergolide (Permax) 0.25 to 1 mg qhs
Bromocriptine (Parlodel) 7.5 mg qhs
Pramipexole (Mirapex) 0.375 to 0.75 mg qhs
Ropinirole (Requip) 0.25 to 1.25 mg qhs

Levodopa (Sinemet) 25/100 to 50/200 qhs
Clonazepam (Klonopin) 1 to 4 mg qhs
Propoxyphene (Darvon) 65 mg qhs
Oxycodone (Oxycontin) 10 to 40 mg qhs
Gabapentin (Neurontin) 300 to 1200 mg qhs

Miscellaneous Disorders

This section briefly discusses those movements from the list in **Step 4** that were not discussed under specific diseases.

Akathisia is most commonly seen as a side effect of certain psychiatric medications.

Asterixis, usually seen bilaterally in the arms, is most commonly a feature of toxic/metabolic states such as liver or renal failure. Patients are often encephalopathic.

Athetosis may appear in a variety of neurologic disorders ranging from cerebral palsy to paroxysmal kinesiogenic choreoathetosis. Athetotic movements may merge with chorea (choreoathetosis).

Ballismus, most commonly unilateral (hemiballismus), is usually the result of a stroke in the contralateral subthalamic nucleus.

Myoclonus may occur anywhere in the body, including palatal myoclonus and ocular myoclonus. Myoclonus may be the result of anoxic ischemic injury (Lance-Adams syndrome), birth injuries, degenerative disorders (Ramsay Hunt syndrome), infections, tumors, strokes, or even medications (levodopa). Hiccups are a physiologic form of myoclonus.

Myokymia, most commonly seen in facial muscles, is often due to pontine lesions, particularly plaques in multiple sclerosis or pontine gliomas.

Epilepsy and Seizure Disorders

Dramatic advances have occurred in the management of epilepsy over the past decade—diagnostically and therapeutically, medically and surgically. Seizures and epilepsy are a prominent component of any neurologist's practice and are a common problem encountered by neurology residents. This chapter covers the basics of epilepsy diagnosis and treatment. Status epilepticus is covered in Chapter 4, and further details of the antiepileptic drugs are covered in Appendix B.

Epilepsy is defined as recurrent (two or more) unprovoked seizures. It occurs in 0.5% to 1% of the population. Nearly 10% of the population will experience at least one seizure in their lifetime.

SEIZURE CLASSIFICATION

Seizures are divided into *primary generalized* seizures (seen in all parts of the cortex simultaneously) and *partial-onset* seizures (localization-related; starting in one region, with or without spread) (Table 25–1). These types are then subdivided into *idiopathic* (presumably genetic) and *symptomatic/cryptogenic* (with an underlying cause). The most common seizure types are described here.

Primary Generalized Seizures

Primary Generalized Tonic-Clonic (Grand Mal) Seizures

Primary generalized tonic-clonic (GTC) seizures are characterized by the absence of an aura, an ictal cry due to forced inhalation, a tonic phase with stiffening of all extremities lasting approximately 30 seconds, followed by gradual progression into a clonic phase, also lasting approximately 30 seconds. Postictal stertorous breathing with gradual awakening extends over many minutes. Often incontinence or tongue biting occurs. Diffuse myalgias are common post-ictally. Although there is typically no aura, there may be a few myoclonic jerks at the start with retained awareness.

TABLE 25–1 **ILAE* Seizure Classification (Simplified)**

I. Localization-related seizures (i.e., focal, partial-onset)
  a. Simple partial seizures (no impairment of consciousness)
    i. With motor symptoms
    ii. With somatosensory or special sensory symptoms
    iii. With autonomic symptoms
    iv. With psychic symptoms
  b. Complex partial seizures (with impaired consciousness)
    i. Beginning as simple partial-onset
    ii. With impaired consciousness at onset
  c. Secondary generalized (secondary GTC)
II. Primary generalized seizures
  a. Absence
    i. Typical absence
    ii. Atypical absence
  b. Myoclonic
  c. Clonic
  d. Tonic
  e. Tonic-clonic (primary GTC)
  f. Atonic
III. Unclassifiable

*International League Against Epilepsy.

Primary or secondary GTCs usually result in a transient postictal lactic acidosis with low HCO_3 and elevated CK, which lasts for 12 to 24 hours. An elevated prolactin (at least three times the baseline prolactin level at similar time of day if drawn 5 to 30 minutes after the convulsion) may be useful in distinguishing it from a non-epileptic event).

Absence (Petit Mal) Seizures

Absence seizures are sudden-onset, brief (approximately 10 seconds) staring spells with immediate recovery. They can occur many times per day, and eye flutter is common. EEG shows *generalized spike and wave discharges.* Typical absence seizures show 3 Hz generalized spike and wave in a very regular pattern and usually occur in neurologically normal children (i.e., in primary generalized epilepsy). Atypical absence seizures tend to be longer, with a less clear onset and offset, show less regular and slower generalized spike and wave (1 to 2.5 Hz) on EEG, and are usually associated with underlying neurologic abnormalities (i.e., in symptomatic generalized epilepsy). Longer absence seizures (20 to 30 seconds) often have associated automatisms that can mimic complex partial seizures.

Myoclonic Seizures

These seizures are characterized by brief, lightning-like muscle jerks. The movements may be symmetric, asymmetric, or multifocal, with no impairment of consciousness. EEG usually shows a *generalized polyspike and wave discharge.*

Tonic Seizures

In these seizures sudden bilateral symmetric tonic posturing is brief, with rapid recovery. Brief impairment of consciousness is typical. EEG usually shows sudden, diffuse, low-voltage, fast activity (beta) or background attenuation. These seizures are usually seen in neurologically abnormal patients, especially children, and especially in those with *Lennox-Gastaut syndrome* (see below).

Partial-Onset Seizures

These seizures are divided into *simple* partial seizures (SPS), with completely retained awareness during the event (although patients may be aphasic), and *complex* partial seizures (CPS), with impairment of awareness. Partial seizures may progress to *secondary generalized tonic-clonic seizures.* If there is no known aura or focal feature at the onset of a convulsion, it is not possible to distinguish primary GTC from secondary GTC without an EEG. An *aura* is a sensation experienced by the patient at the onset of a partial seizure such as a smell, déjà vu, dizziness, or nausea. Auras are actually simple partial seizures with sensory or experiential symptoms only. These are brief and either resolve (SPS) or progress. Some patients have a prolonged sensation lasting many hours prior to their seizures, referred to as a *prodrome;* these feelings are often nonspecific and difficult to describe.

Temporal Lobe Seizures

These seizures are the most common type seen in adults. They are usually accompanied by an aura, often an epigastric rising sensation. Other common auras include indescribable cephalic sensations, smells, and déjà vu. Seizures tend to last 1 to 3 minutes and consist primarily of quiet unresponsive staring. There are frequently oral automatisms (chewing, lip smacking) as well as manual automatisms (picking at clothes, rubbing, patting, etc.). There is often contralateral dystonic posturing of the arm and hand (due to basal ganglia spread). Postictally, there is usually postictal nose wiping near the seizure offset (with the ipsilateral hand as the other hand remains impaired) and some confusion and lethargy lasting at least a few minutes. Patients may not be aware of their seizures. With seizures arising from the dominant hemisphere (usually the left), there is frequently postictal aphasia for at least 1 minute. In nondominant hemisphere seizures, recovery of speech is usually rapid, although the patient may remain confused.

Frontal Lobe Seizures

These seizures usually have no aura or postictal phase and are shorter than temporal lobe seizures (often 15 to 40 seconds in duration).

They tend to occur in sleep. Prominent motor manifestations are often seen, including rhythmic unilateral clonic activity if involving the primary motor cortex; this activity may march across the body as it spreads within the motor homunculus ("Jacksonian march"). There may also be frantic restless movements, bicycling of the legs, incontinence, and vocalizations such as screaming. Asymmetric tonic posturing is common if the supplementary motor area is involved. Bilateral motor manifestations can occur with full retained awareness and memory. It is often difficult to distinguish a frontal lobe seizure from a nonepileptic psychogenic seizure.

Occipital Lobe Seizures

These seizures may begin with a visual aura, either simple (spots or lights) if from the primary visual cortex, or complex (formed visual hallucinations including detailed scenes, usually stereotyped from spell to spell) if from the temporo-occipital region. Occipital seizures can spread either to the temporal lobe, causing a typical temporal lobe CPS, or above the Sylvian fissure, causing motor manifestations that can be difficult to distinguish from a frontal lobe seizure.

Parietal Lobe Seizures

These seizures are the least common. They may begin with a sensory aura and can rarely begin with contralateral pain. They will often spread to either the temporal or frontal lobe, with corresponding symptomatology.

EPILEPSY SYNDROME CLASSIFICATION

Once the seizure type is determined, an effort is made to see whether a patient fits a particular epilepsy syndrome, which may be useful both prognostically and therapeutically. Syndromes incorporate history, seizure type, neurologic status, and EEG findings. The ILAE (International League Against Epilepsy) classification is shown in Table 25–2. The most common syndromes are described here.

Primary Generalized Syndromes

Childhood Absence Epilepsy

In childhood absence epilepsy (CAE), typical absence seizures, often many per day (can be hundreds), begin between ages 4 and 10 years (peak 6 to 7 years) and usually resolve by puberty; they rarely persist into adulthood. Treatment of choice is **ethosuximide** or **valproic acid.** A significant minority (up to 40%) develop convulsions as well (rare and easily controlled).

Juvenile Absence Epilepsy

In juvenile absence epilepsy, typical absence seizures begin between ages 10 and 17 years (peak at 12 years), with fewer seizures per day

TABLE 25–2 **ILAE* Epilepsy Syndrome Classification**

I. Localization-related syndromes (focal, partial-onset)
  a. Idiopathic (with age-related onset)
    i. Benign childhood epilepsy with centrotemporal spikes (a.k.a. benign Rolandic epilepsy of childhood, or BREC)
    ii. Childhood epilepsy with occipital paroxysms
    iii. Primary reading epilepsy
  b. Symptomatic/cryptogenic
    i. By lobe of onset (frontal, temporal, parietal, or occipital)
    ii. Chronic progressive epilepsia partialis continua of childhood (including Rasmussen's encephalitis)
    iii. Epilepsies characterized by seizures with specific modes of precipitation
II. Generalized syndromes
  a. Idiopathic
    i. Benign neonatal familial convulsions
    ii. Benign neonatal convulsions
    iii. Benign myoclonic epilepsy in infancy
    iv. Childhood absence epilepsy (CAE; pyknolepsy)
    v. Juvenile absence epilepsy (JAE)
    vi. Juvenile myoclonic epilepsy (JME)
    vii. Epilepsy with grand mal (GTC) seizures upon awakening
    viii. Other
    ix. Epilepsies with seizures precipitated by specific modes of activation
  b. Cryptogenic or symptomatic (in order of age)
    i. West syndrome (infantile spasms)
    ii. Lennox-Gastaut syndrome
    iii. Epilepsy with myoclonic-astatic seizures
    iv. Epilepsy with myoclonic absences
  c. Symptomatic
    i. Nonspecific etiology
      1. Early myoclonic encephalopathy
      2. Early infantile epileptic encephalopathy with suppression burst
      3. Other symptomatic generalized epilepsies (common)
    ii. Specific etiology
III. Undetermined whether focal or generalized
  a. With both generalized and focal seizures
    i. Neonatal seizures
    ii. Severe myoclonic epilepsy in infancy
    iii. Epilepsy with continuous spike-waves during slow wave sleep
    iv. Acquired epileptic aphasia (Landau-Kleffner syndrome)
    v. Other
  b. Without unequivocal focal or generalized features (e.g., nocturnal GTCs, unclear whether primary or secondary)
IV. Special syndromes
  a. Situation-related seizures
    i. Febrile convulsions
    ii. Isolated seizures or isolated status epilepticus
    iii. Seizures occurring only during acute or toxic event (alcohol/drugs, hypoglycemia, nonketotic hyperglycemia)

*International League Against Epilepsy.

than in CAE. Most patients also have convulsions (approximately 80%), and some have occasional myoclonic seizures (15%). **Valproate** is the treatment of choice, although newer antiepileptic drugs (AEDs) such as lamotrigine are being used more commonly to avoid valproate-related adverse effects and teratogenicity. Although a relatively benign syndrome, it is more likely to persist into adulthood than CAE.

Juvenile Myoclonic Epilepsy

In juvenile myoclonic epilepsy, onset typically occurs at ages 12 to 18 years (peak at 14 to 15 years). It is a common, often missed syndrome that consists of morning myoclonic jerks and primary GTCs; some patients have preceding absence seizures (10% to 33%). It is important to ask about morning myoclonus (twitching, clumsiness, or spilling things) to make this diagnosis, as many patients with this syndrome assume that everybody has myoclonic jerks. The seizures tend to occur shortly after awakening, and GTCs are often preceded by an increased frequency of myoclonic jerking. Sleep deprivation, alcohol, and photic stimulation all precipitate seizures. Family history is positive for epilepsy in 25%. The most effective treatment is **valproic acid,** although several newer AEDs such as lamotrigine, levetiracetam, zonisamide, and topiramate are also used commonly. Recognizing the syndrome is important, as myoclonic seizures (and less commonly absence) can be exacerbated by carbamazepine, oxcarbazepine, and phenytoin. Seizures are usually well controlled in JME, but most patients (>90%) need lifelong medication. EEG shows primary generalized spike and wave in 95%, usually at a fast rate (approximately 4 to 5 Hz generalized spike and wave and generalized polyspike and wave; this is also known as *atypical spike and wave,* to distinguish it from the 3-Hz discharges of CAE and from the slow spike and wave of Lennox-Gastaut syndrome). A photoparoxysmal response is common (approximately one third of patients with JME). *Epilepsy with grand mal seizures upon awakening* is a related syndrome, but without the myoclonic jerks.

Symptomatic Generalized Epilepsy Syndromes

Lennox-Gastaut Syndrome

LGS is characterized by early onset (at ages 1 to 8 years, peak between 3 and 5 years) of multiple seizure types. Almost all patients are developmentally delayed and have multiple seizure types including tonic seizures, drop attacks (can be due to atonic, tonic, or myoclonic seizures; also called "astatic seizures" as a group), GTCs, and atypical absence seizures. EEG in LGS usually shows generalized slow spike and wave (<2.5 Hz), multifocal epileptiform discharges, and diffuse slowing. LGS is often refractory to multiple medications. Approximately one third of these patients have a preceding diagnosis of *West syndrome* (developmental delay, infantile spasms, and hypsarrhythmia on EEG). Prognosis is poor in general.

Localization-Related Epilepsy Syndromes, Symptomatic/Cryptogenic

Temporal Lobe Epilepsy

Temporal lobe epilepsy is the most common syndrome seen in adults and is the form most amenable to surgery. It is often associated with an early life risk factor such as meningitis, head trauma, or febrile seizures. There is a particular association of prolonged febrile seizures, temporal lobe epilepsy, and hippocampal sclerosis (also known as mesial temporal sclerosis, or MTS) both pathologically and on MRI. MRI in these patients shows hippocampal atrophy (best seen on oblique coronal T1 images or STIR) and increased signal (best seen on coronal FLAIR or T2 images). Patients with an early risk factor, MTS, documented temporal lobe seizures, and interictal temporal lobe spikes on EEG are excellent candidates for temporal lobectomy, with >80% of patients becoming seizure-free postoperatively.

Localization-Related Epilepsy Syndromes, Idiopathic

Benign Rolandic Epilepsy of Childhood

This is an idiopathic focal epilepsy with usual onset at 4 to 10 years old (peak at 8 to 9 years; range 2 to 13 years). This syndrome is characterized by simple partial seizures beginning with oropharyngeal symptoms (inability to speak, unilateral facial twitching, drooling), often progressing to a hemiconvulsion and secondary GTC, often nocturnal. EEG shows stereotyped centrotemporal spikes, unilateral (60% to 70% with one EEG) or bilateral, activated by sleep (restricted to sleep in one third of these patients). Generalized spike and wave may be present as well (in 10% to 20%). The disease remits by puberty in most patients. If seizures rarely occur, treatment may not be needed. If seizures and EEG are classic, there is no need to image; this is the only focal epilepsy that does not require neuroimaging. **Carbamazepine** and **gabapentin** are the most commonly used AEDs.

Situation-Related Epilepsies

Febrile Seizures

Febrile seizures occur in approximately 4% of the population, onset being between age 6 months and 6 years, peaking at 18 to 24 months. One third have recurrent febrile seizures that are more likely to recur if the first febrile seizure occurs before 1 year of age. Later epilepsy occurs in 2% to 4% overall; this risk is lowest for *simple febrile seizure* (single convulsion at onset of fever, no lateralizing features, <15 minutes in duration, neurologically normal child), and most febrile seizures fit this category. The risk is higher for *complex febrile seizure* (focal, multiple, prolonged, or neurologically impaired). There is no need to treat, image, or obtain EEG in a child with a simple febrile seizure.

NEW-ONSET SEIZURES

Evaluation of New-Onset Seizures

The history should concentrate on both acute and chronic remote risk factors for seizures as listed in Table 25–3. In adults aged 20 to

TABLE 25–3 **Evaluation of New-Onset Seizures**

I. **History/examination:** look/ask for evidence of the following:
   A. *Acute risk factors*
      Trauma
      Alcohol
      Illegal drugs (especially cocaine, amphetamine)
      Medications: see Table 4–1; also withdrawal from
         benzodiazepines or barbiturates
      Metabolic:
         Low: glucose, sodium, oxygen, calcium, magnesium
         High: glucose, osmolality, BUN
      Infections, especially CNS infections; ask about HIV status and
         risk factors
      Stroke
   B. *Chronic/remote risk factors*
      Cerebral palsy/mental retardation
      Head trauma
      CNS infections
      Family history of epilepsy
      Febrile convulsions, especially if complex
      Neurocutaneous syndromes (examine skin)
      Prior unrecognized seizures, including absence and myoclonic
         jerks
II. **Laboratory Tests**
   CBC with differential blood count
   Basic metabolic panel
   Calcium
   Magnesium
   Phosphate
   LFTs
   Urine toxicology screen
   Serum toxicology
   Ethanol level (usually 0 when seizing)
   HIV testing when appropriate
III. **Imaging**
   Head CT scan with contrast, or brain MRI (preferred)

60, the most common causes, listed in order of frequency, are trauma, infection, metabolic/drugs, tumor, and vascular. For adults over 60 years old, the most common causes, in order, are vascular (stroke is by far the most common), tumor/metastasis, trauma, metabolic, and infection.

If there is an acute symptomatic explanation for the seizure, the underlying etiology should be corrected. Although usually generalized, focal seizures may also be seen with systemic metabolic abnormalities, especially hyper- or hypoglycemia, including *epilepsia partialis continua* (continuous simple partial seizures consisting of focal clonic jerking; common with nonketotic hyperosmolar hyperglycemia). These seizures are best treated by correcting the metabolic abnormality, as they are refractory to anticonvulsants unless this has been done.

If the patient is neurologically normal and has returned to baseline, MRI with and without gadolinium and EEG should be arranged. If MRI is not available and follow-up is questionable, a head CT scan with and without contrast should be obtained before discharge. It is particularly important to image those who are older, immunosuppressed, or at risk for HIV. The only patients with new-onset seizures who do not require any imaging are children with febrile convulsions or those with clear benign Rolandic or primary generalized epilepsy diagnosed by history *and* confirmed by EEG.

Lumbar punctures are rarely helpful in patients with new-onset seizures who have returned to baseline. This excludes patients with evidence of infection or those who may be immunosuppressed.

Risk of Seizure Recurrence

In patients with normal examination, a single seizure, and normal MRI and EEG, the chance of recurrence is approximately 25% to 30% over the next 2 to 3 years. Treatment is usually not recommended in these patients, in order to avoid chronic potentially harmful medication use when the majority will not need it. If the patient is neurologically abnormal or has epileptiform discharges on EEG, the risk goes up significantly (approximately 50% if one factor is present, higher if both are present), and use of anticonvulsants is usually recommended. In general, the use of AEDs will cut the risk of recurrence in half.

The decision to treat or not should be individualized and discussed with the patient. It is important to ask all about prior possible seizures including myoclonic, absence, and partial. All patients should be advised about seizure precipitants such as alcohol use and sleep deprivation. They should also be counseled about seizure safety, including not driving or swimming alone until a full evaluation has been performed. They should be educated about other possible spells that may represent seizures.

If a person has two unprovoked seizures (i.e., epilepsy), the chance of having a third is approximately 70% to 80%, and treatment is almost always recommended.

MEDICAL TREATMENT OF EPILEPSY

General Principles

In general, the first antiepileptic drug (AED) should be continued until the patient is seizure-free or experiencing adverse effects. If the first AED fails, another first-line drug should be tried in monotherapy prior to attempting combination therapy. Choice of AED should be based on the seizure type and epilepsy syndrome as well as practical factors. Medication that can be taken once daily may be necessary for patients with poor memory or noncompliance. Coexisting conditions should be taken into account. For example, valproate and topiramate are also effective for migraine prophylaxis; valproate, carbamazepine, oxcarbazepine, and lamotrigine are effective for bipolar and related disorders; gabapentin and several other AEDs are effective for neuropathic pain; and gabapentin is effective for restless legs syndrome. Patients with severe liver disease may want to take gabapentin or levetiracetam, as these AEDs are not metabolized in the liver. Patients with multiple drug allergies may do best with gabapentin, levetiracetam, valproate, or topiramate, as these AEDs almost never cause allergic reactions. Those with osteoporosis should probably avoid phenytoin (exacerbates bone loss), those who are overweight may prefer topiramate or zonisamide, and those who need to gain weight may prefer valproate or gabapentin.

Although no new medications for epilepsy were approved between 1978 and 1993, eight new AEDs were approved between 1993 and early 2000 (in chronologic order, felbamate, gabapentin, lamotrigine, topiramate, tiagabine, levetiracetam, oxcarbazepine, and zonisamide). Pregabalin was approved in 2005. In general, these newer AEDs have fewer adverse effects and drug interactions than the older AEDs. Felbamate use is restricted to epileptologists due to potentially fatal aplastic anemia or hepatitis in approximately 1 in 5000 patients; it remains a useful medication, especially for patients with Lennox-Gastaut syndrome.

Primary Generalized Epilepsy

The drug of choice for most primary generalized epilepsy syndromes remains valproic acid, although some epileptologists are using lamotrigine, especially in young women (to avoid the weight gain, alopecia, hormonal effects, and teratogenicity that can occur with valproate). Some of the other newer anticonvulsants are also effective, such as topiramate, levetiracetam, and zonisamide. Ethosuximide is used for absence seizures but is ineffective for other seizure types. Acetazolamide and clonazepam can be useful adjuncts as well, although tolerance to these drugs is common. Carbamazepine, oxcarbazepine, and phenytoin can exacerbate myoclonic and absence seizures but can be effective for primary GTC seizures. Primidone and phenobarbital are effective but less well tolerated.

Localization-Related Epilepsy

The first-line treatment for localization-related (partial-onset) epilepsy is no longer clear, as multiple agents are appropriate. All of the newer anticonvulsants are approved for partial epilepsy. Although not all are approved for monotherapy, there is no reason to suspect that any of them will not be effective as such. Carbamazepine, oxcarbazepine, and lamotrigine are common first-line agents. The latter two have been shown in small trials to be as effective as and better tolerated than the older AEDs. Because of its safety and tolerability, gabapentin is a good choice for mild epilepsies such as BRE. Levetiracetam and gabapentin are also reasonable options in the medically ill or elderly patients owing to their safety, ease of use, and lack of interactions. The other newer anticonvulsants are also reasonable first-line treatment in select patients (though not felbamate).

Newer Forms of Antiepileptic Drugs

1. **Cerebyx (fosphenytoin)** is an IV formulation that is rapidly dephosphorylated to phenytoin in the bloodstream. It can be given three times as fast as IV phenytoin, as it is available at a normal pH rather than the highly alkaline and toxic pH of IV phenytoin. This form is much gentler on veins and safer with extravasation. Blood pressure must still be monitored closely, including for at least 10 to 15 minutes after IV load, as phenytoin continues to be formed. This drug has replaced IV phenytoin in most academic centers, especially for use in status epilepticus and in children.
2. **Carbatrol (carbamazepine, long-acting)** is available as a capsule containing three different carbamazepine preparations: enteric release, immediate release, and delayed release. Dosing twice a day with Carbatrol is equivalent to dosing four times a day with Tegretol. It is available in 200 mg and 300 mg capsules.
3. **Tegretol XR (carbamazepine, long-acting)** is available in 100, 200, and 400 mg capsules. Medication is slowly released from a pinhole in the tablet via osmotic forces. The tablet itself will be excreted intact in the stool, and this should be explained to the patient (to avoid patient's misconception that the pill is not being absorbed and possibly stopping the medication).
4. **Depacon (IV valproate)** is an IV preparation of valproate that is extremely well tolerated. It is approved for administration at a rate of 3 mg/kg/minute for up to a 15 mg/kg dose, but seems to be safe even faster (up to 5 to 6 mg/kg/min) and at higher doses (up to 50 to 60 mg/kg in a patient on an enzyme-inducing AED such as phenytoin or phenobarbital). It may play an important role in treating status epilepticus, especially when nonconvulsive (see Chapter 4).

5. **Diastat (rectal diazepam)** is a convenient gel preparation of rectal diazepam (Valium) that can be given via prepackaged syringes by caregivers at home. This drug is excellent for patients with clusters (acute repetitive seizures) or prolonged seizures.

Common Errors in Treatment

1. **Following serum levels rather than clinical response**

   A valproate level of 130 mg/L (typical therapeutic range is 50 to 100 mg/L) may be just right for a given patient as long as the drug is not clinically toxic. Similarly, a phenytoin level of 8 mg/L (therapeutic range, 10 to 20 mg/L) may be adequate for some patients. Seizure control and clinical toxicity should be used as the primary end point, with serum levels as an adjunct.

2. **Missing the diagnosis of primary generalized epilepsy**

   If atypical absence spells are treated as complex partial seizures, many of the selected medications (e.g., phenytoin, carbamazepine) will not work and may even exacerbate seizures. Similarly, if the primary GTC seizures of juvenile myoclonic epilepsy are treated as secondary generalized seizures with carbamazepine, myoclonic jerks and absence seizures may be exacerbated. It is important to ask about morning myoclonus and absence spells.

3. **Missing the diagnosis of psychogenic nonepileptic seizures (a.k.a. pseudoseizures).**

   It can be very difficult to distinguish epileptic spells from psychogenic nonepileptic seizures (PNES) by history. PNES are psychogenic spells that mimic epileptic seizures and are usually a form of conversion disorder (unconscious behavior rather than conscious malingering, which is rare). Risk factors include prior physical or sexual abuse and psychiatric disease, although these may not be present. To complicate matters, some patients have both epileptic seizures and PNES. Video/EEG monitoring is required to make this diagnosis. For this reason alone, any patient with persistent spells that have not responded to AEDs, especially if the EEG and imaging are negative, should be referred for video/EEG monitoring. Approximately 30% of patients admitted to epilepsy monitoring units have nonepileptic spells, most of which are PNES.

4. **Missing the diagnosis of nonepileptic physiologic spells**

   For refractory spells, always consider other physiologic episodes such as arrhythmias/syncope (especially if slumping is present; syncope commonly leads to a few myoclonic jerks or brief tonic stiffening), movement disorders (e.g., paroxysmal dyskinesias), sleep disorders (e.g., REM behavior disorder, somnambulism), or panic attacks (usually lasting longer than partial seizures and with retained awareness, although differentiation can be difficult). Again, recording episodes (with video, EEG, ECG, and possibly EMG or sleep parameters) is the key to accurate diagnosis.

5. **Missing the diagnosis of epilepsy**

Frontal lobe seizures are frequently misdiagnosed as psychogenic spells, a sleep disorder, or paroxysmal nocturnal dystonia, as they tend to be nocturnal with rapid recovery, and EEGs are often normal (including ictally). Temporal lobe seizures with fear and autonomic symptoms may be misdiagnosed as panic attacks.

6. **Causing toxicity with high unbound (free) drug levels**

The free, or unbound, portion of a drug is the active component. Free levels are most important to measure with phenytoin because of its high protein binding (90%) and saturation kinetics (small increases in dose or free fraction will lead to dramatic increase in blood level at higher levels). Free phenytoin toxicity is common in patients with chronic illness (including liver and kidney failure, due to low albumin) and in patients on other highly protein bound drugs, *especially valproate* (also tiagabine and benzodiazepines). It is not unusual for patients with refractory seizures to be given high doses of phenytoin, followed by a load of valproate, leading to very high unbound phenytoin levels. This combination can cause lethargy, myoclonus, and even exacerbation of seizures.

7. **Not being aware of important drug interactions**

Valproate (a P450 enzyme inhibitor) dramatically slows the metabolism of lamotrigine, leading to higher risk of severe rash if not dosed properly (should be started at 25 mg every other day). Erythromycin and calcium-channel blockers are also P450 inhibitors that frequently lead to AED toxicity (erythromycin causing carbamazepine toxicity is the most notorious combination). Pregnancy and oral contraceptives can dramatically lower lamotrigine levels. Table 25–4 gives further examples of medications that can influence AED levels. Antacids and sucralfate can block the absorption of AEDs, especially phenytoin. Finally, remember to check for medications that can lower the seizure threshold (see Table 4–1).

8. **Delaying surgical evaluation**

If spells persist after trying two AEDs, video/EEG monitoring and evaluation at a tertiary center is warranted to confirm the diagnosis of epilepsy and consider surgery, especially in temporal lobe epilepsy. Mesial temporal sclerosis (MTS) can be identified reliably on MRI via hippocampal atrophy and increased signal but requires oblique thin-cut coronal views in multiple sequences and expertise that is often lacking outside of tertiary centers. MTS is rarely recognized on routine brain MRI. When MTS is seen on MRI in a patient with

TABLE 25–4 **Important P450 Enzyme Inhibitors and Inducers**

Enzyme inducers can cause decreased effectiveness of Coumadin, oral contraceptives, theophylline, antihypertensives, antibiotics, haloperidol, steroids, cyclosporine, chemotherapeutics, some SSRIs, and many AEDs.		
Carbamazepine	Primidone	
Ethanol (chronic use)	Rifampin	
Carbamazepine	Theophylline	
Phenytoin		
Phenobarbital		
Enzyme inhibitors can cause toxicity or elevated levels of Coumadin, oral contraceptives, theophylline, antihypertensives, antibiotics, haloperidol, steroids, cyclosporine, chemotherapeutics, some SSRIs, and many AEDs.		
Felbamate	Antifungals	Cimetidine
Clarithromycin	Valproate	Clarithromycin
Ca^{2+}-channel blockers	Erythromycin	Isoniazid
Antifungals	Propoxyphene	
Fluoxetine	Ethanol	
Azithromycin		

temporal lobe epilepsy, temporal lobectomy is likely to result in prolonged seizure freedom. Similarly, cortical dysplasia is difficult to recognize on MRI but is a common cause of intractable seizures and often amenable to surgical treatment.

EPILEPSY SURGERY

Focal Resections

There have been dramatic improvements in epilepsy surgery in the past decade, especially in patients with temporal lobe epilepsy. Carefully selected patients with temporal lobe epilepsy (discussed previously) have an 80% cure rate. All patients with lesions associated with epilepsy (most commonly low-grade tumors or vascular malformations) are also good candidates for surgery, with a postoperative seizure-free rate of approximately 90%. Patients with normal MRIs are a more difficult group, although surgery remains a possibility.

Other Neurosurgical Options

When resection of a single seizure focus is not possible, there are multiple other surgical options. *Corpus callosotomy* can be useful in preventing drop attacks and associated injuries. *Hemispherectomy* is highly effective and often beneficial in patients with hemimegalencephaly, Rasmussen's encephalitis, or other severe unilateral epilepsies. *Multiple subpial transections* are a technique used in eloquent regions of the brain where resection cannot be done. In this procedure, horizontal fibers are transected to prevent lateral spread of seizures, whereas vertical pathways are maintained to allow continued functioning of vertically oriented cortical columns.

Gamma knife radiosurgery is being used, primarily in clinical trials, for treatment of medial temporal lobe epilepsy and epilepsy associated with small deep lesions such as hypothalamic hematomas. Finally, brain stimulation trials are in progress, including deep brain stimulation of the anterior nucleus of the thalamus and responsive neurostimulation at the site of seizure onset upon real-time detection of seizure activity with an implanted intracranial device.

OTHER TREATMENT OPTIONS

Ketogenic Diet

This treatment is most useful in children with severe epilepsies. This high-fat, low-carbohydrate diet causes the brain to rely on ketones for energy. This diet is effective for multiple seizure types, with approximately 30% of patients becoming seizure-free and another 30% showing marked improvement. Adverse effects are fairly common, and maintaining the diet can be labor-intensive.

Vagus Nerve Stimulator

This option requires a minor surgery that is similar to having a pacemaker implant, although the wires are placed around the left vagus nerve. Stimulation is typically set for 30 seconds on and 5 minutes off initially, although parameters are adjustable via a computer/wand interface. The mechanism of action is unclear but is thought to involve modulation of a wide neuronal network, including the limbic system, via the nucleus solitarius. Vagus nerve stimulation (VNS) decreases seizures by an average of 30% in multiple seizure types. Approximately 30% will have a significant reduction in seizures; it is very rare for patients to become seizure-free. Efficacy seems to increase over time. Patients may activate stimulation themselves with a hand-held magnet when they feel an aura. Side effects are usually minimal but include change in voice and cough during stimulation. VNS is also effective for treatment of depression.

PREGNANCY AND SEIZURES

All fertile women with epilepsy should be taking folate (1 mg per day; 4 mg per day if planning pregnancy) in order to decrease the risk of neural tube defects in the fetus. All older anticonvulsants are known to be teratogenic. Infants of mothers with epilepsy have a malformation rate of 4% to 6% (versus 2% in the general population). Thus, approximately 95% of mothers with epilepsy will have normal babies.

Teratogenicity is minimized by using a *single drug at the lowest effective dose*. Drug of choice should be based on the patient's seizure syndrome and drug response, independent of the pregnancy. Drugs should not be changed after conception, as this leads to multiple drug exposure. The greatest risk to the fetus from AEDs is in the first trimester. Seizures during pregnancy can also be harmful, especially later in pregnancy. Recent evidence suggests that valproate and phenobarbital have the greatest potential harm to the fetus (teratogenicity or effect on IQ). Lamotrigine appears relatively safe, with a malformation rate of approximately 3% in monotherapy; data on the other newer AEDs is inadequate at present to reach any conclusions. Pregnant women with epilepsy are encouraged to register with the national AED pregnancy registry during their first trimester (1-888-233-2334).

Screening for neural tube defects and other anatomic abnormalities is usually recommended at 16 to 18 weeks with serum triple screen and anatomic fetal ultrasound. It is also recommended that patients be placed on oral vitamin K (10 mg/day from 36 weeks through delivery) to prevent neonatal peripartum hemorrhage due to vitamin K deficiency, particularly in those on enzyme-inducing AEDs (carbamazepine, phenytoin, primidone, phenobarbital) and perhaps valproate, although this has never been proven to be of benefit.

SEIZURES IN SPECIAL SITUATIONS

Perioperative Seizures

Approximately 3% to 6% of patients undergoing supratentorial craniotomy will develop seizures perioperatively, and 8% to 17% will have new-onset seizures within the first year. Patients at highest risk for perioperative seizures include those with large meningiomas, ruptured aneurysms with parenchymal blood, large arteriovenous malformations, and traumatic ICH.

Patients usually recommended for prophylactic perioperative AEDs (usually phenytoin or fosphenytoin) are listed in Table 25–5. **Phenytoin/fosphenytoin dosing: load 20 mg/kg; maintenance is 5 mg/kg per day;** keep levels between 10 and 25 mg/L. Although not evidence-based, levetiracetam is also commonly used in the perioperative or inpatient setting due its ease of use, lack of allergic reactions, and lack of drug interactions.

If no seizures have occurred, AEDs should be discontinued after the patient has recovered from surgery, usually within 2 weeks.

Head Trauma

Patients with significant head trauma who are at increased risk for seizures include those with intracranial bleeding, depressed skull

TABLE 25–5 **Neurosurgical Conditions for Which Short-Term* Perioperative AED Prophylaxis Is Reasonable**

Aneurysms

Subarachnoid hemorrhage and unclipped aneurysm
Unruptured aneurysm only if significant cortical retraction is required
Arteriovenous malformations

Neoplasms

Supratentorial: all
Sellar region: only if significant cortical retraction is required (not posterior fossa tumors)

Infections

Abscess
Subdural empyema
Intracerebral hematoma, spontaneous, supratentorial, requiring evacuation
Subdural hematoma, chronic, requiring craniotomy

Trauma

Any brain injury that requires neurosurgical intervention

*"Short term" refers to less than 2 weeks unless there is persistently raised ICP or an unstable vascular lesion such as an unclipped aneurysm.

fracture, penetrating wound, Glasgow Coma Scale score <10, and early seizures. These patients should receive phenytoin for 1 week prophylactically. Phenytoin does not appear to be effective in preventing the first seizure after this and may impair rehabilitation.

Stroke

Approximately 4% (2% to 6%) of patients with acute infarcts will have early seizures, most within 24 to 48 hours; 3% to 19% with supratentorial hemorrhage have seizures (14% if cortical intracerebral hemorrhage, 4% if deep, 8% if subarachnoid hemorrhage). Late epilepsy after ischemic stroke is seen in 5% to 10% overall and significantly higher in those with early seizures. Prophylactic AEDs are not recommended in general, although short-term use (in the acute setting only) should be considered with large supratentorial strokes with elevated ICP, especially if hemorrhagic, when a seizure could precipitate herniation. Also, see section on nonconvulsive seizures in the critically ill below.

Alcohol

Alcohol-related seizures usually occur approximately 24 hours after the last drink, although they can occur at any time in chronic alcoholics. Alcohol-related seizures should be treated by abstinence; AEDs tend to be ineffective, and patients who continue to drink are usually noncompliant. Prescribing AEDs to alcoholics is usually counterproductive, because frequent withdrawal from the medications can exacerbate seizures, and the combination of AEDs and alcohol can be particularly toxic to the liver. If seizures persist unrelated to alcohol use, chronic AEDs are usually indicated; many of these cases are post-traumatic epilepsy.

Renal Failure

Daily doses of medications should be given after dialysis (on dialysis days); checking free and total levels before and a few hours after dialysis can be helpful. Most medications do not need dramatic adjustment in dose; the exceptions are AEDs with significant renal clearance (gabapentin, topiramate, levetiracetam, zonisamide, and phenobarbital).

Hepatic Failure

Because most AEDs are metabolized by the liver, they must be given "low and slow." Free phenytoin levels should be followed. Avoid valproate in general. Seizures are not often a major problem in patients with liver failure. Consider medications with minimal or no hepatic metabolism (gabapentin and levetiracetam).

Nonconvulsive Seizures in the Critically Ill

Recent studies have shown that many critically ill patients have seizures that can be detected only by EEG monitoring. When continuous EEG monitoring is performed in comatose ICU patients, approximately 20% will have some form of nonconvulsive seizures or status epilepticus; the rate is approximately 10% in medical ICU patients and 30% in neuro-ICU patients. In the vast majority of patients, the seizures are purely electrographic and would be otherwise undetectable without EEG monitoring. Routine (as opposed to 24-hour continuous) EEGs will miss the seizures in approximately half of patients. Risk factors for nonconvulsive seizures in the critically ill include any prior clinical seizure (recent or remote), acute or chronic brain lesions, young age (<18), coma, and abnormal eye movements (nystagmus, deviation, or hippus).

After seemingly successful treatment of convulsive status epilepticus, 20% of patients will still be seizing on EEG. Thus, EEG is mandatory in patients who do not awaken rapidly after convulsive status epilepticus and are in unexplained coma.

Pediatric Neurology

A developmental, social, and family history should be obtained for every pediatric patient seen as an emergency. The guardians' understanding of any preexisting diseases and of the cause of the current events should also be elicited. At a first glance, determine the degree of neurologic compromise by estimating the level of alertness of the child and the need for rapid intervention. Then, direct the interview towards assessing the child's baseline neurologic performance and how the current event departs from it. Infants become more cooperative when they are spoken to in a pleasant voice, and children are less intimidated when the examiner appears to ignore them at first. When possible, children should be examined while resting on their caretaker's lap and should be engaged in conversation and play. Careful observation and holding of normal-appearing children may reveal unsuspected tone anomalies (Fig. 26–1) but should be reserved for the end of the examination. Both intellectual and motor milestones should be documented (Table 26–1). The basic anthropometric measures (weight, length, and, most important, head circumference) should also be charted. Normative growth charts are available from the National Center for Health Statistics, Hyattsville, MD 20782 (http://www.cdc.gov/growthcharts/).

BIRTH TRAUMA

Large (over 4500 g) infants, use of instrumentation during delivery, uncommon fetal presentations, augmented delivery, and first vaginal delivery are all associated with neurologic birth trauma. **Clavicular fracture,** the most common form of trauma, is diagnosed by palpation and, if needed, by radiographs. Spontaneous recovery is the rule. **Brachial plexus injuries** are common in babies with low Apgar scores. Erb (proximal) palsy involves cervical roots C5, C6, and sometimes C7 and results in a "waiter's tip" appearance, with the shoulder held in adduction and internal rotation, the elbow in extension and pronation, and the fingers in flexion (Fig. 26–2). Total plexus lesion is often misnamed as Klumpke (which is the distal) paralysis and is much less frequent. All plexus roots are affected, with

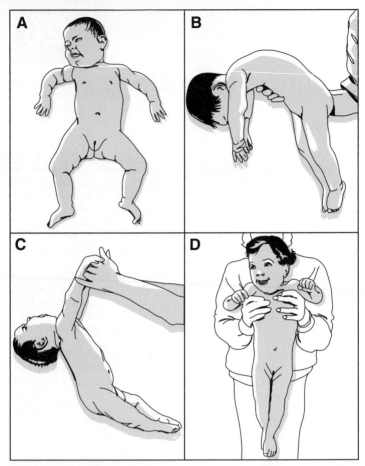

Figure 26–1 Examination of tone. *A* to *C*, Severe hypotonia in an infant with spinal muscular atrophy. *A*, Hypotonic frog-legged posture with arms adducted, legs in external rotation, and knee flexion. All limbs make contact with the examination table. *B*, Ventral suspension revealing limp arms and legs and poor neck extension. *C*, Pulling maneuver demonstrating significant head lag and extended legs. *D*, Hypertonicity after periventricular leukomalacia. The thumbs are in a "cortical" position, and the legs display "scissoring."

TABLE 26–1 **Normal Developmental Milestones**

Age (Months)	Milestones
1 to 1½	Head control; identification of familiar persons
4	Smiling; attempts at lifting up the head briefly
6	Reaching for objects; rolling from prone to supine
8	Transfer between hands; sitting with support; combination of syllables
10	Standing held; fine grasp
12	Walking supported; two- or three-word vocabulary
15	Walking unsupported
18	Command following
24	Phrases
36	Handedness develops

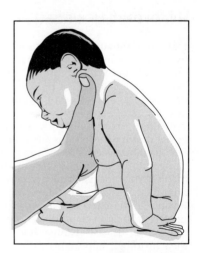

Figure 26–2 Erb palsy in a newborn. The limb is adducted and internally rotated

occasional Horner syndrome from T1 root lesion and hemidiaphragmatic paralysis from C4 injury. EMG shows a diminished number of motor units and fibrillations after 2 to 3 weeks. MRI is informative when suspecting root avulsion, which carries a poor prognosis. The outcome of Erb palsy is good, with marked recovery in 88% and 92% of cases by 4 and 12 months, respectively. Physical therapy is instituted in the second week, and MRI and surgical exploration may be considered in infants who do not improve by the third month.

Spinal cord injury, sometimes caused by rotation of the head during forceps or forceful extraction, may be difficult to appreciate in low-Apgar-score infants. Long-term sequelae include hydromyelia and myelomalacia. C1-C2 subluxation, however, is more common and follows a benign course. Atlantoaxial rotatory subluxation may cause torticollis. When caudal dysraphism is suspected, lumbosacral ultrasounds may be obtained until the sixth month of life. Thereafter, MRI is preferred for diagnosis.

Tentorial subdural hematoma that resolves within the first weeks of life occurs predominantly in neonates who are extracted with vacuum. **Subgaleal hemorrhage** is palpable as a soft collection that crosses skull sutures and may cause progressive anemia and consumption coagulopathy. **Cephalohematoma** is confined to the subperiosteum and therefore respects suture lines. It is firm to palpation and self-limited. Both should be differentiated from **caput succedaneum** caused by subcutaneous edema involving the presenting part during delivery.

HYPOTONIC NEWBORN

Extreme prematurity and **sepsis** are the leading causes of newborn hypotonia. When encephalopathy due to ischemia, Down syndrome, Prader-Willi syndrome, or neurotransmitter disorders has been excluded, attention must be turned to the spinal cord, nerve, or muscle as the cause of hypotonia. **Infantile spinal muscular atrophy** may occasionally present in the newborn period and is sometimes accompanied by arthrogryposis or respiratory failure. Lower motor neuron signs and tongue fasciculations are present. The first diagnostic step is the genotyping of the SMN gene for deletions. **Congenital myotonic dystrophy** can be associated with diaphragmatic hernia and is usually maternally inherited in an autosomal-dominant fashion. Therefore, mothers should be examined for myotonia. **Neonatal myasthenia gravis** is due to placental antibody transfer from a mother afflicted by myasthenia gravis or inflammatory bowel disease. **Congenital myopathies** are characterized by their histologic appearance (with nemaline, central cores, or myotubules), whereas the **metabolic myopathies** mitochondrial DNA depletion syndrome, Pompe disease (with cardiomegaly, macroglossia, and anterior horn cell dysfunction), and cytochrome C oxidase deficiency exhibit specific metabolic abnormalities useful for diagnosis. **Congenital muscular dystrophies** may be associated with cerebral dysgenesis and signs of severe encephalopathy including seizures and hydrocephalus. The **congenital myasthenic syndromes** are caused by mutations in the neuromuscular junction apparatus, and some can manifest with diminished pupillary reactivity or recurrent apnea (the latter sometimes becoming prominent later in childhood), in addition to fatigability and weakness. Often times, an unexplained elevation of serum AST and ALT (originating from muscle instead of liver) in a weak infant (or a child) is the first clue to a myopathy until CK is eventually measured.

CEREBROVASCULAR COMPLICATIONS OF PREMATURITY

Premature infants are susceptible to intraventricular hemorrhage, periventricular hemorrhagic infarction, and periventricular leukomalacia. All are diagnosed by ultrasonography, which can be performed for as long as the anterior fontanelle remains open. **Intraventricular hemorrhage** is associated with extreme prematurity (or birth weight below 1500 g) and occurs within the first few days of life. It is divided into grades I (germinal matrix), II (intraventricular blood that does not distort the ventricular system), III (blood that causes ventricular enlargement), and IV (parenchymal infiltration). Higher grade hemorrhages cause hydrocephalus, manifested as an abrupt increase in head circumference and a bulging fontanelle. Decreased tone or spontaneous movements, loss of pupillary reactivity, apnea, hypotension, and anemia may be associated features. Serial lumbar punctures relieve the hydrocephalus in some cases; the remainder necessitate ventriculoperitoneal or ventriculosubgaleal shunt. Long-term outcome correlates with the degree of parenchymal damage.

Periventricular hemorrhagic infarction, which must be distinguished from intraventricular hemorrhage type IV, is a venous infarct probably caused by compression of terminal veins located under the germinal matrix of the lateral ventricles. The infarct involves the dorsal and lateral aspect of the lateral ventricle and is usually asymmetric, evolving into a cavity that communicates with the ventricle. It is associated with a significant mortality rate and with spastic hemiparesis in survivors.

Periventricular leukomalacia affects the white matter of the centrum semiovale. It is caused by perfusion failure at the border zone between the long penetrator vessels branching off the middle cerebral artery that enter the brain from its surface and the basal lenticulostriate arteries (short penetrators). It may cause spastic quadriparesis with predominant lower extremity involvement or paraplegia (see Fig. 26–1). The lesions tend to cavitate, causing a typical Swiss cheese ultrasound appearance of the white matter.

NEONATAL SEIZURES

Newborns do not display generalized seizures, possibly owing to immature myelination; they may, however, exhibit shifting focality when the epileptogenic process affects the brain diffusely. Causes of neonatal and early infantile seizures are listed in Table 26–2. Except in rare cases, neonatal convulsions are not a benign phenomenon. Newborns and infants younger than 3 months of age with unexplained new-onset seizures should be evaluated and treated for infection until blood, urine, and CSF cultures are negative for at least

TABLE 26–2 **Causes of Neonatal and Early Infantile Seizures**

Sepsis and meningitis
Intrauterine infection (TORCH)
Drug effect or withdrawal
Cerebral dysgenesis
Ischemic encephalopathy
Intraventricular hemorrhage of prematurity
Other intracranial hemorrhages
Biotinidase deficiency
Folinic-acid responsive seizures
Pyridoxine dependency
Glycine encephalopathy
Neonatal maple syrup urine disease
Hypoparathyroidism and hypocalcemia
Menkes disease
Cerebral venous thrombosis
Tuberous sclerosis
Fukuyama muscular dystrophy
Muscle-eye-brain disease
Infantile neuronal ceroid lipofucsinosis
Incontinentia pigmenti
Urea cycle defects
Familial benign neonatal seizures
Organic acidemia
Ketotic hyperglycinemia
Neonatal adrenoleukodystrophy and other leukodystrophies
Gaucher disease type 2
GM_1 gangliosidosis
Herpes simplex encephalitis
Sulfite oxidase deficiency
Glucose transporter type 1 deficiency
Pyruvate dehydrogenase deficiency
Pyruvate carboxylase deficiency

2 days even without fever. In the absence of infection or of cerebral structural abnormality detectable by imaging, the single most important diagnostic procedure is the lumbar puncture. CSF protein levels can be as high as 150 mg/dl in normal newborns, but glucose should never fall below 40 mg/dl. Several polymorphonuclear cells may also be found in the CSF after delivery. A small volume of extra CSF may be stored on ice for specialized analyses for up to 16 hours. Continuous video-EEG monitoring may reveal unsuspected ictal events and background rhythm abnormalities in neonates. Management also includes emergent evaluation of electrolytes and **phenobarbital,** given as a **20 mg/kg IV** load, followed by **5 mg/kg** daily orally or IV. Two repeat loading doses of **10 mg/kg** may be administered for refractory seizures. To avoid respiratory depression, care must be taken not to add a benzodiazepine while administering

phenobarbital. **Fosphenytoin** at a loading dose of **20 mg/kg IV** may substitute or be added to phenobarbital. Intractable seizures may warrant a trial (followed by a course) of pyridoxine, folinic acid, and biotin.

INFANTILE SPASMS

West syndrome (infantile spasms) is an age-specific epilepsy that affects predominantly infants between 4 and 6 months of age. The spasms are seizures characterized by an initial contraction phase (manifested as flexion of the neck, abduction of the shoulders, and flexion of the hips) followed by a more sustained tonic phase. They occur in clusters of increasing frequency and duration. They may be predominantly flexor, extensor, or mixed flexor-extensor spasms, and they may be asymmetric. The EEG eventually demonstrates hypsarrhythmia, and onset of spasms is frequently associated with neurodevelopmental regression. Infantile spasms are classified as either symptomatic or cryptogenic by the International League Against Epilepsy. The symptomatic group is recognized by their coexistence with prior encephalopathy (as revealed by psychomotor retardation, neurologic signs, radiologic abnormalities, or other types of seizures). Prenatal causes include chromosomal abnormalities, inborn errors of metabolism, and neurocutaneous syndromes (such as tuberous sclerosis, cortical malformations, and intrauterine infections). Perinatal causes include ischemic encephalopathy and birth trauma. Postnatal causes include CNS trauma, infection, and intracranial hemorrhage. The smaller cryptogenic group is characterized by the lack of prior encephalopathy or of known cause, and it is associated with a better long-term outcome. Both **ACTH IM** and **vigabatrin** are effective first-choice agents, administered in a variety of dosing regimens.

FEBRILE SEIZURES

Febrile seizures occur in children between 6 months and 5 years of age in association with fever without nervous system infection. Although they may display any type of semiology, they usually are generalized tonic-clonic or tonic. They recur for a second time in one third of children, and of those, one half may experience further episodes. Early age at the time of seizure onset, preexisting neurologic anomalies, persistence for more than 15 minutes, or focal features all increase the likelihood of subsequent epilepsy and warrant investigation by EEG and MRI. The main management decisions are whether to perform a lumbar puncture to rule out infection and whether to prescribe prophylactic antiepileptics. When in doubt, a lumbar puncture should be performed. Recurrent febrile seizures do not necessitate the use of prophylactic anticonvulsants but may be treated with **5 mg rectal diazepam gel.**

DISORDERS THAT RESEMBLE SEIZURES

Syncope may be followed by automatisms and be pallid (thought to represent an exaggerated autonomic response) or cardiogenic (which may be due to congenital heart disease or long QT syndrome). **Breath-holding spells** occur between 6 months and 2 years of age and are preceded by vigorous crying and followed by brief apnea and cyanosis. **Sandiffer syndrome,** caused by gastric reflux, can mimic tonic seizures and be accompanied by autonomic dysfunction. **Hyperexplexia** results in loss of tone in response to a sudden stimulus with preserved consciousness. Excessive startle is a feature of some cerebral degenerations such as Tay-Sachs disease. **Benign myoclonus of infancy** occurs as an isolated phenomenon in a normal neurologic substrate and disappears by 12 months of age. Isolated **apnea** is rarely a seizure manifestation but can be prominent in nonketotic hyperglycinemia. **Paroxysmal dyskinesias** may be elicited by movement (kinesogenic) or occur at rest (nonkinesogenic). **Spasmus nutans** is a benign condition that usually occurs before 1 year of age and disappears within 2 years. It includes head nodding, torticollis, and nystagmus. When monocular nystagmus is the presenting sign, MRI must be performed to exclude optic nerve glioma. **Oculogyric crises** may last from seconds to hours and can be caused by a variety of agents that interfere with neurotransmitter function or by aromatic L-amino acid decarboxylase deficiency.

INFECTIONS OF THE CENTRAL NERVOUS SYSTEM

Meningitis, encephalitis, and cerebral abscess are the most common CNS infections in children. The signs of meningitis may be absent in children who are younger than 3 years of age or neutropenic (absolute neutrophil count below 1000 per mm³). In the newborn, the most common organisms are group B *Streptococcus, Escherichia coli,* and *Listeria monocytogenes. Citrobacter* spp. cause cerebral abscesses via hemorrhagic necrosis; in general, these abscesses should not be drained. During infancy and preschool age, the responsible agents are *Haemophilus influenzae, Neisseria meningitidis,* and *Streptococcus pneumoniae* and in school age, *N. meningitidis* and *S. pneumoniae.* Treatment of meningitis in infants and children should include **dexamethasone 0.15 mg/kg every 6 hours** for 4 days. For empiric antibiotic coverage, see Table 21–2. Sequelae of meningitis include hydrocephalus, mental retardation, epilepsy, and hearing loss. Except for *Citrobacter* infection, meningitis does not cause abscess, and therefore, predisposing cardiopulmonary conditions should be investigated in every case of cerebral abscess.

FULMINANT ENCEPHALOPATHIES OF INFANCY AND CHILDHOOD

Several inflammatory disorders may first manifest with fever, depressed consciousness, seizures, meningeal signs, and CSF pleocytosis in the absence of infection. **Acute disseminated encephalomyelitis** preferentially affects children over 2 years of age and follows trivial infections, immunizations, or the administration of certain drugs by 2 to 21 days. The lesions are widespread, with preferential white matter and occasional gray matter and peripheral nerve involvement. However, CT abnormalities may be undetectable until the second week after onset. MRI is abnormal from the beginning of the neurologic illness, and up to 60% of the lesions enhance with gadolinium. A polymorphonuclear pleocytosis is commonly found in CSF, which later becomes mononuclear. The CSF glucose level is normal, and the protein is elevated. The course may be polyphasic, particularly in patients treated with steroids. **Postinfectious cerebellitis** can present with acute and profound cerebellar dysfunction, often following the resolution of a trivial infectious illness. **Neuromyelitis optica** (Devic disease) is associated with optic neuritis and necrotizing myelitis occurring either simultaneously or in succession, often without CSF oligoclonal protein bands and often accompanied by cerebral white matter demyelinating plaques. **Acute toxic encephalopathy** is more common in children younger than 2 years and may also be preceded by banal infections. It causes cerebral edema without inflammation. The CSF is under high pressure but its composition is normal. **Acute hemorrhagic encephalitis** is the least common postinfectious and postvaccinal disorder. The pathologic process consists of a small-vessel necrotizing vasculitis of gray and white matter with circulating atypical lymphocytes and albuminuria. The CSF pleocytosis occurs at the expense of polymorphonuclear cells. **Serum sickness** occurs as an adverse drug reaction, accompanied by CSF polymorphonuclear, lymphocytic, or eosinophilic pleocytosis, elevated protein, and sometimes, peripheral eosinophilia. Numerous immune-modulating agents can cause a similar picture. CT is usually normal. **Systemic lupus erythematosus** occasionally presents with aseptic meningitis, epilepsy, or psychosis. **Behçet disease** may also present with meningitis or seizures caused by vasculitis in association with orogenital ulcers and uveitis. **Metabolic encephalopathies** are an important consideration even when acute encephalopathy presents without preexisting evidence of an abnormal neurologic substrate. Among these, organic acidemias, Leigh syndrome (subacute necrotizing encephalopathy), aminoacidopathies, urea cycle disorders, fatty acid oxidation defects, and mitochondrial encephalomyopathy with ragged red fibers and strokelike episodes (MELAS) must be considered. Analysis of serum glucose, carnitine metabolites, amino acids, ammonia, creatine kinase and lactate, of urinary ketones and other organic acids, and of CSF amino acids, lactate, and pyruvate constitutes an effective initial screening strategy. A dietary trigger may sometimes be identified, as may be a mild prior infection. In the neonate, prompt retrieval of the cursory newborn screening results is mandatory, although not all disorders are screened in all locations (for a U.S. listing, consult http://genes-r-us.uthscsa.edu/resources/newborn/state.htm).

PEDIATRIC STROKE

Fetal stroke is rare and may be the consequence of maternal alloimmune thrombocytopenia, intrauterine cocaine exposure, or trauma, evolving into porencephaly. In the **neonate,** cardiovascular malformations, elevated plasma homocysteine, polycythemia, factor-V Leiden mutation, protein C or S deficiency, prothrombin mutation, placental embolism, and institution of extracorporeal membrane oxygenation are associated with stroke. Typically, the signs of hemispheric infarction are short-lived (except when complicated by seizures) and do not manifest again until approximately 6 months of age, when hemiparesis becomes clinically detectable. Transthoracic (as opposed to transesophageal) echocardiography is sufficient to diagnose most cardiac malformations, including persistent foramen ovale. **Older children** are also susceptible to stroke from cardiogenic emboli. In addition, Fabry disease (associated to skin angiokeratomas and neuropathy), Moyamoya disease (caused by dysplastic large intracranial vessels leading to compensatory proliferation of malformed capillaries), a common entity in both Asian children and in patients with sickle cell disease, and arterial dissection (as the consequence of neck trauma) are all causes of childhood stroke. Children with sickle cell disease are particularly prone to recurrent "silent" infarcts (generally affecting the deep frontal white matter) starting from infancy and causing intellectual decline or poor scholastic achievement. When the medial cerebral artery flow velocity is elevated beyond 200 cm/sec in transcranial Doppler measurements, the risk of stroke is very significant unless transfusions are instituted. Conditions mimicking stroke include MELAS (in older children) and alternating hemiplegia of childhood (with onset during infancy), the latter sometimes caused by a disorder of energy metabolism.

VENTRICULOPERITONEAL SHUNT MALFUNCTION

Permanent drainage of CSF is accomplished by ventriculojugular, ventriculoatrial, ventriculouretheral, or, most commonly, by ventriculoperitoneal shunt. The most common cause of congenital or infantile-onset hydrocephalus is aqueductal stenosis, followed by late sequelae of intracranial hemorrhage or infection. Proximal shunt malfunction is caused by either disconnection or obstruction of the intracranial portion of the shunt by hemorrhage or protein. Distal shunt fracture or tip occlusion with viscus perforation or penetration through the retroperitoneal or abdominal fascia may also occur. Complete malfunction in the infant manifests as irritability, feeding difficulties, an enlarged head, and a tense fontanelle. In the older child, it first causes headache, vomiting, and progressive depression of consciousness. Seizures may seldom occur, and they suggest shunt infection. An infected shunt additionally causes fever but rarely local signs of infection. Partial shunt malfunction is insidious, develops over weeks or months, and causes poor cognition (first manifested as school difficulties), papilledema, sixth nerve and upgaze palsies, hyper-reflexia, and lower extremity hypertonicity. The evaluation involves a radiographic shunt series to assess the continuity and position of the system, a head CT to determine ventricular size (most helpful when prior scans are available for comparison), and tapping of the shunt reservoir by a neurosurgeon with measurement of the pressure if distal malfunction is suspected. All CSF samples should be routinely analyzed and cultured. If malfunction cannot be excluded, admission for observation is warranted. When it is suspected or confirmed, urgent neurosurgical consultation is required. Infected shunts should generally be removed as soon as infection is found and temporary ventriculostomy considered. The term, overshunting refers to low CSF pressure due to excess drainage. It may cause subdural hematoma and postural headaches that are alleviated when the patient is in a supine position.

TUMORS

The mode of presentation of brain tumors depends on volume and location, infiltration of brain and meninges, and development of hydrocephalus. In infancy, they may cause irritability, failure to thrive, developmental arrest and regression, poor feeding, vomiting, and macrocephaly. In childhood, they may not produce localizing neurologic signs but cause instead progressive and recurrent episodes of headache, ataxia, and vomiting as well as a rapid increase in head circumference. **Supratentorial hemispheric** tumors, most commonly low-grade astrocytomas and malignant gliomas, may produce focal neurologic deficits and seizures. **Supratentorial midline** tumors such as low-grade gliomas, craniopharyngiomas, and pineal tumors may compress the optic chiasm, producing visual disturbances; may affect the hypothalamus, altering endocrine function, appetite, and behavior; and may cause Parinaud syndrome or obstructive hydrocephalus. **Infratentorial** tumors cause a variety of symptoms: diffuse brain stem glioma causes cranial neuropathies and long tract signs; cerebellar astrocytomas, medulloblastomas, and ependymomas produce ataxia, hydrocephalus, and vomiting.

On occasion, highly inflammatory demyelinating lesions may be difficult to differentiate from tumors, and brain biopsy is recommended. **Neuroblastomas** are extraneural tumors (most commonly abdominal) that in two thirds of cases are associated with neurologic complications such as metastasis, carcinomatous meningitis, and paraneoplastic opsoclonus-myoclonus. The latter causes erratic, conjugate eye movements ("dancing eyes") and irritability. Emergency **management** of brain tumors includes CT followed by staging MRI including the spine for tumors that are suspected to expand multifocally. **Dexamethasone,** administered **at 0.1 mg/kg four times a day,** relieves symptoms caused by peritumoral edema. Neurosurgical consultation for biopsy, resection, or relief of hydrocephalus must be obtained.

HEAD INJURY

Initial management of minor accidental head trauma requires establishing the likelihood of cerebral injury and the need for CT scanning of the head. In general, children with a normal examination who have fallen out of bed onto a hard surface, who wore protective equipment such as a helmet, or who were injured more than 6 hours prior to the examination have not sustained cerebral damage. Similarly, brief amnesia, headache, vomiting up to three times, and scalp laceration (alone or in combination) do not suggest brain injury. On the other hand, in the presence of seizures, alteration of consciousness, skull fracture (including raccoon eyes or Battle signs), or focal neurologic deficit, cerebral injury must be suspected. **Diagnosis** of suspected brain injury relies on CT. Skull radiographs are not sufficient. **Management** of suspected brain injury with normal CT includes admission to the hospital for a 24- to 48-hour observation period. The neurologic status should be assessed periodically. A CT demonstrating hemorrhage or significant contusion must be repeated in 6 to 12 hours, along with prompt evaluation of coagulation. **Fosphenytoin IV** may be administered when CT is abnormal and neurosurgical consultation must be considered. Skull radiographs and palpation should be performed 2 months after skull fracture in children younger than 2 years of age to detect fracture expansion with arachnoid herniation.

CHILD ABUSE

Shaken-baby syndrome should be suspected in injured infants and children younger than 3 years of age. The history is usually vague, and trivial head trauma disproportionate to the degree of injury is commonly invoked by the perpetrators. Abused children may fail to thrive and are sometimes admitted to the hospital solely for that reason. While hospitalized, these children quickly grow and gain weight.

Extracranial lesions include finger marks over the chest and limbs, bruising, burns, lacerations, and skeletal fractures, particularly those involving the lateral ribs and metaphyses of long bones. The lesions may have been inflicted at different times, as manifested by a yellowish discoloration of the older skin lesions. **Intracranial injuries** are subdural hematoma, subarachnoid hemorrhage with a preference for the interhemispheric fissure, loss of gray-white matter differentiation due to axonal shearing, cerebral contusion, skull fracture, and retinal hemorrhages. Layering of subdural blood is indicative of trauma of different ages after coagulopathy has been excluded. **Clinical presentation** includes lethargy, irritability, seizures, meningeal signs, vomiting, poor feeding, apnea, a bulging fontanelle, and coma.

The **differential diagnosis** includes the retinal hemorrhages seen in up to 40% of vaginally delivered newborns (which resolve within 1 month), coagulopathy, sepsis, osteogenesis imperfecta (with blue sclerae, dental anomalies, short stature, and angulation of healed fractures), glutaric aciduria type I (with developmental delay, hypotonia, cerebral opercular hypotrophy, and chronic subdural collections), Menkes disease (in males), benign subdural fluid collections of infancy (usually bifrontal), and accidental trauma.

The **diagnosis** must be parsimoniously pursued and the legal authorities alerted; it requires head CT scanning including bone windows, a radiographic skeletal survey, fundoscopy after mydriasis, coagulation profile (platelet count, PT, PTT), urinary organic acids, and serum copper (in males). Photographs of all visible injuries should be taken. Cerebral gradient ECHO MRI aids with the identification of hemorrhage of different ages. Lumbar puncture performed to evaluate cases confounded with sepsis reveals a bloody fluid. Ophthalmologic consultation should document any retinal findings.

BRAIN DEATH

Determination of brain death in a child younger than 1 year of age represents a special challenge, as the developing brain possesses a greater potential for recovery than the adult brain does. **Requisites** for the diagnosis of brain death include knowing the cause of coma, documentation of normothermia, normotension, and a normal metabolic and toxicologic profile, including the absence of prescribed agents that depress the nervous system. **Examination** must reveal coma, apnea, mid positioned or dilated unreactive pupils, absence of oculocephalic and caloric reflexes, absent corneal reflexes, absent gag reflex, flaccidity, and absence of spontaneous movements. In preterm infants before the thirty-second gestational week, most brain stem reflexes remain undeveloped and therefore may not be assessed. The respiratory drive in response to sustained apnea may also develop as late as the thirty-third week. Structural lesions in the posterior fossa that may resemble brain death include tumors, subdural hematoma, and Dandy-Walker and Chiari malformations and should be ruled out by imaging. **Adjunctive** diagnostic methods include radioisotopic cerebral blood flow determination, cerebral angiography, and EEG. In neonates, however, cerebral flow may persist after brain death, and it is only of diagnostic value when absent. Age-related brain death **criteria** may be locally legislated and may include:

1. For patients over 1 year
   Two examinations spaced 12 to 24 hours
   EEG and cerebral blood flow determinations optional
2. For patients 2 months to 1 year
   Two examinations and EEGs 24 hours apart *or*
   One examination with an EEG and a cerebral blood flow
       study
3. For patients 7 days to 2 months
   Two examinations and EEGs 48 hours apart

The latter criteria may be extended to term newborns younger than 7 days of age, but consensus has not been reached. In anencephaly, adjunctive techniques such as EEG and cerebral blood flow studies are not needed, and they may be impractical for anatomic reasons; the diagnosis is therefore clinical.

Dementia

Memory dysfunction may be variable in its presentation and ranges from the highly functioning senior citizen complaining of forgetfulness to the patient brought in by a relative for bizarre behavior and confusion. **Amnesia** is defined as a pure loss of memory without other cognitive dysfunction. **Dementia** implies chronic, progressive cognitive loss including chronic loss of memory to a degree sufficient to interfere with occupational or social performance. Dementia should not be confused with **delirium,** which is an acute, global disorder of thinking and perception characterized by impaired consciousness and inattention (see Chapter 8). **Retrograde amnesia** refers to loss of memory for events before a specific point in time. **Anterograde amnesia** is the inability to lay down new memory. Memory is often categorized into **immediate recall** (seconds), **short-term memory** (minutes to hours), and **long-term memory** (days to years), with short-term memory being the most vulnerable to pathologic processes, both in acute amnestic states and in dementia syndromes. The hippocampi and parahippocampal structures, and dorsomedial thalamus along with the dorsolateral prefrontal cortex, have been implicated in short-term memory function. Verbal memory is mediated predominantly by the left hemisphere, and visuospatial memory is mediated by the right hemisphere.

The differential diagnosis of dementia can be categorized as follows:

V (**vascular**): cerebral infarction, multiple strokes, diffuse white-matter ischemia, bilateral thalamic infarctions, amyloid angiopathy

I (**infectious**): syphilis, chronic meningitis (tubercular or fungal), AIDS, progressive multifocal leukoencephalopathy, herpes simplex encephalitis, Creutzfelt-Jacob disease, subacute sclerosing panencephalitis, Whipple's disease

T (**traumatic**): subdural hematoma, dementia pugilistica, head injury

A (**autoimmune**): CNS vasculitis, multiple sclerosis, systemic lupus erythematosus (SLE), Hashimoto's encephalopathy

M (**metabolic/toxic**): renal failure, hepatic failure, hypothyroidism, hypercalcemia, benzodiazepine and other tranquilizer intoxication, chronic alcohol use (Wernicke-Korsakoff syndrome), vitamin B_{12} deficiency, nicotinic acid deficiency (pellagra), lead exposure, carbon monoxide exposure

I **(idiopathic/inherited):** Alzheimer's disease, Huntington's disease, Parkinson's disease dementia, dementia with Lewy bodies, frontotemporal dementia, progressive supranuclear palsy, cortical basal ganglionic degeneration, transient global amnesia

N **(neoplastic):** brain tumor, paraneoplastic limbic encephalitis, meningeal carcinomatosis, postradiation effects

S **(seizure, psychiatric, structural):** complex partial seizure, postictal state, depression (pseudodementia), normal-pressure hydrocephalus

Examination of the Demented Patient

Dementia can be screened for with the standardized Mini–Mental State Examination (MMSE). A score less than 28 out of 30 in a younger person or less than 24 out of 30 in an older person is abnormal. The MMSE yields a quantitative score, which can be used to monitor the patient over time.

1. Higher Cortical Function
   a. Alertness and attentiveness
      Have the patient count backward from 20 to 1 or recite the months of the year backward. Serial sevens (serially subtracting 7 from 100) can be used also, but the test may be influenced by education level.
   b. Aphasia
      Check for the following:
      (1) Fluency
          Listen for effortful, nonfluent speech with loss of grammar and syntax, not just word-finding difficulties.
      (2) Naming
          Anomia is a nonspecific finding common to all types of aphasia but may be the only language function affected in Alzheimer's disease.
      (3) Auditory comprehension of single and multistep commands
          For example, use commands such as "Show two fingers" or "With your eyes closed, tap your right knee with two fingers of your left hand."
      (4) Repetition of unfamiliar phrases
          When testing repetition, avoid stock phrases such as "no ifs, ands, or buts," which may be overlearned, practiced utterances. Using a sentence such as "The spy fled to Greece" for testing both repetition and reading aloud may yield a clinically important dissociation (e.g., conduction aphasia versus pure alexia).
      (5) Reading aloud

(6) Writing

Have the patient write his or her name, a dictated sentence, and a spontaneous sentence.

(7) Listen for phonemic paraphasias (substitution of one phoneme for another within a word: e.g., "tadle" for "table") or semantic paraphasias (substitution of one semantically related word for another: e.g., "door" for "window").

c. Memory

Check for immediate recall by asking the patient to repeat number strings (digit span). Reciting fewer than six numbers forward or four numbers backward is abnormal for younger patients; reciting fewer than six numbers forward or three numbers backward is abnormal for patients over 65 years of age. Check short-term memory by asking the patient to repeat three words and then to recall them after 5 minutes. Long-term memory and fund of knowledge can be tested by asking the current month and year or the patient's address and phone number and by asking the patient to name present and past presidents, mayors, or sports players. Be sure to take into account education level and interests (the patient may follow sports but not politics, or vice versa).

d. Calculations

Ask the patient to do two-digit addition or multiplication, based on his or her education level, or to tell you how many quarters are in $1.75.

e. Hemineglect

Have the patient bisect a horizontal line. Average deviation from the true midline greater than 10% on six lines is abnormal. Ask the patient to perform a target cancellation task (e.g., to circle all letter "a"s in an array of letters); look for left-right asymmetry in targets missed.

f. Apraxia

Apraxia is impairment of the execution of a learned or imitated movement in the absence of weakness, sensory loss, or incoordination. Ask the patient to pantomime or imitate striking a match or opening a lock with a key. Abnormal performance on this task (ideomotor apraxia) may be seen in Alzheimer's disease and other dementias. In more severe dementia, inability to use real objects in a sequence of acts may be seen (ideational apraxia), for example, inability to put on and button a shirt.

g. Drawing

Have the patient copy a complex figure, for example, interlocking pentagons or the Rey Complex Figure shown in Figure 27–1. Dyspraxia for drawing (constructional apraxia) may be found in dementia. Evidence of hemine-

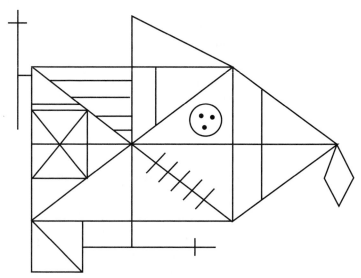

Figure 27–1 Rey Complex Figure.

glect may also be picked up by this test (e.g., the left side of the drawing is incomplete or less organized than the right).

2. Motor

Look for signs of hemiparesis that may suggest a focal lesion such as subdural hematoma, stroke, or tumor. Adventitial movements such as myoclonus, chorea, and tremor often accompany degenerative dementias, particularly in the later stages. Signs of parkinsonism should suggest dementia with Lewy bodies, progressive supranuclear palsy, or Parkinson's disease dementia, but may also be seen in Alzheimer's disease or in patients treated with neuroleptics.

3. Coordination and gait

Ataxia may be present with Wernicke-Korsakoff syndrome. A magnetic gait, characterized by hesitancy and shuffling in initiation of gait and difficulty in turning 180 degrees, is seen in normal-pressure hydrocephalus (triad of urinary incontinence, gait dysfunction, and dementia).

4. Signs of frontal lobe dysfunction

Frontal lobe dysfunction may produce a disinhibition of motor and behavioral functions, signaled by the appearance of frontal release signs such as persistent blinking when the examiner taps the forehead just above the bridge of the nose (Myerson's or glabellar sign) or the snouting, rooting, grasp,

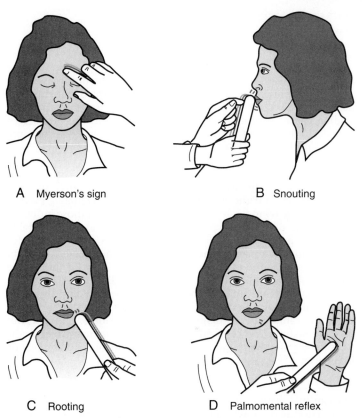

A   Myerson's sign

B   Snouting

C   Rooting

D   Palmomental reflex

Figure 27–2 Frontal release signs. *A*, Myerson's sign. Patient displays persistent blinking (does not habituate) to repeated taps to the brow above the bridge of the nose. *B*, Snouting. Patient purses lips reflexively in response to tapping with a pen or tongue blade. *C*, Rooting. Patient's lips and mouth deviate toward a light scratch to the side of the mouth. *D*, Palmomental reflex. Patient's chin twitches when the palm is scratched.

and palmomental reflexes (Fig. 27–2), although these responses are not always due to disturbances of the frontal lobes. Other tests that may indicate frontal lobe dysfunction are the go-no-go test, where the examiner gives the patient two different tasks to perform in response to two different cues ("If I show you one finger then you show me two, and if I show you two fingers then you show me none"), or the Luria three-step hand motion sequence.

PRIMARY NEURODEGENERATIVE DISORDERS

Alzheimer's Disease

Alzheimer's disease (AD) is the most common neurodegenerative dementia, representing anywhere from 50% to 80% of patients with dementia. AD is on par with cerebrovascular disease as the third leading cause of death in the United States, and the number of patients in the United States with AD is expected to increase to more than 13 million by 2050.

Risk Factors

The most important risk factor for AD is age. AD rarely presents before age 65, and the prevalence doubles approximately every 5 years from age 65 to 85, to as high as 35% to 40% in those individuals over age 85. A small percentage of AD (<5%) is attributable directly to genetic causes, including mutations in the genes for amyloid precursor protein and the presenilins, and tends to present at an earlier age. The e4 allele of the apolipoprotein E (ApoE) gene has also been established as a susceptibility allele for AD. Despite the strong evidence linking ApoE e4 homozygosity and increased risk for AD, ApoE genotyping is not routinely done due to lack of predictive value. The vast majority of AD is considered sporadic, but an increased prevalence of family history in patients with sporadic AD suggests that the sporadic form may also be mediated by genetic influences.

Clinical Presentation

The cardinal feature of AD is the insidious onset of **memory loss,** with associated slowly progressive decline in other cognitive domains. Patients and family members often have difficulty dating the onset of memory decline due to its slow progression, and instead may report a fairly sudden onset of symptoms, likely related to a worrisome event, such as getting lost or leaving a pot on the stove. A careful history, with specific attention paid to changes in performance status, evokes the more protracted course of cognitive and functional decline. It is important to confirm the history with one or more family members, because patients with memory loss often lack insight into the extent of their impairment. Memory loss is initially manifest as forgetfulness for new information, such as names or recent events, but with progression of the disease more remote memories are also lost. Initial **language decline** is characterized by dysnomia and overall reduced conversational output. Language becomes progressively dysfluent, with eventual compromise of comprehension, and in later stages can progress to near mutism. **Visuospatial disorientation** may initially present as misplacing objects or difficulty drawing complex figures. Functionally, patients often are noted to have worsening directions ability. Driving ability becomes impaired, and, with progression of the disease, patients can become disoriented in previously familiar locations. Other aspects of cognitive decline often seen in early AD include **difficulty with calculation** (often manifest as difficulty handling money or balancing a checkbook) and **executive dysfunction** (leading to impaired organizational skills and impaired judgment). In contrast to the progressive cognitive deficits, social and interpersonal skills are relatively preserved, although with disease progression these functions are also compromised. **Behavioral changes** and **perceptual disorders** are also characteristic of AD. Delusions are common, often manifesting as paranoia, including fear of others causing harm or stealing. Behavioral disturbances such as disinhibition, agitation, wandering, and sleep disturbance are more common in advanced stages of AD and can lead to significant strain on caregivers. These symptoms, in combination with the progressive loss of basic independent skills such as feeding, bathing, and toileting, often lead to placement of late-stage AD patients in nursing homes. Survival of patients with AD is variable, but life expectancy can be shortened due to complications of severe cognitive decline, such as malnutrition, dehydration, and infections.

Diagnosis

The diagnosis of AD is made clinically. The list of criteria for diagnosis of Alzheimer's dementia found in the DSM-IV states that there must be a gradual onset and continuing decline of cognitive function from a previously higher level, resulting in impairment of social and occupational function, that there is an impairment in recent memory as well as impairment in at least one other cognitive domain (including language, praxis, visual processing, construction, spatial abstraction, and executive function), and that these deficits are not due to any other psychiatric, neurologic, or systemic diseases and do not occur exclusively in the setting of delirium. A thorough history should include full functional and psychiatric assessments. Outside of mental status testing, most AD patients will have a relatively normal neurologic examination, and any major or lateralizing abnormalities should be more fully investigated. Many AD patients will exhibit some degree of paratonia or extrapyramidal rigidity. A thorough general examination should be performed to exclude any evidence of systemic disease that could be contributing to cognitive impairment. Routine blood work and ancillary tests to rule out other treatable disorders should be done (see diagnostic testing above). CSF analysis is not routinely performed in patients presenting with gradual cognitive decline after the age of 65 but is done to rule out treatable diseases in younger patients, in whom a diagnosis of AD would be less common. Brain MRI or CT should be done to rule out any structural abnormalities or hydrocephalus. Functional neuroimaging studies such as PET or SPECT showing characteristic posterior parietotemporal hypometabolism is consistent with but does not establish the diagnosis, since the same patterns may be observed in patients without AD. There is no "diagnostic" imaging test available at this time. A diagnosis of AD is considered *probable* or *possible* depending on the presence of typical or atypical clinical features. The diagnosis can only be *proven* with histopathologic evidence of amyloid plaques and neurofibrillary tangles in brain specimens obtained from autopsy (or biopsy, which is rarely indicated).

Treatment

There are no curative or disease-modifying treatments currently available for AD, but there are a number of medications that have been shown to have modest but significant symptomatic benefit. The mainstays of medical therapy to treat memory dysfunction are the centrally acting cholinesterase inhibitors donepezil (Aricept), rivastigmine (Exelon), and galantamine (Reminyl), which reduce the breakdown of acetylcholine in brain synapses. Enhancement of CNS cholinergic tone may have positive effects on learning and memory. For symptomatic treatment of memory dysfunction in mild, moderate, and severe AD, start one of the three agents listed below:

Donepezil 5 mg qAM, increase to 10 mg qAM in 4 weeks, as tolerated

Rivastigmine 1.5 mg bid, increase to 6 mg bid over 4 weeks, as tolerated

Galantamine 4 mg bid, increase to 12 mg bid over 8 weeks, as tolerated

Watch for gastrointestinal side effects, weight loss, increased confusion, or insomnia. For treatment of moderate to severe AD, memantine (Namenda), an N-methyl-D-aspartate receptor antagonist, may also have some symptomatic benefit. **Start memantine at 5 mg qd and increase by 5 mg weekly to a target dose of 10 mg bid.** Vitamin E has been reported to delay functional decline but must be prescribed with caution, especially in those patients with bleeding diatheses or those who are subject to frequent falls. Other agents may also be particularly useful for treating other symptomatic and behavioral manifestations of AD (Table 27–1). The selective serotonin reuptake inhibitors are helpful for treatment of concomitant depression and sleep disturbances. The atypical antipsychotics are also often used to treat more severe behavioral disturbances and hallucinations, but these agents must be used with caution in the elderly due to the risk of sedation and extrapyramidal side effects, as well as the increased risk of cardiovascular and cerebrovascular disease.

Frontotemporal Dementia

First described in 1892 by Arnold Pick, frontotemporal dementia (FTD) comprises a set of neurodegenerative syndromes characterized by circumscribed atrophy of the frontal and/or temporal lobes.

TABLE 27–1 **Medications That May Be Associated with Memory Impairment**

Benzodiazepines	Chlorpromazine
Anticonvulsants (overdose)	Cyclosporine
Corticosteroids	Anticonvulsants (overdose)
Isoniazid	Interleukins
Benzodiazepines	Interferons
Barbiturates	Methotrexate
Bromides	Clioquinol (antifungal)

These disorders are linked by the presence of focal, severe fronto-temporal atrophy and common histopathologic features, including spongiform degeneration, ballooned neurons either with tau or ubiquitin inclusions (Pick bodies), or the absence of any defining histopathology (dementia lacking distinctive histology). FTD can present as either a behavior-dominant or a language-dominant syndrome, with language-dominant presentations further subdivided into a primary defect in language expression, also called primary progressive aphasia (PPA), and a primary defect in comprehension and word meaning, also called semantic dementia (SD). Although memory and spatial ability may become affected in FTD patients over time, these areas of cognition are relatively spared early on in the disease process. FTD prevalence is much lower than AD, with frequencies ranging from 1% to 15% of overall dementia patients. FTD tends to present at a younger age than AD (mean age 50 to 65 years). In this age group, prevalence of AD and FTD are similar. Abrupt onset with ictal events and a recent history of head trauma are exclusion features. Two related disorders, progressive supranuclear palsy (PSP), and cortical basal ganglionic degeneration (CBD), can present with cognitive impairment and motor symptoms. There are genetic associations of FTD with both parkinsonism and ALS, and FTD patients should be clinically screened for these conditions.

Behavioral FTD

This syndrome is characterized by early **progressive personality change** and **early decline in social interpersonal conduct.** Emotional blunting, impairment in personal conduct, and early loss of insight into these changes are also cardinal features of the disease. Associated behavioral changes such as decline in grooming and personal hygiene, disinhibition, mental inflexibility, hyperorality and hypersexuality (Klyver-Bucy syndrome), perseveration, and utilization behavior (unrestrained exploration of objects in the environment) are supportive of the diagnosis. Alterations in speech and language are also frequently seen, with decreased spontaneous speech, stereotypy, perseveration, echolalia, and mutism.

Neuroimaging showing marked frontal and anterior temporal atrophy, hypometabolism, and/or hypoperfusion is part of the diagnostic criteria.

Primary Progressive Aphasia

The core diagnostic feature of primary progressive aphasia (PPA) is the insidious onset and gradual progression of **loss of speech fluency,** with associated **anomia, phonemic paraphasias,** and **agrammatism** (inappropriate word order and simplified sentence structure). Word meaning is preserved early in the disease, but stuttering, oral apraxia, impaired repetition, alexia, and agraphia are often present. With time, patients become mute and can develop behavioral changes similar to behavioral FTD. Imaging reveals early left (dominant) perisylvian atrophy, usually more anterior than posterior.

Semantic Dementia

In semantic dementia (SD), the language disorder is characterized by **fluent but empty spontaneous speech with loss of word meaning.** SD patients often present with word-finding difficulties and also exhibit anomia, which stems from a fundamental loss of semantic knowledge about the item, leading to deficient object recognition with the associated naming defect. Semantic paraphasias are often present. Neuroimaging shows structural and/or metabolic changes of the left (dominant) anterior temporal lobe. With disease progression, more anterior language deficits and behavioral changes become evident.

Progressive Supranuclear Palsy

Progressive supranuclear palsy (PSP) is characterized by **vertical gaze palsy** with predominant downgaze abnormality, **axial rigidity,** and **postural instability.** Progressive cognitive impairment mainly involving the frontal lobes tends to evolve during the course of the disease. PSP does not tend to respond to treatment with levodopa.

Cortical Basal Ganglionic Degeneration

The clinical syndrome of cortical basal ganglionic degeneration (CBD) is progressive cognitive impairment with associated **asymmetric rigidity, apraxia, cortical sensory loss,** and **pyramidal dysfunction.** Patients may manifest the phenomenon of alien limb, where the limb seems to move without voluntary control, but this feature is not essential to the diagnosis. Myoclonus and focal limb dystonia are associated clinical features. Like PSP, this syndrome is poorly responsive to levodopa treatment, and management is supportive.

Treatment of FTD and Related Syndromes

As in AD, there are no treatments yet that affect the course of FTD. Treatment is symptomatic and focuses mainly on modulation of the

TABLE 27–2 **Medications Commonly Used to Treat Symptoms Associated with Dementia**

Symptom	Medication	Starting Dose	Typical Effective Dose
Agitation, disinhibition, wandering, psychosis, or other severe behavioral symptoms	Quetiapine	12.5 mg qhs	25 mg qhs to 100 bid
	Risperidone	0.5 mg qhs	0.5 mg qhs to 1.5 mg bid
	Olanzapine	2.5 mg qhs	2.5 mg qhs to 10 mg bid
	Haloperidol	0.5 mg prn	0.5 mg to 3 mg per day
Depression or emotional lability	Fluoxetine	10 mg qd	10 mg to 40 mg qd
	Sertraline	25 mg qd	50 mg to 100 mg qd
	Paroxetine	10 mg qd	10 mg to 40 mg qd
	Citalopram	10 mg qd	10 mg to 60 mg qd
	Nortriptyline	10 mg qhs	10 mg to 75 mg qhs
Anxiety or obsessive/compulsive behavior	SSRI	See above	
	Lorazepam	0.5 mg qhs	0.5 mg qhs to 1 mg tid
	Buspirone	2.5 mg qhs	2.5 mg to 10 mg bid-tid
	Clomiprimine	10 mg qd	10 mg qd to 25 mg tid
Insomnia	Trazodone	25 mg qhs	50 mg to 200 mg qhs
	Zolpidem	5 mg qhs	5 to 10 mg qhs
	Melatonin	3 mg qhs	3 to 12 mg qhs

behavioral syndrome in order to improve functional status and caregiver burden (Table 27–2). Paroxetine, trazodone, and selegiline have all been used with some success. A recent study of rivastigmine in FTD suggests that there may be a modest symptomatic benefit, but cholinesterase inhibitors are not routinely used in the treatment of FTD at this time.

Dementia with Lewy Bodies

Dementia with Lewy bodies (DLB) is a syndrome marked by **early dementia, fluctuations in cognition and level of consciousness, and visual hallucinations,** with **subsequent development of parkinsonism.** The cognitive impairment is characterized by varying degrees of memory impairment, executive dysfunction, spatial disorientation, visuospatial impairment, apathy, and bradyphrenia (slowed thought processes). Misidentification errors, where patients fail to recognize once familiar people such as friends and family, often occur. DLB patients may not recognize their own reflection in a mirror and may develop Capgras syndrome, where they do not recognize a spouse but instead develop a fixed belief that the spouse has been replaced by an identical-appearing impostor. Fluctuations are a defining hallmark of DLB, where for periods of time cognition and arousal can be near normal, whereas other periods are distinguished by marked confusion and hypersomnolence. Neuropsychiatric features of the disorder include visual hallucinations that are often well formed and vivid, whereas auditory or other types of hallucinations are uncommon. Parkinsonism becomes apparent after cognitive symptoms (bradykinesia, hypomimia, and rigidity). Action or postural tremor is as common in DLB as is resting tremor. Another feature that supports this diagnosis is the presence of a sleep disorder, such as excessive daytime somnolence, insomnia, restless legs syndrome, or periodic limb movements of sleep. **REM sleep behavior disorder** (RBD), where there is a loss of muscle atonia during REM sleep, with associated complex motor behavior while dreaming, is often seen in DLB patients. Patients often act out their dreams, which may lead to self-inflicted injuries or injuries to bed partners. Autonomic dysfunction, including orthostatic hypotension, impotence, urinary incontinence, and constipation, may also be present. Structural neuroimaging does not tend to show any specific abnormalities, but functional neuroimaging may show decreased occipital hypometabolism and hypoperfusion, which is significantly different from the pattern seen in AD. The histopathologic hallmark of DLB is the presence of Lewy bodies, intraneuronal inclusions composed of α-synuclein aggregates, in areas of cerebral cortex. There are no disease-modifying treatments available yet for DLB, and management is targeted toward modification of symptoms. Cholinesterase inhibitors have been used with success in symptomatic treatment of memory impairment but should not be used in those patients with severe autonomic dysfunction or other contraindications. Typical neuroleptics are contraindicated due to a propensity for increased neuroleptic sensitivity and irreversible parkinsonism. Atypical agents should be used with caution. Motor symptoms may improve with carbidopa/levodopa and dopamine agonists, but these agents may worsen psychotic features. **For treatment of RBD, clonazepam 0.25 mg to 1 mg qhs** can be used, and patients should also be counseled on how to make the bedroom safer.

Parkinson's Disease Dementia

Patients with Parkinson's disease are at risk for developing cognitive impairment that is similar in character to that seen in DLB. Parkinson's disease dementia is differentiated from DLB by the **time** course of the onset of dementia, which appears early in DLB and later, if at all, in PD, although there may be some overlap. Overlap is also present in the histopathology of these disorders, which are both characterized by the presence of Lewy bodies in the cerebral cortex. Symptomatic treatment is similar to that of DLB.

Huntington's Disease

The cognitive impairment seen in early Huntington's disease (HD) tends to be mild, but usually includes forgetfulness and concentration difficulty. With time, more severe memory decline, learning difficulty, slowing of information processing, executive dysfunction, language decline, and apraxias may become evident. Associated neurobehavioral changes such as agitation, depression, social withdrawal, impulsivity, outbursts, obsessive-compulsive behaviors, and sleep disturbances may be observed. There are no treatments for the cognitive decline seen in HD. Treatment of the behavioral symptoms is driven by the given symptoms. Typical or atypical neuroleptics such as **haloperidol, quetiapine,** or **risperidone** are helpful for severe agitation or psychosis, but should be used with caution due to adverse effects. Depression and obsessive-compulsive behaviors may respond to fluoxetine, paroxetine, or other SSRI medications.

OTHER IMPORTANT DEMENTIA SYNDROMES

Vascular Dementia

Cognitive impairment as a result of stroke or cerebrovascular disease is a well-known phenomenon. Vascular dementia (VaD), as described by the NINDS-AIREN criteria, describes cognitive decline consisting of impairment of memory plus two additional cognitive domains, with **evidence of significant cerebrovascular disease** on neurologic examination and imaging, and a **relationship between the dementia and the cerebrovascular disease.** The strokes observed with neuroimaging must be relevant to the diagnosis of dementia, including multiple infarcts such as multiple basal ganglia and white matter lacunes, strategically placed infarcts, for example, in the thalamus, anterior limb of the internal capsule, or medial temporal lobes, or extensive periventricular white matter lesions. The relationship between onset of cognitive decline and cerebrovascular disease can be inferred by either abrupt onset, onset within 3 months of a recognized stroke, or a fluctuating, stepwise progression of cognitive deficits. In general, VaD patients show greater impairment of executive functioning with relatively less memory and visuospatial impairment than AD patients, possibly due to increased involvement of subcortical structures in VaD. Neurologic examination often reveals deficits compatible with previous infarcts. Documenting infarcts on neuroimaging is essential to the diagnosis. Histopathology reveals atherosclerotic and microvascular ischemic changes in addition to infarcts. It is not rare for amyloid plaques and neurofibrillary tangles to be identified in the brains of VaD patients as well, indicating a mixed dementia pattern. Treatment focuses on reduction of modifiable risk factors for cerebrovascular disease, including hypertension, hyperlipidemia, and hyperglycemia, although there is some evidence that cholinesterase inhibitors may be helpful as well. An antiplatelet agent should also be given if not contraindicated.

Normal Pressure Hydrocephalus

The classic triad of **gait disturbance, urinary incontinence,** and **cognitive dysfunction** should prompt further evaluation for normal pressure hydrocephalus (NPH). NPH is a poorly understood condition where communicating hydrocephalus develops in elderly patients without clear obstruction to CSF outflow. Typically the classic magnetic gait, characterized by small steps with feet dragging across the floor and shuffling, presents prior to cognitive change. The dementia seen in NPH tends to involve memory and executive function, with a slowing of cognitive processes thought to be related to subcortical dysfunction. The coexistence of urinary incontinence with gait disorder in patients without significant signs of dementia is particularly suspicious for NPH, whereas other dementia patients tend to develop incontinence and gait abnormalities late after dementia onset. Ventriculomegaly out of proportion to brain atrophy is the classic finding on neuroimaging studies, but this finding can be hard to assess in the setting of advanced atrophy. CSF analysis is essential, both to exclude other causes of hydrocephalus and to clinically confirm the diagnosis of NPH. Videotaped observation of the patient before and after removal of a large volume of CSF (30 ml) should document clear improvement in gait, and this finding should be reproducible. Patients with documented gait improvement after multiple large-volume taps should be referred for a shunt. Cognitive changes less frequently reverse with shunting.

Creutzfeldt Jacob Disease (CJD)

The most frequent of the human prion diseases, CJD is a **rapidly progressing form of dementia that typically leads to death in less than 1 year,** and thus differentiates it from the neurodegenerative disorders described above. Most cases in the United States are sporadic, although iatrogenic forms have been described. The new variant form of CJD has been described in the United Kingdom and Canada in patients who had consumed beef products from cattle infected with bovine spongiform encephalopathy (BSE), and likely represents transmission of BSE to humans. In sporadic CJD, mental deterioration is characterized by memory and concentration impairment, and associated behavioral abnormalities, apathy, and depression are common. **Myoclonus** is an important feature observed in the vast majority of CJD patients, especially provoked by startle. Other associated features include visual disturbance, cerebellar dysfunction, and pyramidal or extrapyramidal involvement. In addition to the clinical syndrome, the diagnosis is supported by brain MRI, which shows increased T2 signal in the striatum and linearly in the cortex (cortical ribboning), seen best with DWI. EEG shows a characteristic pattern of periodic, synchronous, sharp wave complexes, although these may be negative early in the disease course. Identification of 14-3-3 protein in CSF is also supportive, although this test may have relatively poor sensitivity. When considering the diagnosis of CJD, it is important to rule out other causes of a more rapidly progressive dementing disorder. A careful history should focus on previous head trauma, environmental toxins, prescription and recreational drug use, HIV, Lyme disease, and other infectious disease risk factors. In addition to the routine studies done to evaluate for metabolic and other infectious etiologies, workup should also include testing for autoimmune, connective tissue, and paraneoplastic disorders. CSF analysis should include PCR testing for HSV and other viral encephalitides, and cytology or flow cytometry to evaluate for a neoplastic process. Diagnosis is confirmed by histopathologic evaluation of brain tissue, which demonstrates spongiform degeneration, neuronal loss, gliosis, and positive immunostaining for prion proteins. There is no treatment available for CJD at this time, although quinacrine is being actively studied as an antiprion agent.

Vitamin B_{12} Deficiency

Cognitive effects of cobalamin deficiency may include memory impairment, slowed information processing, irritability, depression, and psychosis. Diagnosis is confirmed by low vitamin B_{12} levels in the blood or elevated homocysteine and/or methylmalonic acid levels in patients with low normal B_{12} levels. Treatment consists of **B_{12} replacement of 1000 μg IM daily for 2 weeks, followed by 1000 μg IM monthly.**

HIV-Associated Dementia (AIDS Dementia Complex)

HIV-associated dementia, an AIDS-defining condition, presents as a subcortical dementia, initially with slowed processing speed and mild memory impairment. The syndrome later progresses to involve multiple cognitive domains, including language, executive function, affect, and praxis. **Zidovudine (AZT) 200 mg every 4 hours** has been shown to improve cognitive function over placebo. The standard treatment of HIV-associated dementia is highly active antiretroviral therapy (HAART) combined with aggressive treatment of affective symptoms. Treatment with tricyclic antidepressants and psychostimulants such as **methylphenidate 10 to 30 mg daily** in divided doses and **dextroamphetamine tapering up from a dose of 5 mg daily** in divided doses may help specifically with symptoms of apathy and abulia.

Wernicke-Korsakoff Syndrome

Wernicke-Korsakoff syndrome is a nutritional thiamine deficiency occurring in chronic alcoholics. The acute component (Wernicke's encephalopathy) is characterized by inattentiveness, lethargy, truncal ataxia, and ocular dysmotility (nystagmus—horizontal with or without a vertical or rotary component; and gaze palsy—horizontal or lateral rectus palsy, progressing to complete external ophthalmoplegia). Other signs of nutritional deficiency may be present, such as skin changes or redness of the tongue. If left untreated, the condition is fatal in 10% of patients. Treatment is **thiamine 100 mg IV, IM, or PO daily for 3 days,** along with magnesium and multivitamins. These patients should also be watched carefully for any signs of alcohol withdrawal or delirium tremens, or evidence of hepatic encephalopathy, which may also affect cognitive status. Although the ataxia, inattentiveness, and ocular dysmotility may resolve, the more purely amnestic Korsakoff's syndrome persists in greater than 80% of patients. Korsakoff's syndrome is characterized by moderate to severe anterograde amnesia and patchy long-term memory loss. Unlike patients with TGA, patients with Korsakoff's syndrome are not distressed by their amnesia. Confabulation is often present. Even with good nutrition, the amnesia of Korsakoff's syndrome rarely resolves. Histopathologic examination shows cell loss and degenerative changes in the dorsomedial thalami, the mamillary bodies, the periaqueductal midbrain, and the Purkinje cell layer of the cerebellar vermis.

Transient Global Amnesia

Patients with TGA are middle-aged or older, often with hypertension, prior ischemic episodes, or atherosclerotic heart disease, but are otherwise healthy. Typically, they are brought in by a relative or friend because they are "confused." On examination, there are no focal neurologic deficits. Cognitive function and language are intact, except for profound anterograde amnesia and retrograde amnesia for the preceding several hours or days. Patients typically appear agitated and will repeat the same question over and over, such as "What am I doing here?" The anterograde amnesia clears gradually after minutes to hours and usually resolves completely within 24 to 48 hours. A residual retrograde amnesia for the hours immediately surrounding the event is often permanent. TGA often appears in the setting of an emotional or physical stress. The pathophysiology is unknown; both epileptic mechanisms and vascular mechanisms have been proposed. The differential diagnosis includes unwitnessed head trauma or seizure, drug intoxication, stroke, dissociative states, and Wernicke-Korsakoff syndrome. The EEG is usually negative. MRI should be obtained to evaluate for a seizure-producing lesion or infarct. The condition is self-limiting and there is no specific treatment, although some physicians have advocated using **aspirin 325 mg per day** for secondary prophylaxis. Recurrence occurs in less than one fourth of the patients.

Muscles of the Neck and Brachial Plexus

Muscle	Action to Test	Roots*	Nerve
Deep neck	Flexion, extension, rotation of neck	C1, C2, C3, C4	Cervical
Sternocleidomastoideus	Rotation of head to contralateral shoulder	XI, C2, C3	Spinal accessory
Trapezius	Elevation of the shoulders	XI, C3, C4	Spinal accessory
Diaphragm	Inspiration	C3, C4, C5	Phrenic
Serratus anterior	Forward shoulder thrust	C5, C6, C7	Long thoracic
Rhomboideus minor	Adduction and elevation of scapula	C4, C5	Dorsal scapular
Levator scapulae	Elevation of scapula	C4, C5	Dorsal scapular
Supraspinatus	Abduction of arm (0 to 90 degrees)	**C5**, C6	Suprascapular
Infraspinatus	Lateral arm rotation	**C5**, C6	Dorsal scapular
Deltoideus	Abduction of arm (>30 degrees)	**C5**, C6	Axillary
Teres minor	Medial arm rotation	C4, C5	Axillary
Biceps brachii	Flexion of supinated forearm	**C5**, C6	Musculocutaneous
Brachialis	Flexion of pronated forearm	C5, C6	Musculocutaneous
Teres major	Medial rotation and adduction of arm	C5–C7	Subscapular
Latissimus dorsi	Adduction of arm	C6, **C7**, C8	Thoracodorsal
Flexor carpi ulnaris	Ulnar flexion of hand	C7, **C8**, T1	Ulnar
Flexor digitorum profundus (ulnar part)	Flexion of distal phalanx of fingers 4 and 5	**C8**, T1	Ulnar
Adductor pollicis	Adduction of thumb	C8, T1	Ulnar
Abductor digiti minimi manus	Abduction of little finger	C8, T1	Ulnar
Flexor digiti minimi brevis manu	Flexion of little finger	C8, **T1**	Ulnar
Interossei	Abduction (dorsal) or adduction (palmar) of fingers	C8, T1	Ulnar

***Boldface** letters indicate primary innervation.

Continued

Muscle	Action to Test	Roots*	Nerve
Lumbricales 3 and 4	Flexion of proximal phalanges and extension of two distal phalanges (fingers 4 and 5)	C8	Ulnar
Flexor digitorum superficialis	Flexion of middle phalanx fingers 2 to 5, flexion of hand	C7, **C8**, T1	Median
Pronator teres	Pronation of forearm	C6, C7	Median
Flexor carpi radialis	Radial flexion of hand	C6, C7	Median
Palmaris longus	Wrist flexion	C6, C7	Median
Abductor pollicis brevis	Abduction of thumb metacarpal	C7, C8, **T1**	Median
Flexor pollicis brevis	Flexion of proximal phalanx of thumb	C8, **T1**	Median
Opponens pollicis	Opposition of thumb	C8, **T1**	Median
Lumbricales 1 and 2	Flexion of proximal phalanx and extension of distal phalanges (fingers 2 and 3)	C8, **T1**	Median
Flexor digitorum superficialis	Flexion of middle phalanx fingers 2 to 5, flexion of hand	C7, C8, T1	Median
Pronator teres	Pronation of forearm	C6, C7	Median
Flexor carpi radialis	Radial flexion of hand	C6, C7	Median
Palmaris longus	Wrist flexion	C7, C8, T1	Median
Abductor pollicis brevis	Abduction of thumb metacarpal	C8, T1	Median
Flexor pollicis brevis	Flexion of proximal phalanx of thumb	C8, T1	Median

Muscle	Action to Test	Roots*	Nerve
Flexor digitorum profundus (radial part)	Flexion of distal phalanx of fingers 2 and 3; flexion of hand	C7, C8	Median (anterior interosseous nerve)
Flexor pollicis longus	Flexion of distal phalanx of thumb	C7, C8	Median (anterior interosseous nerve)
Triceps brachii	Forearm extension	C6, **C7**, C8	Radial
Brachioradialis	Forearm flexion (with thumb pointing upwards)	**C6**, C7	Radial
Extensor carpi radialis	Radial hand extension	**C6**, C7	Radial
Supinator	Forearm supination	**C6**, C7	Radial
Extensor digitorum	Extension of hand and phalanges of fingers 2 to 5	**C7**, C8	Radial (posterior interosseous nerve)
Extensor carpi ulnaris	Ulnar hand extension	**C7**, C8	Radial (posterior interosseous nerve)
Abductor pollicis longus	Abduction of thumb metacarpal	**C7**, C8	Radial (posterior interosseous nerve)
Extensor pollicis brevis and extensor pollicis longus	Thumb extension and radial wrist extension	**C7**, C8	Radial (posterior interosseous nerve)
Extensor indicis	Index finger extension and hand extension	**C7**, C8	Radial (posterior interosseous nerve)

***Boldface** letters indicate primary innervation.

Muscles of the Perineum and Lumbosacral Plexus

Muscle	Action to Test	Roots	Nerve
Iliopsoas	Hip flexion	L1, **L2**, * **L3**	Femoral and L1, L2 and L3
Sartorius	Hip flexion and lateral thigh rotation	L2, L3	Femoral
Quadriceps femoris	Leg extension	L2, **L3, L4**	Femoral
Adductor longus	Thigh adduction	L2, **L3**, L4	Obturator
Adductor brevis	Thigh adduction	L2, L3, L4	Obturator
Adductor magnus	Thigh adduction	L3, L4	Obturator
Gracilis	Thigh adduction	L2, L3, L4	Obturator
Obturator externus	Thigh adduction and lateral rotation	L3, L4	Obturator
Gluteus medius and gluteus minimus	Thigh adduction and medial rotation	**L4, L5**, S1	Superior gluteal
Tensor fasciae latae	Thigh adduction	L4, L5	Superior gluteal
Gluteus maximus	Hip extension	**L5, S1**, S2	Inferior gluteal
Biceps femoris	Knee flexion (and assistance with thigh extension)	L5, S1, S2	Sciatic (trunk)
Semitendinosus	Knee flexion (and assistance with thigh extension)	L5, S1, S2	Sciatic (trunk)
Semimembranosus	Knee flexion (and assistance with thigh extension)	L5, S1, S2	Sciatic (trunk)
Tibialis anterior	Foot dorsiflexion and inversion	L4, **L5**	Deep peroneal
Extensor digitorum longus	Extension of toes 2 to 5 and foot dorsiflexion	**L5**, S1	Deep peroneal
Extensor hallucis longus	Great toe extension and foot dorsiflexion	**L5**, S1	Deep peroneal
Extensor digitorum brevis	Extension of toes	**L5**, S1	Deep peroneal
Peroneus longus and peroneus Brevis	Foot eversion (and assistance with plantar flexion)	**L5**, S1	Superficial peroneal
Tibialis posterior	Foot plantar flexion and inversion	**L5**, S1	Tibial
Flexor digitorum	Foot plantar flexion and flexion of toes 2 to 4	S2, S3	Tibial
Flexor hallucis longus	Foot plantar flexion and flexion of terminal phalanx of great toe	S1, S2	Tibial
Gastrocnemius	Knee flexion and ankle plantar flexion	**S1** (S2)	Tibial
Soleus	Ankle plantar flexion	**S1** (S2)	Tibial
Perineal muscles and sphincters	Voluntary contraction of the pelvic floor	S2, S3, S4	Pudendal

*__Boldface__ letters indicate primary innervation.

Brachial Plexus

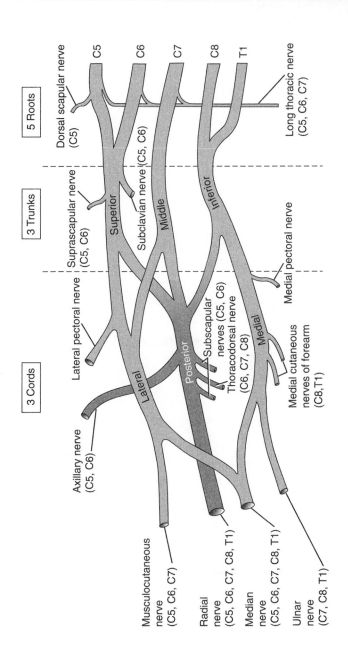

Lumbar Plexus

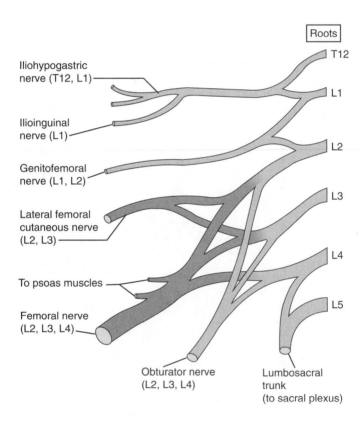

Roots

T12

Iliohypogastric
nerve (T12, L1)

L1

Ilioinguinal
nerve (L1)

L2

Genitofemoral
nerve (L1, L2)

L3

Lateral femoral
cutaneous nerve
(L2, L3)

To psoas muscles

L4

Femoral nerve
(L2, L3, L4)

L5

Obturator nerve
(L2, L3, L4)

Lumbosacral
trunk
(to sacral plexus)

Sensory Dermatome Map

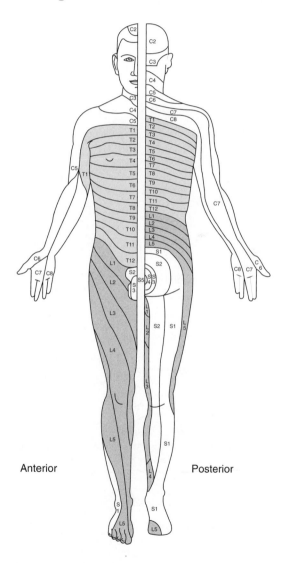

Anterior   Posterior

Surface Map of the Brain

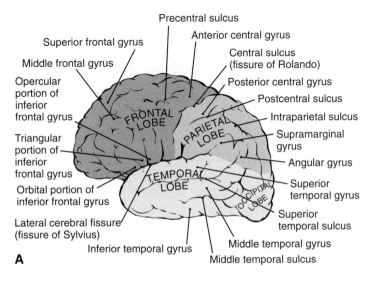

A

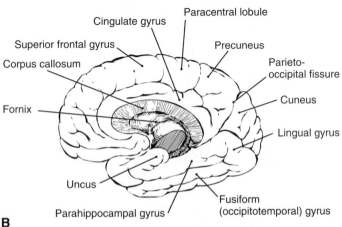

B

Nuclei of the Brainstem

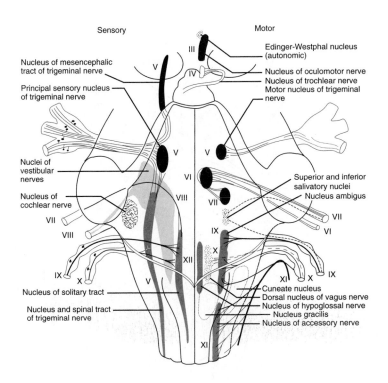

Surface Anatomy of the Brainstem

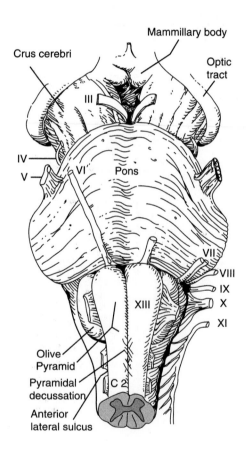

On-Call Formulary: Commonly Prescribed Medications in Neurology

ACETAZOLAMIDE (Diamox) *(Chapters 11, 14, 21)*

Indications	Pseudotumor cerebri, seizures, paroxysmal symptoms of multiple sclerosis
Actions	Carbonic anhydrase inhibitor, a weak diuretic that may reduce cerebrospinal fluid (CSF) volume and intracranial pressure
Side effects	Paresthesias, tinnitus or hearing dysfunction, anorexia, nausea, vomiting, diarrhea, polyuria
Dose	250 mg to 500 mg two times a day

ACYCLOVIR (Zovirax) *(Chapters 5, 21)*

Indications	Herpes simplex encephalitis
Actions	Antiviral
Side effects	Local phlebitis, renal insufficiency, encephalopathy
Comments	Requires generous concurrent IV hydration to minimize risk of renal insufficiency
Dose	10 mg/kg IV over 1 hr, q8h

ALPROSTADIL (Edex) *(Chapter 21)*

Indications	Erectile dysfunction in multiple sclerosis and spinal cord injury
Actions	Relaxes arterial smooth muscle, producing vasodilation, resulting in penile engorgement
Side effects	Hypotension, hematoma, ecchymosis, erectile pain, bleeding, headache, back pain, flulike symptoms, hypertension, sinusitis; rare: penile fibrosis, priapism
Comments	Avoid use in patients with history of sickle cell trait, leukemia, multiple myeloma, and in patients taking anticoagulants
Dose	2.5 to 40 µg intracavernous injection prior to intercourse

AMANTADINE (Symmetrel) *(Chapter 25)*

Indications	Parkinson's disease
Actions	Antiviral agent that also increases dopamine release, blocks dopamine reuptake, and stimulates dopamine receptors
Side effects	Livedo reticularis, ankle edema, confusion, hallucinations, insomnia
Comments	More effective for akinesia and rigidity, less effective for tremor; best used for 6 months to a year as monotherapy in patients with mild to moderate Parkinson's disease; may delay need for initiation of levodopa
Dose	100 to 300 mg two times a day

AMITRIPTYLINE (Elavil) *(Chapters 14, 17, 21)*

Indications	Neuropathic pain, migraine prophylaxis, depression
Actions	Inhibitor of membrane pump responsible for uptake of norepinephrine and serotonin, anticholinergic effects; unknown mechanism for action on neuropathy and migraine
Side effects	Drowsiness, paresthesias, urinary retention, dry mouth, dizziness, constipation, blurred vision, confusion, cardiac conduction block, arrhythmias, rare: seizures, myocardial infarction, stroke, bone marrow suppression
Comments	Sedative effect may limit use for migraine and neuropathy to evening doses; monitor CBC
Dose	25 to 75 mg every day at nighttime for migraine and peripheral neuropathy; up to 150 mg daily in divided doses may be required for antidepressant effect

AMPICILLIN/SULBACTAM (Unasyn) *(Chapter 6)*

Indications	Bacterial meningitis
Actions	Combination antibacterial
Side effects	Rash, diarrhea, fungal superinfection
Dose	1.5 g (1g ampicillin, 0.5 g sulbactam) IV q6h

AMPHOTERICIN B (Amphocin, AmbiSome, Abelcet) *(Chapter 21)*

Indications	Fungal meningitis
Actions	Antifungal
Side effects	Fever, chills, nausea, headache, dyspnea, renal insufficiency, injection site reaction, muscle cramps, vomiting
Comments	Liposomal and lipid complex preparations (Ambisome and Abelcet) are available with better side effect profiles
Dose	1.5 mg/kg per day IV for 4 to 6 weeks

ARGININE VASOPRESSIN (Pitressin) *(Chapters 9, 18)*

Indications	Diabetes insipidus, refractory hypotension after brain death
Actions	Antidiuretic hormone analog

Side effects	Vasopressin infusion combined with free water administration can lead to dilutional hyponatremia
Comments	Causes renal free water retention and peripheral vasoconstriction
Dose	Acute diabetes insipidus: 6 to 10 U IV push, every 6 hours. Maintenance therapy for hypotension of diabetes insipidus: 1 to 4 U/hr

ASPIRIN (Ecotrin, Ascriptin, Bayer) *(Chapter 24)*

Indications	Secondary stroke prevention
Actions	Platelet aggregation inhibitor
Side effects	Dyspepsia, gastrointestinal bleeding
Comments	Reduces risk of recurrent stroke by 10% to 20% compared with placebo
Dose	81 or 325 mg once a day

ASPIRIN/EXTENDED RELEASE DIPYRIDAMOLE (Aggrenox) *(Chapter 24)*

Indications	Secondary stroke prevention
Actions	Platelet aggregation inhibitor
Side effects	Headache, dizziness, nausea, abdominal pain, dyspepsia
Comments	Reduces risk of recurrent stroke by 10% compared with either agent alone, or 24% compared with placebo
Dose	25 to 200 mg twice a day

ATENOLOL (Tenormin) *(Chapter 16)*

Indications	Recurrent vasovagal syncope
Actions	Beta 1-adregenergic (cardiac-selective) blocker
Side effects	Bradycardia, lightheadedness, nausea, bronchospasm
Dose	50 to 100 mg PO qd

ATROPINE *(Chapter 15)*

Indications:	Reversal of edrophonium, reversal of organophosphate poisoning
Actions	Anticholinergic (muscarinic) antagonist
Side effects	Dry mouth, palpitations, dilated pupils, tremor
Comments	Caution in patients over 40; may precipitate acute glaucoma, convert pyloric stenosis to obstruction, or urinary retention in prostate hypertrophy
Dose	0.4 mg IV

AZATHIOPRINE (Imuran) *(Chapter 15)*

Indications	Myasthenia gravis (long-term management)
Actions	Immunosuppressant
Side effects	Leukopenia, thrombocytopenia, nausea, vomiting, increased secondary infection risk
Comments	Adequate immunosuppression is reflected by mild decrease in white blood cell count and increase in mean corpuscular volume
Dose	100 to 250 mg per day

BACLOFEN (Lioresal) (Chapters 21, 25)

Indications	Dystonia, spasticity of multiple sclerosis
Actions	γ-Aminobutyric acid agonist, antispasmodic
Side effects	Confusion, sedation, increased muscle weakness
Comments	Can be given via intrathecal pump for severe cases
Dose	10 to 20 mg three times a day (up to 240 mg/day in some cases)

BENZTROPINE (Cogentin) (Chapter 25)

Indications	Parkinsonism, extrapyramidal reactions
Actions	Anticholinergic
Side effects	Dry mouth, constipation, urinary retention, tachycardia, psychosis
Comments	Effective for Parkinsonian tremor
Dose	Start 0.5 mg once or twice daily, increase 0.5 mg a day every 5 days to max 6 mg a day

BETHANECHOL (Urecholine) (Chapter 21)

Indications	Urinary retention due to neurogenic atonic bladder
Actions	Cholinergic agonist that stimulates parasympathetic muscarinic receptors
Side effects	Cramps, nausea, diarrhea, lacrimation, hypotension, sweating
Comments	Antidote for overdose is atropine 0.6 mg IV
Dose	10 to 50 mg PO three to four times a day

BIPERIDEN (Akineton) (Chapter 25)

Indications	Parkinsonism, extrapyramidal reactions
Actions	Anticholinergic
Side effects	Dry mouth, constipation, urinary retention, tachycardia, psychosis
Comments	Helpful for extrapyramidal reactions caused by neuroleptic agents
Dose	2 mg one to three times a day

BOTULINUM TOXIN (Botox) (Chapter 25)

Indications	Focal dystonia, blepharospasm
Actions	Neuromuscular blocking agent
Side effects	Increased muscle weakness
Comments	Antibody-mediated tolerance may develop over time
Dose	1.25 to 2.50 units per injection site

BROMOCRIPTINE (Parlodel) (Chapters 20, 25)

Indications	Parkinson's disease, neuroleptic malignant syndrome, prolactinoma
Actions	Dopamine agonist
Side effects	Nausea, headache, dizziness, fatigue, vomiting
Comments	May delay the need for levodopa
Dose	2.5 mg to 10 mg three times a day

CABERGOLINE (Dostinex)   *(Chapters 22)*

Indications	Prolactinoma
Actions	Dopamine agonist
Side effects	Orthostatic hypotension, nausea, dizziness, fatigue, increased libido
Comments	Not FDA-approved
Dose	0.25 to 1.0 mg PO once or twice a week

CALCIUM GLUCONATE   *(Chapter 8)*

Indications	Hypocalcemia
Actions	Calcium replacement
Side effects	Bradycardia, syncope, chalky taste
Dose	10 to 20 ml (1 to 2 g) of 10% calcium gluconate IV in 100 ml D5W over 30 minutes

CAPSAICIN (Zostrix)   *(Chapter 18)*

Indications	Painful peripheral neuropathy
Actions	Topical analgesic; probable substance P mediator in sensory neurons
Side effects	None significant
Comments	Now available without prescription
Dose	0.025% or 0.075% cream, apply topically three to four times a day

CARBAMAZEPINE (Tegretol)   *(Chapters 21, 24, 26)*

Indications	Partial and generalized seizures, trigeminal neuralgia, neuropathic pain
Actions	Reduces polysynaptic responses and blocks post-tetanic potentiation
Side effects	Double or blurred vision, dizziness, drowsiness, vertigo, ataxia, gastrointestinal upset, diarrhea, rare agranulocytosis, syndrome of inappropriate antidiuretic hormone, rash, hyponatremia, hypersensitivity, rare: cardiac arrhythmias, bone marrow suppression, cutaneous eruptions
Comments	Half-life of 10 to 35 hours; drug levels needed for anticonvulsant use are 4 to 12 μg/ml; raises levels of phenytoin, lowers levels of valproate. Monitor CBC, Na^{++}
Dose	300 to 1600 mg daily in divided doses three to four times a day; usual starting dose is 200 mg three times a day; Tegretol XR (100, 200, 400 mg caps) can be given twice a day

CEFTRIAXONE (Rocephin)   *(Chapters 5, 8, 21)*

Indications:	Bacterial meningitis, alternative for CNS Lyme disease
Actions	Antibacterial
Side effects	Diarrhea, LFT elevations
Dose	2 g IV every 12 hours

CLINDAMYCIN (Cleocin)   *(Chapters 6, 21)*

Indications	Toxoplasmosis (with pyrimethamine) in patients with sulfa allergies
Actions	Antimicrobial
Side effects	Abdominal pain, colitis
Dose	600 mg IV or PO four times a day

CLONAZEPAM (Klonopin)   *(Chapter 25)*

Indications	Tourette's syndrome, tics, anxiety, seizures
Actions	Benzodiazepine sedative-hypnotic drug
Side effects	Sedation
Comments	May be habit forming
Dose	1 to 10 mg per day, divided, two to three times a day

CLOPIDOGREL (Plavix)   *(Chapter 24)*

Indications	Secondary stroke prevention
Actions	Platelet aggregation inhibitor
Side effects	Dyspepsia, thrombotic thrombocytopenic purpura (rare)
Comments	Also reduces risk of fatal and nonfatal vascular events in patients with MI or peripheral vascular disease
Dose	75 mg once a day

CYPROHEPTADINE (Periactin)   *(Chapter 14)*

Indications	Migraine prophylaxis
Actions	Serotonin and histamine antagonist
Side effects	Dizziness, drowsiness, decreased coordination
Comments	Second line of therapy; contraindicated with monoamine oxidase inhibitors, closed-angle glaucoma, pyloric or bladder obstruction
Dose	4 to 8 mg PO three times a day

DANTROLENE (Dantrium)   *(Chapter 20)*

Indications	Neuroleptic malignant syndrome
Actions	Direct-acting skeletal muscle relaxant
Side effects	Pulmonary edema, thrombophlebitis
Comments	Approved by Food and Drug Administration for use in malignant hyperthermia; use in neuroleptic malignant syndrome described in medical literature
Dose	1 to 10 mg/kg IV every 4 to 6 hours

DEXAMETHASONE (Decadron)   *(Chapters 5, 7, 21, 23)*

Indications	Spinal cord compression, neoplasm or abscess of the brain or spinal cord, acute bacterial meningitis, multiple sclerosis acute relapses
Actions	Anti-inflammatory agent
Side effects	Peptic ulcer disease, sodium and fluid retention, hypertension, hyperglycemia, myopathy, impaired wound healing, avascular necrosis of femoral or humeral heads, endocrine abnormalities

Comments	Reduces vasogenic edema but not cytotoxic edema
Dose	For spinal neoplasm: 100 mg IV bolus; for intracranial mass: 4 to 10 mg IV every 6 hours

DIAZEPAM (Valium)   *(Chapters 4, 8, 21)*

Indications	Seizures, anxiety, alcohol withdrawal
Actions	Benzodiazepine
Side effects	Sedation, hypotension, respiratory depression, paradoxical agitation
Comments	May be administered IV, PO, or rectally as a gel; patients with history of benzodiazepine use or ethanol abuse may have cross-tolerance, requiring higher doses; habit forming with chronic use
Dose	For ongoing seizure or status epilepticus: 5 mg IV push, repeat every 5 minutes up to 20 mg; for ongoing seizures at home, rectal gel 2.5, 5, 10, or 20 mg via syringe; for agitation, anxiety, spasticity, or ethanol withdrawal: 2 to 10 mg PO or IV every 4 hours

DIPHENHYDRAMINE (Benadryl)   *(Chapter 18)*

Indications	Acute drug-induced dystonic reaction, insomnia
Actions	Antihistamine and anticholinergic
Side effects	Drowsiness, dizziness, dry mouth, urinary retention
Comments	Avoid use in elderly, confused patients: may have CNS side effects
Dose	For dystonic reaction: 50 mg IV or IM, may repeat after several minutes; for insomnia: 25 to 50 mg PO per day at night

DOCUSSATE SODIUM (Colace)   *(Chapter 21)*

Indications	Constipation
Actions	Stool softener
Side effects	Diarrhea, cramps, throat irritation, rash, electrolyte disorders
Comments	Contraindicated in bowel obstruction and undiagnosed abdominal pain
Dose	100 mg three times daily with meals

DONEPEZIL HYDROCHLORIDE (Aricept)   *(Chapter 18)*

Indications	Alzheimer's disease
Actions	Cholinesterase inhibitor
Side effects	Nausea, diarrhea
Comments	May promote GI bleeding in patients with peptic ulcer disease
Dose	5 mg to 10 mg PO per day

DOXYCYCLINE   *(Chapter 21)*

Indications:	Lyme disease
Actions	Antibacterial
Side effects	Anorexia, nausea, vomiting

Comments   For CNS Lyme disease doxycycline should be used only
                    if there is isolated facial palsy with normal CSF
Dose   100 mg PO two times a day

DULOXETINE (Cymbalta)   *(Chapter 17)*

Indications   Diabetic peripheral neuropathy
Actions   Selective serotonin and norepinephrine reuptake
                    inhibitor
Side effects   Nausea, somnolence, dizziness, fatigue
Dose   60 mg PO qd

EDROPHONIUM (Tensilon)   *(Chapter 15)*

Indications   Evaluation for myasthenia gravis
Actions   Short-acting anticholinesterase (cholinergic action)
Side effects   Nausea, bradycardia, arrhythmias
Comments   Atropine 0.4 mg should be kept at the bedside to reverse
                    adverse cholinergic side effects
Dose   2 mg IV test dose, then 8 mg IV after 45 seconds

ENOXAPARIN   *(Chapter 15)*

Indications   DVT prophylaxis in immobilized hospital patients;
                    thromboembolic stroke prevention
Actions   Anticoagulant (low-molecular-weight heparin)
Side effects   Hemorrhage
Comments   May be used as a bridge to oral anticoagulation when
                    indicated in cardioembolic stroke
Dose   For DVT prophylaxis 40 mg SQ QD; as bridge to
                    Coumadin 1 mg/kg SQ Q12h

ERGOTAMINE (Dihydroergotamine or DHE 45 IV or IM Injection; with Caffeine: Cafergot, Wigraine)   *(Chapter 14)*

Indications   Migraine (abortive therapy)
Actions   Alpha-adrenergic/serotonin antagonist; cranial
                    vasoconstrictor
Side effects   Precordial tightness, myalgias, paresthesias, nausea
Comments   DHE 45 may require pretreatment with metoclopramide
                    10 mg IV or IM and promethazine 50 mg IV as
                    antiemetic; contraindicated in complicated migraine or
                    patients with coronary artery disease
Dose   1 tablet PO at onset, then repeat every 30 minutes up to
                    6 tabs; alternatively, 1 suppository per rectum, may
                    repeat one time; DHE 45: 1 mg IV or IM, repeat in 1
                    hour if needed

ETHOSUXIMIDE (Zarontin)   *(Chapter 26)*

Indications   Absence seizures
Actions   Anticonvulsant
Side effects   Drowsiness, gastrointestinal (GI) upset, anorexia,
                    headache, dizziness, hiccups

Comments	Pediatric population
Dose	250 mg PO per day (ages 3 to 6), 500 mg PO per day if over 6 years of age

FELBAMATE (Felbatol)   *(Chapter 26)*

Indications	Adjunctive therapy for Lennox-Gastaut syndrome
Actions	Anticonvulsant
Side effects	Aplastic anemia (can be fatal), hepatotoxicity, anorexia, headache, insomnia, somnolence
Comments	Use only with written informed consent due to risk of potentially fatal hepatotoxicity
Dose	400 mg PO three times a day, taper up to 3600 mg per day; in pediatric patients: begin 15 mg/kg per day

FLUCONAZOLE (Diflucan)   *(Chapter 21)*

Indications	Fungal meningitis (mild)
Actions	Antifungal
Side effects	Headache, rash, vomiting, elevated LFTs/hepatitis
Comments	Severe meningitis cases need to be treated with amphotericin
Dose	400 to 800 mg PO daily

FLUDROCORTISONE (Florinef)   *(Chapter 16)*

Indications	Orthostatic hypotension
Action	Potent mineralocorticoid
Side effects	Volume overload, congestive heart failure, hypertension, edema
Comments	The lowest possible effective dose should be used
Dose	0.1 mg PO one to three times per day

FLUMAZENIL (Romazicon)   *(Chapters 5, 10)*

Indications	Benzodiazepine overdose
Actions	Benzodiazepine antagonist
Side effects	Agitation, anxiety, dizziness
Comment	May precipitate seizures
Dose	0.5 mg IV

FOLINIC ACID   *(Chapter 21)*

Indications	Adjunctive therapy in toxoplasmosis
Actions	Reduces hematologic toxicity of toxoplasmosis antimicrobials
Dose	10 to 20 mg PO every day

FOSCARNET   *(Chapter 21)*

Indications	CMV retinitis, CMV central nervous system infection in HIV patients
Actions	Antiviral
Side effects	Renal impairment, electrolyte disturbances

Comments   Second-line therapy after gancyclovir for CNS infection
Dose   60 mg/kg IV every 8 hours for 14 days

FOSPHENYTOIN   *(Chapter 4)*

Indications   Status epilepticus
Actions   Anticonvulsant
Side effects   Nystagmus, ataxia, cardiac arrhythmias, hypotension
Comments   Phenytoin prodrug that is rapidly converted to
                phenytoin within minutes; causes less hypertension than
                IV phenytoin; can also be given IM
Dose   15 to 20 mg/kg IV load infused at 50 mg per minute

FRESH FROZEN PLASMA   *(Chapter 5)*

Indication   Reversal of oral anticoagulant therapy in patients with
                acute intracranial hemorrhage
Actions   Replaces the essential vitamin K-dependent coagulation
                factors II, VII, IX, and X
Side effects   Fluid overload, congestive heart failure, allergic
                transfusion reaction, anaphylaxis, transfusion-related
                acute lung injury
Comments   Requires serial monitoring of INR to establish successful
                reversal of anticoagulation
Dose   15 ml/kg (usually 4 to 6 200 ml units)

GABAPENTIN (Neurontin)   *(Chapters 4, 21)*

Indications   Adjunctive therapy in adult epilepsy, neuropathic pain
Actions   Anticonvulsant
Side effects   Somnolence, dizziness, ataxia, fatigue, nystagmus,
                drowsiness, weight gain, rare: leukopenia
Comments   Useful for partial-onset seizures; renally cleared with no
                drug interactions, and very safe; FDA approved for
                painful diabetic peripheral neuropathy
Dose   Taper from 100 to 300 mg PO three times a day
                over a few days; average dose is 300 to 900 mg three
                times a day to a maximum of 1600 mg three times
                a day

GANCICLOVIR (Cytovene)   *(Chapter 21)*

Indications   CMV retinitis, CNS CMV infection in HIV patients
Actions   Antiviral
Side effects   Fever, leukopenia, thrombocytopenia diarrhea
Dose   5 mg/kg IV every 12 hours

GLATIRAMER (Copaxone)   *(Chapter 21)*

Indications   Relapsing-remitting multiple sclerosis
Actions   Immune modulator
Side effects   Injection-site pain, systemic reaction with chest pain,
                vasodilation

Comments	Reduces frequency and severity of MS episodes; in 10% of patients, transient weakness, flushing, and palpitations may occur after injection
Dose	20 mg injected SC every day

GLYCOPYRROLATE (Robinul) *(Chapter 15)*

Indications	Control of secretions in myasthenia gravis or bulbar amyotrophic lateral sclerosis
Actions	Anticholinergic (antimuscarinic) agent
Side effects	Anticholinergic: decreased sweating, urinary retention, tachycardia, blurred vision
Dose	1 to 2 mg PO three times a day

HALOPERIDOL (Haldol) *(Chapters 8, 25)*

Indications	Psychosis, acute agitation, Tourette's syndrome, Huntington's disease
Actions	Antipsychotic neuroleptic butyrophenone
Side effects	Sedation, extrapyramidal effects (acute or with chronic use), galactorrhea, jaundice, neuroleptic malignant syndrome
Comments	Extrapyramidal effects may occur acutely or with chronic use
Dose	For agitation or acute psychosis: 2 to 10 mg IM, may repeat every hour; for chronic agitation or psychosis: 0.5 to 2 mg PO two to three times a day

HEPARIN *(Chapters 6, 11, 24)*

Indications	Acute embolic or progressing stroke, transient ischemic attack
Actions	Antithrombin effect; acts in conjunction with antithrombin III
Side effects	Hemorrhage, thrombocytopenia
Comments	Monitor aPTT, usually to a target of 1.5 to 2 times control
Dose	20,000 units in 500 ml D5W at 20 ml per hour (800 units per hour maintenance, no bolus)

HYPERTONIC SALINE SOLUTION
(2%, 3%, 23.4% Sodium Chloride-Acetate Solution) *(Chapter 5)*

Indications	Control of elevated intracranial pressure, treatment of acute symptomatic hyponatremia
Actions	Reduces brain edema by shifting water from the intracellular to the intravascular fluid compartment
Side effects	Congestive heart failure, fluid overload, rebound hyponatremia and brain swelling after discontinuation
Comments	2% and 3% infusions are generally given to establish and maintain a state of hypernatremia (target sodium 150 to 155 mEq/L) and hyperosmolality (target osmolality 300 to 320 mOsms/L). Infusions should be slowly tapered over 48 hours and sodium not allowed to fall >12 mEq/L

over 24 hours. The anion is a 50-50 mixture of chloride and acetate to avoid hyperchloremic metabolic acidosis. Highly concentrated 23.4% solution comes in 30 ml vials and is given as bolus therapy through a central line for acute ICP control.

Dosage	2% and 3% solutions: 1 ml/kg/hr
	23.4% solution: 0.5 to 2.0 ml/kg

IMMUNE GLOBULIN (IVIG)   (Chapters 17, 20, 21)

Indications	Guillain-Barré syndrome (GBS), chronic inflammatory demyelinating polyneuropathy (CIDP), myasthenia gravis, acute disseminated encephalomyelitis
Actions	Immunosuppressive
Side effects	Renal failure, aseptic meningitis, anaphylaxis, hyperviscosity syndrome, leukopenia
Comments	Hydrate patient well to avoid renal toxicity
Dose	For GBS: 0.4 g/kg IV per day for 5 days; for CIPD 0.4 g/kg IV weekly

INTERFERON BETA-1A (Avonex)   (Chapter 21)

Indications	Relapsing-remitting multiple sclerosis
Actions	Cytokine, immune modulator
Side effects	Flulike symptoms, muscle ache, fevers, chills, liver function abnormalities, leukopenia, thyroid function abnormalities, depression
Comments	Reduces frequency and severity of MS episodes; use with caution in patients with depression or seizures
Dose	30 µg injected IM once a week

INTERFERON BETA-1A (Rebif)   (Chapter 21)

Indications	Relapsing-remitting multiple sclerosis
Actions	Cytokine, immune modulator
Side effects	Flulike symptoms, muscle ache, fevers, chills, liver function abnormalities, leukopenia, thyroid function abnormalities, depression
Comments	Reduces frequency and severity of MS episodes; use with caution in patients with depression or seizures
Dose	22 µg or 44 µg injected SC three times weekly

INTERFERON BETA-1B (Betaseron)   (Chapter 21)

Indications	Relapsing-remitting multiple sclerosis (MS)
Actions	Antiviral, immunoregulatory agent
Side effects	Injection site pain and inflammation, influenza-like symptoms, headache
Comments	Reduces frequency and severity of MS episodes
Dose	0.3 mg (9.6 million IU [one vial]) SC every other day

ISONIAZID   (Chapter 21)

Indications	Tuberculous meningitis
Actions	Antimicrobial

Side effects	Paresthesias, peripheral neuropathy
Comment	Need to give concomitant pyridoxine (vitamin B_6)
Dose	300 mg per day

LABETOLOL (Normodyne, Trandate) *(Chapters 5, 9)*

Indications	Control of acute hypertension
Actions	Combined beta and alpha receptor antagonist
Side effects	Hypotension, bradycardia, bronchospasm
Comments	Arterial BP monitoring is recommended
Dose	For acute BP control: 10 to 80 mg IV push every 10 to 15 minutes, to a maximal total dose of 240 mg. For infusion 2 to 8 mg/min adjusted to target BP level

LACTULOSE *(Chapter 8)*

Indications	Hepatic encephalopathy
Actions	Diarrheal, reduces ammonia-producing intestinal flora
Comments	Follow ammonia level as indicator of efficacy during treatment
Dose	15 to 45 ml two to four times per day

LAMOTRIGINE (Lamictal) *(Chapters 21, 26)*

Indications	Partial-onset or generalized epilepsy, neuropathic pain
Actions	Anticonvulsant
Side effects	Rash (including Stevens-Johnson syndrome), dizziness, ataxia, nausea, vomiting, somnolence, headache, insomnia; rare: bone marrow suppression, hepatic failure, pancreatitis
Comments	Dose must be reduced with concurrent phenytoin, carbamazepine, or phenobarbital; risk of rash is especially high when given with valproic acid, or in children; monitor CBC and LFTs
Dose	Start 50 mg PO per day for 14 days, then 50 mg two times a day for 14 days, up to 150 mg to 250 mg two times a day

LEVETIRACETAM (Keppra) *(Chapter 26)*

Indications	Add-on for partial-onset seizures in adults
Actions	Antiepileptic
Side effects	Sedation, dizziness, behavioral, infection (mostly mild URIs)
Comment	Primarily renal excretion; no drug interactions; may help for primary generalized seizures also
Dose	1000 to 3000 mg daily divided twice a day; start at 500 mg twice a day

LEVODOPA-CARBIDOPA (Sinemet, Sinemet CR) *(Chapter 25)*

Indications	Parkinson's disease
Actions	Levodopa is converted to dopamine in the basal ganglia; carbidopa inhibits dopamine production (dopa decarboxylation) in the periphery

Side effects	Dyskinesias: dystonia, chorea; confusion, paranoia
Comments	Dosing highly dependent on clinical response; top number denotes milligrams of carbidopa, bottom number denotes milligrams of levodopa; controlled-release preparation (CR) may mediate on/off changes; available in 10/100, 25/100, 25/250, and 50/200 (CR)
Dose	Start with 25/100 tablets three times a day, taper up as clinically indicated

LIDOCAINE PATCH 5% (Lidoderm transdermal patch) *(Chapter 17)*

Indications	Postherpetic neuralgia
Action	Local anesthetic, inhibits sodium channels
Side effects	Local skin irritation
Comment	Apply only to intact skin
Dose	Apply to cover painful areas, may use up to three patches at a time, for up to 12 hours daily

LORAZEPAM (Ativan) *(Chapters 4, 8)*

Indications	Ongoing seizure or status epilepticus, anxiety
Actions	Benzodiazepine sedative, anxiolytic; anticonvulsant
Side effects	Drowsiness, respiratory depression
Comments	Habit forming
Dose	For status epilepticus: 0.1 mg/kg IV given versus repeated 2-mg boluses; for anxiety 0.5 to 2 mg PO two times a day

MANNITOL (Osmitrol) *(Chapters 9, 12)*

Indications	Increased intracranial pressure
Actions	Osmotic diuretic
Side effects	Hypotension, dehydration, hyponatremia, hyperosmolar renal tubular damage, CHF exacerbation
Comments	Rebound intracranial hypertension with prolonged administration; monitor serum osmolality, electrolytes, and fluid balance
Dose	0.25 to 1.5 g/kg of 20% solution (20 g per 100 ml), repeat every 1 to 6 hours according to ICP values and clinical exam

MECLIZINE (Antivert) *(Chapter 13)*

Indications	Benign positional vertigo, labyrinthitis
Actions	Antihistamine
Side effects	Drowsiness, dry mouth, blurred vision
Comments	Efficacy in about 50% of patients
Dose	12.5 to 25 mg PO three times a day

MEMANTINE (Namenda) *(Chapter 27)*

Indications	Moderate to severe Alzheimer's disease
Actions	NMDA antagonist
Side effects	Dizziness, headache, constipation, confusion

| Comments | Generally used in combination with a cholinesterase inhibitor |
| Dose | Start memantine at 5 mg qd and increase by 5 mg weekly to a target dose of 10 mg bid |

METHYLPHENIDATE (Ritalin) *(Chapter 21)*

Indications	Narcolepsy, attention deficit disorder, fatigue, and lassitude of multiple sclerosis
Actions	Stimulant
Side effects	Dependency, nervousness, insomnia, nausea, anorexia, abdominal pain, dyskinesia, rash, blood pressure changes, seizures, arrhythmias, angina; rare: leucopenia, thrombocytopenic purpura, toxic psychosis, cutaneous eruptions
Comment	Second-line therapy for lassitude of multiple sclerosis
Dose	5 to 15 mg up to 3 times; last dose before 6 PM

METHYLPREDNISOLONE (Solu-Medrol) *(Chapters 11, 14, 20, 21)*

Indications	Traumatic spinal cord injury, multiple sclerosis relapse, inflammatory optic neuritis, pseudotumor cerebri
Actions	Anti-inflammatory/immunosuppressive agent
Side effects	Peptic ulcer disease, sodium and fluid retention, hypertension, hyperglycemia, psychosis, insomnia, increased appetite, myopathy, impaired wound healing, avascular necrosis of femoral or humeral heads, endocrine abnormalities
Comments	Stronger mineralocorticoid effect than dexamethasone or prednisone
Dose	For multiple sclerosis and inflammatory optic neuritis: 1 g IVSS per day for 5 to 10 days, followed by prednisone taper; for traumatic cord injury: 30 mg/kg IV bolus over 15 minutes, then 45-minute pause, and then 5.4 mg/kg per hour continuous IV infusion over next 23 hours; for pseudotumor cerebri: 250 mg IVSS four times a day

METHYSERGIDE (Sansert) *(Chapter 14)*

Indications	Migraine prophylaxis
Actions	Serotonin antagonist
Side effects	Retroperitoneal and pleuropulmonary fibrosis, nausea, vomiting, drowsiness, insomnia, hallucinations
Comments	Should not be used for 2 to 6 months after 6 months of use
Dose	2 mg PO one to three times a day

MIDAZOLAM (Versed) *(Chapters 4, 15)*

Indications	Agitation while on ventilator, refractory status epilepticus
Actions	Short-action benzodiazepine sedative-hypnotic
Side effects	Drowsiness, respiratory depression, hypotension

Comments	Rapid acting, with very short half-life
Dose	For sedation: 1 to 2 mg IV/IM every 30 to 60 minutes; for status epilepticus: 0.1 to 0.3 mg/kg IV push load, then maintenance of 0.05 to 0.4 mg/kg per hour

MIDODRINE (ProAmatine) *(Chapter 16)*

Indications	Orthostatic hypotension
Actions	Alpha receptor agonist
Side effects	Supine hypertension, paresthesias, pruritus
Comments	Last dose should be given no later than 6 PM to avoid nocturnal supine hypertension
Dose	10 mg PO three times per day

MITOXANTRONE (Novantrone) *(Chapter 21)*

Indications	Relapsing and progressive multiple sclerosis
Actions	Chemotherapeutic agent breaks DNA in actively dividing cells
Side effects	Dose-dependent cardiotoxicity, congestive heart failure, arrhythmias, hepatotoxicity, serious infections, myelosuppression, hypotension, nausea, diarrhea, constipation, dyspnea, elevated alkaline phosphatase, urine discoloration, cough; menstrual irregularities, amenorrhea, fatigue, anorexia, alopecia, urinary tract infection; rare: anaphylaxis, secondary leukemia, interstitial pneumonitis, renal failure, hemorrhage, tissue necrosis caused by extravasation
Comments	Used primarily for multiple sclerosis patients who have experienced disease progression despite treatment with interferon beta or glatiramer acetate; monitor left ventricular function every 6 months, check CBC and LFTs prior to each dose and check CBC 14 days after each dose
Dose	12 mg/m^2 every 3 months for up to 2 years; cumulative lifetime total dose 140 mg/m^2; alternative schedule 5 mg/m^2 every month

MODAFINIL (Provigil) *(Chapter 21)*

Indications	Narcolepsy, fatigue in MS, abulia
Actions	Stimulant
Side effects	Headache, nausea, diarrhea, dry mouth, anorexia
Comments	May impair thinking or motor skills
Dose	100 to 200 mg PO once to twice a day

NALOXONE (Narcan) *(Chapter 5)*

Indications	Suspected narcotic coma
Actions	Narcotic antagonist
Side effects	Nausea, vomiting, may precipitate withdrawal in narcotic addicts
Comments	Reversal of narcotic coma may wear off after 1 to 2 hours

Dose	0.4 to 2.0 mg IV, IM, or SC every 5 minutes to a maximum dose of 10 mg

NARATRIPTAN (Amerge) *(Chapter 14)*

Indications	Migraine (abortive therapy)
Actions	Selective serotonin agonist
Side effects	Paresthesias, dizziness, drowsiness, fatigue, throat tightness
Comments	Longer duration of action than other triptans, but slower onset and lower efficacy rate; contraindicated in patients with coronary artery disease
Dose	1 or 2.5 mg, may repeat after 4 hours, maximum 5 mg daily

NEOMYCIN *(Chapter 8)*

Indications	Hepatic encephalopathy
Actions	Antibiotic to reduce ammonia-producing bacteria in the intestines
Side effects	Nausea, diarrhea
Dose	2 to 4 g per day PO

NEOSTIGMINE (Prostigmin) *(Chapter 15)*

Indications	Myasthenia gravis
Actions	Acetylcholinesterase inhibitor
Side effects	Abdominal cramps, diarrhea, salivation, fasciculations
Comments	Has longer duration of action than does pyridostigmine
Dose	15 mg to 90 mg PO four times a day; 0.5 to 1.0 mg IV or IM every 2 to 3 hours

NICARDIPINE (Cardene) *(Chapters 5, 9)*

Indication	Control of acute hypertension
Actions	Dihydropyridine calcium channel blocker
Side effects	Hypotension, reflex tachycardia
Comments	Continuous arterial BP monitoring is recommended
Dose	5 to 15 mg/hr as a continuous IV infusion

NIMODIPINE (Nimotop) *(Chapter 24)*

Indications	Subarachnoid hemorrhage
Actions	Calcium-channel blocker with CNS penetration
Side effects	Hypotension
Comments	Reduces the frequency of delayed ischemia from vasospasm by 30%
Dose	60 mg every 4 hours for 21 days

NATALIZUMAB (Tysabri) *(Chapter 21)*

Indications	Relapsing multiple sclerosis
Actions	Inhibits leukocyte trafficking by binding to $\alpha4\beta1$-integrin expressed on the cell surface of activated lymphocytes

Side effects	Hypersensitivity reaction, anaphylaxis, headache, infusion reaction, fatigue, depression, arthralgia, infections, pharyngitis, rash, menstrual irregularities; rare: progressive multifocal leukoencephalopathy, serious infections
Comments	Withdrawn from market
Dose	300 mg intravenously every month

OXCARBAZEPINE (Trileptal)   *(Chapters 21, 26)*

Indications	Monotherapy or add-on for partial-onset seizures in adults; add-on for children ages 4 years or older; neuropathic pain
Actions	Antiepileptic; sodium-channel blocker
Side effects	Dizziness, sedation, nausea, vomiting, diplopia, rash, fatigue, acne, alopecia, hyponatremia; rare: angioedema, bone marrow suppression, cutaneous eruptions
Comment	Similar to carbamazepine but fewer side effects and drug interactions; active ingredient is the 10-monohydroxy metabolite; monitor CBC, Na^{++}, LFTs
Dose	300 to 3600 mg a day divided in two doses (usually need 150% of carbamazepine dose)

OXYBUTYNIN (Ditropan)   *(Chapter 21)*

Indications	Bladder spasticity (e.g., in multiple sclerosis)
Actions	Smooth muscle antispasmodic, antimuscarinic
Side effects	Palpitations, decreased sweating, dry mouth, dizziness, urinary retention, constipation
Comments	Contraindicated in patients with obstructive uropathy
Dose	5 mg PO three to four times daily

PHENOXYBENZAMINE   *(Chapter 17)*

Indications	Reflex sympathetic dystrophy
Actions	Systemic alpha-adrenergic blocker
Side effects	Postural hypotension, tachycardia, impotence
Comments	Taper up dose until side effects occur
Dose	10 mg two times a day, tapering up to 120 mg per day

PRAMIPEXOLE (Mirepex)   *(Chapter 25)*

Indications	Parkinson's disease
Actions	Dopamine agonist
Side effects	Hallucinations, dizziness, somnolence, nausea
Comments	Can be used alone or in combination with levodopa
Dose	0.125 mg three times daily, increase weekly to a maximum of 1.5 mg three times a day

PREGABALIN (Lyrica)   *(Chapter 17)*

Indications	Peripheral (diabetic) neuropathy, postherpetic neuralgia, central pain syndromes

Actions	Antinociceptive, antiseizure
Side effects	dizziness, somnolence, dry mouth
Dose	150 to 300 mg PO bid

PROTAMINE SULFATE *(Chapter 5)*

Indications	Reversal of heparin-induced coagulopathy in patients with acute intracranial hemorrhage
Actions	1 ml of protamine sulfate neutralizes ~100 units of heparin
Side effects	Hypotension, allergic reaction
Comments	Requites PTT monitoring to assess adequacy of response
Dose	10 to 50 mg slow IV push

PEMOLINE (Cylert) *(Chapter 21)*

Indications	Narcolepsy, abulia after brain injury, attention deficit disorder
Actions	CNS stimulant
Side effects	Insomnia, anorexia, weight loss, seizure, dyskinesias, hallucinations, rare aplastic anemia
Comments	Contraindicated in patients with impaired hepatic function
Dose	18.75 mg PO every day, taper weekly as indicated up to maximum of 75 mg per day

PENICILLAMINE (Cuprimine) *(Chapter 25)*

Indications	Wilson's disease
Actions	Copper chelator
Side effects	Lupus-like rash, polyarteritis, leukopenia, thrombocytopenia, epigastric pain, nausea, diarrhea, nephrotic syndrome, tinnitus, neuropathy
Comments	May precipitate myasthenia gravis
Dose	125 to 1000 mg per day, divided, two to four times a day

PENTOBARBITAL *(Chapters 4, 9)*

Indications	Status epilepticus, increased intracranial pressure
Actions	Anticonvulsant, sedative
Side effects	Respiratory suppression, sedation, hypotension
Comments	EEG monitoring indicated; hypotension may require pressors. Levels of 25 to 35 mg/L are generally sufficient to control intracranial pressure; levels of <5 mg/L are compatible with a clinical diagnosis of brain death
Dose	5 to 20 mg/kg IV load, 1 to 4 mg/kg per hour maintenance

PERGOLIDE (Permax) *(Chapter 25)*

Indications	Parkinson's disease
Actions	Dopamine agonist
Side effects	Nausea, headache, dizziness, fatigue, vomiting

Comments	May delay onset or reduce required dose of levodopa
Dose	0.75 to 3.0 mg per day, divided, three to four times a day

PHENOBARBITAL (Luminal)   *(Chapter 4)*

Indications	Epilepsy, status epilepticus
Actions	Anticonvulsant
Side effects	Sedation, respiratory suppression, hypotension, behavioral changes, hyperactivity
Comments	For chronic therapy, therapeutic range is 20 to 40 µg/ml; lowers levels of phenytoin, carbamazepine, and valproate
Dose	For status epilepticus: 10 to 20 mg/kg IV load infused at 100 mg/min; for epilepsy 60 mg PO two to three times a day; for pediatric patients: 3 to 6 mg/kg per day

PHENYLEPHRINE (Neo-Synephrine)   *(Chapter 5)*

Indications	Low cerebral perfusion pressure
Actions	Alpha receptor agonist
Side effects	Reflex bradycardia, excessive hypertension
Comments	Intra-arterial BP monitoring is recommended. Can be used to raise BP in hemodynamically unstable ischemic stroke syndromes, or in patients with elevated ICP
Dose	10 to 200 µg/min titrated to desired BP target

PHENYTOIN (Dilantin)   *(Chapter 4)*

Indications	Epilepsy, status epilepticus
Actions	Anticonvulsant
Side effects	Nystagmus, ataxia, gingival hyperplasia, hirsutism, rash, adenopathy, liver function test abnormalities
Comments	For chronic therapy, therapeutic range is 10 to 20 µg/ml; lowers levels of carbamazepine and valproate and increases or decreases phenobarbital level
Dose	Typical maintenance dose is 300 mg every day at night

PIMOZIDE (Orap)   *(Chapter 25)*

Indications	Tourette's syndrome
Actions	Piperidine antipsychotic
Side effects	Dry mouth, sedation, dyskinesias, akinesia, behavioral effects, prolongation of QT interval
Comments	None
Dose	Start with 1 mg PO two times a day, up to 2 to 10 mg per day in divided doses

PREDNISONE   *(Chapter 11)*

Indications	Temporal arteritis, Bell's palsy
Actions	Anti-inflammatory agent
Side effects	Peptic ulcer disease, sodium and fluid retention, hypertension, hyperglycemia, myopathy, impaired

wound healing, avascular necrosis of femoral or humeral heads, endocrine abnormalities, increased susceptibility to infection

Comments	Initiate therapy as soon as diagnosis is suspected to avoid irreversible visual loss
Dose	100 mg PO per day, tapered slowly to alternate-day therapy over several weeks

PRIMIDONE (Mysoline) *(Chapters 4, 25)*

Indications	Generalized tonic-clonic epilepsy, essential tremor
Actions	Anticonvulsant
Side effects	Ataxia, vertigo, nausea, anorexia, vomiting, irritability, sedation
Comments	Second line of therapy; metabolized to phenobarbital
Dose	Start with 100 to 125 mg PO once a day, taper up to 250 mg three to four times a day

PROPANTHELINE BROMIDE (Pro-Banthine) *(Chapter 15)*

Indications	Control of secretions in myasthenia gravis
Actions	Antimuscarinic agent
Side effects	Anticholinergic: decreased sweating, urinary retention, tachycardia, blurred vision
Comments	None
Dose	15 mg PO four times a day

PROPOFOL (Diprivan) *(Chapters 4, 9)*

Indications	Refractory status epilepticus, ICP control, sedation in setting of mechanical ventilation
Actions	Alkylphenol sedative-hypnotic agent
Side effects	Apnea, respiratory depression, hypotension, propofol infusion syndrome (metabolic acidosis, hypotension, renal failure), bloodstream infections
Comments	Should only be administered to patients who are intubated. Continuous arterial BP monitoring is recommended. Prolonged high dosages, particularly in children, are not recommended due to an increased risk of propofol infusion syndrome
Dose	Status epilepticus: 1 to 3 mg/kg loading dose, followed by 50 to 250 µg/kg/min. Sedation: 25 to 100 µg/kg/min

PROPRANOLOL (Inderal) *(Chapters 14, 25)*

Indications	Benign essential tremor, migraine prophylaxis
Actions	Nonspecific beta-adrenergic blocker
Side effects	Hypotension, bradycardia, bronchospasm, may mask symptoms of hypoglycemia, impotence
Comments	Avoid use in asthmatics and diabetics
Dose	For tremor: 40 to 240 mg PO per day, divided, three to four times a day; for migraine 20 to 40 mg per day

PSYLLIUM (Metamucil) *(Chapter 21)*

Indications	Constipation
Actions	Increases stool bulk
Side effects	Diarrhea, constipation, cramps, bronchospasm, rhinitis, esophageal obstruction, bowel obstruction
Comments	Contraindicated in bowel obstruction and undiagnosed abdominal pain
Dose	1 to 2 teaspoons three times daily with meals

PYRIDOSTIGMINE (Mestinon) *(Chapter 15)*

Indications	Myasthenia gravis
Actions	Acetylcholinesterase inhibitor
Side effects	Excess salivation, pulmonary secretions, diarrhea
Comments	Muscarinic side effects controlled by glycopyrrolate or propantheline bromide
Dose	Start at 30 mg PO three times a day, up to 120 mg every 3 to 6 hours

RECOMBINANT ACTIVATED FACTOR VII (NovoSeven) *(Chapter 5)*

Indications	Acute coagulopathic intracranial hemorrhage, spontaneous intracerebral hemorrhage
Actions	Promotes rapid hemostasis and clot formation by accelerating thrombin formation on the surface of activated platelets
Side effects	Myocardial infarction, cerebral infarction, venous thromboembolism, disseminated intravascular coagulation
Comments	Use for acute intracranial hemorrhage is currently investigational and considered off-label; Cost is prohibitive, approximately 1 U.S. dollar per microgram
Dose	40 to 80 µg/kg IV push over 1 to 2 minutes; Doses may be rounded to the nearest 1.2, 2.4, or 4.8 mg vial

RILUZOLE (Rilutek) *(Chapter 20)*

Indications	Amyotrophic lateral sclerosis
Actions	Glutamate antagonist
Side effects	Malaise, abdominal pain, nausea, dizziness, circumoral numbness, liver function abnormalities
Comments	May extend survival 60 to 90 days and delay time to intubation; avoid use in patients with liver dysfunction
Dose	50 mg PO two times a day

RIVASTIGMINE (Exelon) *(Chapter 27)*

Indications	Alzheimer's dementia
Actions	Centrally acting cholinesterase inhibitor
Side effects	Nausea, dizziness
Comments	May be first- or second-line therapy after donezepil
Dose	1.5 mg bid, increase to 6 mg bid over 4 weeks, as tolerated

RIZATRIPTAN (Maxalt) *(Chapter 14)*

Indications	Migraine (abortive therapy)
Actions	Selective serotonin agonist
Side effects	Weakness, fatigue, chest or throat pressure, dizziness, somnolence
Comments	Faster acting and slightly more effective than other triptans, but more likely to cause side effects. Contraindicated in patients with coronary artery disease.
Dose	5 to 10 mg, may repeat in 2 hours, maximum 30 mg daily

ROPINIROLE (Requip) *(Chapter 25)*

Indications	Parkinson's disease
Actions	Dopamine agonist
Side effects	Syncope, hallucinations, dyskinesias, nausea, dizziness, somnolence, headache
Comments	May be used alone or in combination with levodopa
Dose	0.25 mg three times daily

SELEGILINE (Eldepryl) *(Chapter 25)*

Indications	Parkinson's disease
Actions	Monoamine oxidase B inhibitor: antioxidant
Side effects	Nausea, dizziness, confusion, hallucinations
Comments	Thought to slow progression of disease
Dose	Taper up to 5 mg PO two times a day

SENNA (Sennakot) *(Chapter 21)*

Indications	Constipation
Actions	Increases peristalsis
Side effects	Nausea, bloating, cramps, flatulence, diarrhea, urine discoloration, melanosis coli; rare: cathartic colon, laxative abuse
Comments	Contraindicated in bowel obstruction and undiagnosed abdominal pain
Dose	6.6 mg sennosides, take 2 to 4 at night

SILDENAFIL (Viagra) *(Chapter 21)*

Indications	Erectile dysfunction in multiple sclerosis and spinal cord injury
Actions	Inhibits phosphodiesterase type 5, enhances effects of nitric oxide-activated increases in cGMP, resulting in penile engorgement
Side effects	Headache, flushing, dyspepsia, nasal congestion, dizziness, rash, priapism; rare: MI, stroke, sudden death, cardiac arrhythmia, hypotension, hemorrhage, hypersensitivity reaction, dyspnea
Comments	Avoid use in patients with history of coronary artery disease
Dose	25 to 100 mg 0.5 to 4 hours prior to intercourse

SUMATRIPTAN (Imitrex)   *(Chapter 14)*

Indications	Migraine (abortive therapy)
Actions	Selective serotonin agonist
Side effects	Coronary vasospasm, tingling, flushing, tightness in jaw, neck, and chest, dizziness, injection site reaction
Comments	Contraindicated in patients with coronary artery disease
Dose	6 mg SC, may repeat in 1 hour, maximum 12 mg per day, 6 doses per month; 25 mg PO, may repeat up to 100 mg in 2 hours

TACRINE (Cognex)   *(Chapter 18)*

Indications	Alzheimer's disease
Actions	Reversible cholinesterase inhibitor
Side effects	Nausea, vomiting, diarrhea, abdominal pain, fatigue, agitation, confusion
Comments	May improve cognitive scores in some patients
Dose	Start 10 mg PO three times a day, tapering up to 30 mg three times a day

TADALAFIL (Cialis)   *(Chapter 21)*

Indications	Erectile dysfunction in multiple sclerosis and spinal cord injury
Actions	Inhibits phosphodiesterase type 5, enhances effects of nitric oxide-activated increases in cGMP, resulting in penile engorgement
Side effects	Headache, dyspepsia, back pain, myalgia, nasal congestion, flushing, limb pain, priapism; rare: angina, MI, stroke, hypotension, hypertension, syncope
Comments	Avoid use in patients with history of coronary artery disease, effects may last up to 36 hours, lower dose in patients with hepatic dysfunction
Dose	5 to 20 mg prior to intercourse

TEMOZOLIDE (Remodar)   *(Chapter 22)*

Indications	Newly diagnosed gliomoblastoma multiforme, refractory anaplastic astrocytoma.
Actions	Cytotoxic alkylating agent which damages DNA in rapidly multiplying cells
Side effects	Leukopenia, thrombocytopenia, alopecia, nausea/vomiting, anorexia, headache, weakness. Women and older patients are at higher risk for complications. During concomitant phase, Bactrim must be given 3 times a week for *Pneumocystitis carinii* prophylaxis, and CBC should be measured weekly. Therapy should be suspended if absolute neutrophil count <1,500/μL or platelets <100,000/μL.
Dosage	75 mg/m^2 PO daily concomitant with radiation treatment for 42 days, followed by maintenance therapy with 150 to 200 mg/m^2 PO daily for 5 days every 28 days over 6 cycles

THIAMINE *(Chapters 4, 8)*

Indications	Coma, thiamine deficiency neuropathy
Actions	Enzymatic cofactor in oxidative metabolism (thiamine pyrophosphate)
Side effects	None
Comments	Give with glucose in setting of coma to prevent Wernicke's encephalopathy
Dose	For coma: 100 mg IV push; 100 mg PO or IM for 3 days

TIAGABINE (Gabitril) *(Chapter 26)*

Indications	Add-on for partial-onset seizures in adults
Actions	Antiepileptic; GABA-reuptake inhibitor
Side effects	Sedation, cognitive dysfunction, dizziness, nausea, vomiting, tremor, anxiety
Comment	Highly protein-bound
Dose	4 to 56 mg daily, divided two to four times a day

TICLOPIDINE (Ticlid) *(Chapter 24)*

Indications	Secondary stroke prevention
Actions	Platelet aggregation inhibitor
Side effects	Neutropenia, diarrhea, rash, nausea, vomiting, thrombotic thrombocytopenic purpura
Comments	Check CBC every 2 weeks during the first 3 months of treatment
Dose	250 mg twice a day

TISSUE PLASMINOGEN ACTIVATOR (t-PA) *(Chapters 6, 24)*

Indications	Hyperacute ischemic stroke
Actions	Thrombolytic
Side effects	Intracerebral hemorrhage
Comments	Must be given within 3 hours of stroke onset; increases chance of full recovery or minimal residual deficit at 3 months by 33%; patients with acute hemorrhage, uncontrolled hypertension (>180/105 mm Hg), or those on anticoagulant therapy should be excluded
Dose	0.9 mg/kg IV (10% IV push, then infuse the remaining 90% over 1 hour), maximum dose 90 mg

TOLCAPONE (Tasmar) *(Chapter 25)*

Indications	Parkinson's disease
Actions	Catechol-*O*-methyltransferase (COMT) inhibitor
Side effects	Fulminant hepatic failure (may be fatal), dyskinesias, nausea, sleep disorders, anorexia, somnolence
Comments	Should be reserved for patients with symptom fluctuations on levodopa who do not respond to other adjunctive agents; withdraw if no substantial benefit is seen after 3 weeks
Dose	100 to 200 mg three times daily

TOPIRAMATE (Topamax)   *(Chapters 21, 26)*

Indications	Add-on for partial-onset or primary generalized seizures, neuropathic pain
Actions	Antiepileptic, weak carbonic-anhydrase inhibitor
Side effects	Sedation, cognitive dysfunction, anorexia, dizziness, paresthesias, ataxia, renal stones, metabolic acidosis, visual disturbance, weight gain, agitation; rare: angle closure glaucoma, bone marrow suppression, cutaneous eruptions
Comment	Probably effective for all seizure types; mostly renal excretion; monitor CBC
Dose	Start 25 to 50 mg per day; maintenance 100 to 600 mg per day divided in two doses; 1 to 10 mg/kg per day in children; also available in sprinkles

TRAMADOL (Ultram)   *(Chapter 21)*

Indications	Analgesia
Actions	Exact mechanism is unknown but parent compound and M1 metabolite bind opiate μ receptors; and parent compound also inhibits reuptake of norepinephrine and serotonin
Side effects	Dizziness, nausea, constipation, headache, somnolence, psychiatric disturbance, urinary retention, withdrawal symptoms; rare: seizures, respiratory depression, angioedema, cutaneous eruptions, serotonin syndrome, orthostatic hypotension, hallucinations
Comment	Useful for neuropathic pain; use with SSRIs or other antidepressants may trigger serotonin syndrome
Dose	50 to 100 mg three times daily

TRIHEXYPHENIDYL HCL (Artane)   *(Chapter 25)*

Indications	Parkinson's disease, idiopathic torsion dystonia
Actions	Anticholinergic
Side effects	Visual blurring, dry mouth, urinary retention
Comments	May be effective in treating parkinsonian tremor; botulinum toxin has largely replaced anticholinergics for the treatment of focal dystonias
Dose	1 to 15 mg PO per day, divided, three to four times a day

VALPROIC ACID (Depakote, Depakene (syrup), Depacon (IV))
                                                   (Chapter 4)

Indications	Partial or generalized seizures, migraine prophylaxis
Actions	Anticonvulsant
Side effects	Nausea, weight gain, hair loss, tremor, hepatitis, agranulocytosis, thrombocytopenia, Stevens-Johnson syndrome
Comments	Therapeutic range is 50 to 100 μg/ml; increases levels of carbamazepine, phenytoin, and lamotrigine

Dose	250 to 2000 mg PO four times a day; 5 to 15 mg/kg IV every 6 hours. Loading dose for status epilepticus is 30 to 60 mg/kg IV

VARDENAFIL (Levitra) *(Chapter 21)*

Indications	Erectile dysfunction in multiple sclerosis and spinal cord injury
Actions	Inhibits phosphodiesterase type 5, enhances effects of nitric oxide-activated increases in cGMP, resulting in penile engorgement
Side effects	Headache, flushing, rhinitis, dyspepsia, dizziness, nausea, arthralgias, elevated CPK, priapism; rare: anaphylaxis, angina, MI, cardiac arrhythmia, hypotension, hypertension
Comments	Avoid use in patients with history of coronary artery disease, lower doses in patients with hepatic dysfunction
Dose	5 to 20 mg 1 hour prior to intercourse

WARFARIN (Coumadin) *(Chapters 6, 24)*

Indications	Stroke prophylaxis in atrial fibrillation or other conditions predisposing to cardioembolism
Actions	Inhibits vitamin K-dependent clotting factors
Side effects	Hemorrhage, rash
Comments	Used for secondary stroke prevention in cardioembolic stroke and in large-vessel atherosclerosis when antiplatelet therapy has failed; used for primary stroke prevention in atrial fibrillation; close monitoring of prothrombin times (PT or International Normalized Ratios [INRs]) required
Dose	Begin with 4 mg PO per day, with dose adjusted according to target PT/INR

ZOLMITRIPTAN (Zomig) *(Chapter 14)*

Indications	Migraine (abortive therapy)
Actions	Selective serotonin agonist
Side effects	Paresthesias, nausea, neck or chest tightness, dry mouth, somnolence
Comments	May be useful for keeping headaches away in patients with early recurrence after sumatriptan; contraindicated in patients with coronary artery disease
Dose	2.5 mg may repeat after 2 hours, maximum 10 mg daily

ZOLPIDEM (Ambien) *(Chapter 18)*

Indication	Insomnia
Action	Sedative
Side effects	Confusion in the elderly
Comments	Do not use for benzodiazepine or ethanol withdrawal
Dose	5 to 10 mg at night

ZONISAMIDE (Zonegran) *(Chapters 21, 26)*

Indications	Add-on for partial-onset seizures in adults; neuropathic pain
Actions	Antiepileptic, weak carbonic anhydrase inhibitor
Side effects	Sedation, dizziness, anorexia, irritability, rash, kidney stones, psychiatric disturbance, withdrawal seizures; rare cutaneous eruptions, bone marrow suppression, heat stroke, pancreatitis
Comments	Sulfa drug; mostly renal excretion; may help for absence seizures and for other generalized seizures; monitor CBC
Dose	100 to 600 mg daily, divided twice a day

Index

Page numbers followed by b indicate boxes; f, figures; n, notes; t, tables.